The Birth Control Clinic in a Marketplace World

Rochester Studies in Medical History

Senior Editor: Theodore M. Brown
Professor of History and Preventive Medicine
University of Rochester

ISSN 1526-2715

*The Mechanization of the Heart:
Harvey and Descartes*
Thomas Fuchs
Translated from the German by
Marjorie Grene

*The Workers' Health Fund in Eretz Israel
Kupat Holim, 1911–1937*
Shifra Shvarts

*Public Health and the Risk Factor:
A History of an Uneven Medical Revolution*
William G. Rothstein

*Venereal Disease, Hospitals and the Urban Poor:
London's "Foul Wards," 1600–1800*
Kevin P. Siena

*Rockefeller Money, the Laboratory and
Medicine in Edinburgh 1919–1930:
New Science in an Old Country*
Christopher Lawrence

Health and Wealth: Studies in History and Policy
Simon Szreter

*Charles Nicolle, Pasteur's Imperial Missionary:
Typhus and Tunisia*
Kim Pelis

*Marriage of Convenience:
Rockefeller International Health and
Revolutionary Mexico*
Anne-Emanuelle Birn

*The Value of Health:
A History of the Pan American
Health Organization*
Marcos Cueto

*Medicine's Moving Pictures:
Medicine, Health, and Bodies in
American Film and Television*
Edited by Leslie J. Reagan, Nancy Tomes,
and Paula A. Treichler

*The Politics of Vaccination:
Practice and Policy in England, Wales, Ireland,
and Scotland, 1800–1874*
Deborah Brunton

*Shifting Boundaries of Public Health:
Europe in the Twentieth Century*
Edited by Susan Gross Solomon, Lion
Murard, and Patrick Zylberman

*Health and Zionism:
The Israeli Health Care System, 1948–1960*
Shifra Shvarts

Death, Modernity, and the Body: Sweden 1870–1940
Eva Åhrén

*International Relations in Psychiatry:
Britain, Germany, and the
United States to World War II*
Edited by Volker Roelcke,
Paul J. Weindling, and Louise Westwood

Ludwik Hirszfeld: The Story of One Life
Edited by Marta A. Balińska and
William H. Schneider
Translated by Marta A. Balińska

*John W. Thompson:
Psychiatrist in the Shadow of the Holocaust*
Paul J. Weindling

*The Origins of Organ Transplantation:
Surgery and Laboratory Science, 1880-1930*
Thomas Schlich

*Communities and Health Care:
The Rochester, New York, Experiment*
Sarah F. Liebschutz

The Neurological Patient in History
Edited by L. Stephen Jacyna and
Stephen T. Casper

The Birth Control Clinic in a Marketplace World
Rose Holz

The Birth Control Clinic in a Marketplace World

Rose Holz

R· UNIVERSITY OF ROCHESTER PRESS

All Rights Reserved. Except as permitted under current legislation, no part of this work may be photocopied, stored in a retrieval system, published, performed in public, adapted, broadcast, transmitted, recorded, or reproduced in any form or by any means, without the prior permission of the copyright owner.

First published 2012
Transferred to digital printing 2013
Reprinted in paperback 2014

University of Rochester Press
668 Mt. Hope Avenue, Rochester, NY 14620, USA
www.urpress.com
and Boydell & Brewer Limited
PO Box 9, Woodbridge, Suffolk IP12 3DF, UK
www.boydellandbrewer.com

hardcover ISBN-13: 978-1-58046-399-7
paperback ISBN-13: 978-1-58046-489-5
ISSN: 1526-2715

Library of Congress Cataloging-in-Publication Data
Holz, Rosemarie Petra, 1968–
    The birth control clinic in a marketplace world / Rose Holz.
        p. cm. — (Rochester studies in medical history, ISSN 1526-2715 ; v. 21)
    Includes bibliographical references and index.
    ISBN 978-1-58046-399-7 (hardcover : alk. paper)
    1. Birth control clinics—United States. 2. Birth control—United States. 3. Family
planning services—United States. 4. Planned Parenthood Federation of America.
I. Title.
    HQ766.5.U5H65 2012
    363.9'60973—dc23   2011049620

A catalogue record for this title is available from the British Library.

This publication is printed on acid-free paper.
Printed in the United States of America.

Parts of chapter 2 appeared in Rose Holz, "Nurse Gordon on Trial: Those Early Days of the Birth Control Clinic Movement Reconsidered," in *Journal of Social History* 39 (Fall 2005): 112–40, and are reprinted here with permission.

Front cover photo: Detail from cover of pamphlet, "In the Beginning . . . ," published by the Margaret Sanger Research Bureau, circa 1940s. (Planned Parenthood Federation of America Records (PPFA I)) Photographer/creator: Planned Parenthood Federation of America, Inc. (Margaret Sanger Research Bureau). Copyright: PPFA has retained copyright, although the Sophia Smith Collection has been authorized to grant permission to researchers to publish. Back cover photo: Entrance to Planned Parenthood clinic at 841 East 63rd Street, Chicago, 1960. (Planned Parenthood Federation of America Records (PPFA II)) Photographer/creator: Planned Parenthood Federation of America. Copyright: PPFA has retained copyright, although the Sophia Smith Collection has been authorized to grant permission to researchers to publish.

to shylette miss violet
and her beloved miss louise
for theirs is a love for the high flying trapeze

to gingersnap their pony
for bravely does he carry them
across the lone prairie

but most especially
to my beloved husband eric
for together we sail
the great blue sea

Contents

Acknowledgments   ix

Introduction   1

1   The Birth of the Clinic   20
2   Rising Above   46
3   Old Habits Are Hard to Break   69
4   New Habits Are Formed   96

Conclusion   146

Notes   159

Bibliography   201

Index   215

Acknowledgments

I'd be lying if I didn't say there were times when I thought this book would never be finished. I'd also be lying if I didn't say that I lived in fear that I would be crushed under the historical weight of the entire Planned Parenthood organization (it's pretty heavy). And I'd be lying again if I didn't say how often it felt as if this were a project I bore alone. Fortunately, I was wrong on all three counts—the book exists, I narrowly escaped, and more than a few people lent a hand, each according to her or his inimitable fashion. For these reasons, many grateful thanks go to the following people, organizations, and occasional inanimate thing for their help along the way:

The archives listed in the bibliography, whose collections I used (and the great people who worked inside), Bill Baird (my favorite birth control radical), the Bake Shop (everybody who worked there too), Gail Bederman (who had faith in my first article), Lisa Bell, Busby Berkeley (oh, the repetition), Owen Brown, Masha Bucur, the Buhs Family (Ervin, Susan, Laura, Edith, Ismael Guerrero, and Peter Thomson), the Cackle Sisters, Johnny Cash (my first love), Henry Darger (fellow xeroxer), Dr. Diamant, the Dictionary (my favorite book to read), Barbara DiBernard (she gets my Christmas cards), Kirk Douglas (because "when I say 'hup,' you better hup"), Frederick Douglass (who whispered in my ear), Bob Dylan, some new friends (Lee Heerten, Sean James, Michaela Kocanda, Lisa Lux, Garrett McConnell, Charlie Rogers, Michelle Tiedje, and Azure Wall), e-mail, Energy Lake Industries, Dawn Flood, Les and Wynn Goodchild, Nurse Adele Gordon, Merle Haggard, Cathy Moran Hajo (more on Cathy in the introduction), Kathryn Harvey, the history departments at the University of Illinois at Urbana-Champaign (UIUC) and University of Nebraska–Lincoln (UNL), Roscoe Holcomb, the Imaginary Institute for Plain Art, the interlibrary loan, the Internet, Margaret Jacobs (great boss and fellow bicycle rider), John G. (for in horror lies hope), Gayle Johnson (who turned in drawings along with her papers), Sandra Johnson (fellow cook and gardener), the Kinks, Dr. Lauer, the libraries at the University of Illinois and the University of Nebraska, Jeff Machota, Sandy Marshall (who did the job I couldn't face: index), the Marx Brothers (especially Harpo), Miss Mayo, Mickey Moran, Nature's Table (the site of my first real education), Willie Nelson, my nephews and nieces, Kathy Oberdeck, Roy Orbison, the outlaws (Karyn Holz, Annette Ellingwood-Holz, Mary Holz, Dave Mosiman, and Dave Drajeske), the Paulukonis family (Rob, Susan, Annie, and Joe), Pony Express Enterprises (Guenther, Trixie, and all the rest of the gang, some of whom have been mentioned already), Rob Prescott (my first favorite teacher), Joy Ritchie, Sarah Webber Rodriguez (who knows the same library call numbers I do), Linda Scott (who told me to look at *The Gift* by Marcel Mauss), Maria Seferian (who gave me a bed to sleep on), Emily Singer, Lauralee Sollinger (who shares my passion for glitter) and the rest of the McNurlen-Sollinger clan (Brian, Max, Sam, and Rosie), Christine Stansell (for believing in this project even though we never met), my students (each and every last one of them), my TAs (who helped me grade large piles of papers and exams), J. R. R. Tolkien (my first favorite writer), Paula Treichler (who said I could write), Vincent Van Gogh, the Velvet Underground, Dan Ward (who showed up at my office clutching a well-worn spiral notebook), Charlotte Wiebe, Brian Wilson, several undergrads who helped with oral history transcriptions (Jill Savage and Jessica Wall—more on Jess in a moment), UNL's Women's and Gender Studies Program (including Glenda Dietrich Moore, Maureen Gallagher, Rachel McClain, Laura Roost, Melissa Swihart Townsend, Catherine Medici-Thiemann, and Lori Weier), and of course Neil Young. Forgive me if I've missed a few. But there still are a few names left, which you'll find in special spot down below.

In terms of money, many grateful thanks also go to UIUC's Department of History and Gender and Women's Studies Program, the American Institute of the History of Pharmacy, the Illinois Historic Preservation Agency, Radcliffe Institute's Schlesinger Library, and the Social Science Research Council (SSRC). So generous was the SSRC that they even gave me the words through which to express my gratitude: "This research was assisted by a fellowship from the Sexuality Research Fellowship Program of the Social Science Research Council with funds provided by the Ford Foundation." It is my firm belief that very kind and thoughtful people must surely exist behind such formal titles because they, for reasons that remain beyond my ken, had faith in my fancies.

Extra special thanks go to the following: To *Leslie Reagan*, who introduced me to the topic of the birth control clinic and the history of medicine, for which I remain eternally grateful, and who also sent the editors at the University of Rochester Press my way. To *Dave Roediger*, who generously listened when I thought nobody would and who put aside his own politics and told me to stick with my defense of the market, even though it probably killed him to say those words. To *Jim Barrett*, a favorite teacher as an undergraduate who then served on my dissertation committee. He also gets my Christmas cards, more perhaps than he dares imagine. To the editors at the University of Rochester Press—*Ted Brown, Suzanne Guiod, Ryan Peterson*, and *Mary Petrusewicz*—who never once uttered the phrase I hate most to hear: "it's just not done that way." It's been a lovely editing ride, so much so that each has a standing invitation for a day sail on our Sea Pearl *Zuma* should they ever find themselves in Nebraska. The same holds true for the two *anonymous reviewers*, who made this a far better manuscript. To the *Holz siblings* (Peter, Stephen, Werner, Gisela, and Erika, all of whom learned to quit asking when this book would finally be done—well, except Erika, who knew I had to finish it). To *Jessica Wall,* who was first my student and then my good friend. How proud I was when she opted for western Nebraska and delighted when she moved further east to Lincoln. To *Mick Powers,* who taught me everything I needed to learn about art and to trust the voices in my head, even (no, especially) when they were a bit scary. Without him, I may never have found the other side. To *Brian Reedy,* who knew all about ponies long before I learned how to ride mine and who is the best "best friend" that Eric and I could ever share. To *Eric Buhs,* who found me when I was twenty and for some reason decided to hang on. I would be completely lost without him, and he knows for better or for worse I'll never let go. And finally, to *Mutti und Papa,* my once penniless German Catholic immigrant parents who endured the Second World War. Thank you for regularly reminding my five siblings and me: "You would be amazed with all that can be made when nothing is all you have." So here's to nothing, *Mutti und Papa,* here's to nothing—because although I know there are many things in this book about which you disapprove, my hope is that in its spirit you find something about which to be proud, be it from heaven above or more earthly places below.

Introduction

It was August 1998. I had been doing research for this book—a history of the Illinois birth control clinic movement—for almost two years. I had read through the records of the local and national Planned Parenthood offices and gathered material from the popular and medical press. I had also begun to conduct a series of oral history interviews with women who had worked in local Illinois clinics. Slowly my research was coming together. Or so I thought, because it was in that warm month of August that I finally followed the advice of historian Leslie Reagan, drove up to Chicago, and visited the archives of the American Medical Association in order to look through its Historical Health Fraud and Alternative Medicine Collection. It was here that I realized I had to shift my thinking entirely. I had to move beyond the messages that the Planned Parenthood organization had long promoted and, to the extent possible, think like someone from an earlier era, long before the organization had established the authority it now enjoys.

The catalyst for this epiphany lay in the sea of records through which I waded, which revealed the massive contraceptive marketplace that was in full swing by the Depression era.[1] After spending several days sifting through the boxes of documents, I found myself growing ever more dizzy with the maze of contraceptive choices before me. Then I came across a document that sent me reeling. "Enclosed find a letter from one Margaret Sanger of New York City," wrote an Indiana physician in June 1924 to the editors of the *Journal of the American Medical Association*, "and another letter written to her after she failed to answer my first. Up to date, I have not heard from her. When I received her letter I put her down as a fake, and now I believe more than ever all she wants out of [myself and others] is the one dollar she ask[ed] for her Dr. Bocker's book. I looked for said Dr. Bocker in the directory. I can not find her. Another fake in my opinion." He then ended his letter with an equally strong statement of condemnation. "I hope the medical profession of America do[es] not sanction Margaret Sanger's motives and I hope that none are fools enough to send the money."[2]

That the doctor was so opposed to Sanger's request that he buy the book by Dr. Bocker, the first physician to run the birth control clinic Sanger established in New York City in 1923, came as no surprise;[3] historians have long described the animosity Sanger faced from the medical profession for her efforts to repeal the 1873 Comstock Act (and similar laws enacted in the decades thereafter) that banned birth control in America.[4] But then I thought, why shouldn't he, or anyone else for that matter, consider her a fake, just another person interested in self-promotion, or just another huckster out to make an easy buck? Or the reverse: what was wrong with wanting to earn a living by engaging in the sale of birth control products as long as your products were good? Suddenly my established perspective had been challenged because now I neither assumed that Sanger and the birth control clinics she and others were establishing were inherently good, nor did I believe that the marketplace was inherently bad. It was important for this conceptual awakening to have happened if I was ever to move beyond the historiography, which often depicted just that.[5] It also didn't hurt that in this collection the documents produced by and critical of Sanger lay alongside documents produced by and critical of the birth control marketplace. Not only did I have a hard time telling the differences between them, but together they also served as a reminder that these documents represented worlds that did not develop in isolation from one another. Thus what follows is an interrogation of the relationship between these two seemingly disparate worlds in their material and their ideological intersections.

Sanger's vision was but one among many and drew its strength not from the birth control marketplace but rather the charity birth control clinic. But because this institution sought at its most fundamental level to make available what were undeniably commercial products, it could never quite break free from this marketplace connection, though at one point it certainly tried. Furthermore, this relationship between the charity clinic and the commercial marketplace was neither fixed nor rigid, but rather fluid and dynamic, and when the clinic rubbed up against the marketplace (as it always somehow did), it did so at times with great friction and at times with great ease. It all depended on how commercial interests fit within the larger mission of the charity birth control clinic movement. For example, the early birth control radicals of the 1910s (like the political and sexual revolutionaries of New York's Greenwich Village with whom the early Sanger associated) found in the birth control marketplace an ally of sorts. With the shift in the 1920s and 1930s of the charity birth control movement to the more conservative circles of doctors and female middle-class reformers, the birth control marketplace was seen more as an adversary. By the late 1950s the relationship had come full circle; pharmaceutical companies occupied an important role in the work of Planned Parenthood.

An examination of the material and ideological intersections between the charity clinic and the marketplace also calls for much-needed theoretical investigation. As I found myself regularly wondering: why was it that when I first looked at the charity birth control clinic and the commercial birth control worlds together, I so readily accepted the virtue of the clinic organizers and the deceit of the entrepreneurs, even when historians themselves have long suggested the presence of less-than-benevolent motivations within the charity clinic movement?[6] Although now I know that good, old-fashioned propaganda is in part to blame for my initial perception—in that the charity clinic movement worked hard during the 1930s to convince the public that its clinics were good because they were born of compassion while commercial providers were bad because they were driven by the pursuit of profit—why was this such an effective strategy in the first place? It would seem, then, that something about charity work in and of itself carries weight, then and today. But something about business carries weight too. And the more I looked at the charity clinic and the commercial worlds together, the more I questioned the relevance, authority, and values automatically accorded to each, prompting me to ask even more questions. What does it mean to engage in the charitable provision of birth control (by way of the clinic)? What does it mean to engage in its commercial provision (by way of the market)? And how in turn could these meanings be used as sources of power—to oppress, to resist oppression, and even sometimes to be used as weapons against each other or as powerful tools to borrow from each other? Clearly something very deep was at work because the conventional wisdoms from which I was drawing were getting in the way of finding satisfactory answers. Consequently, if I was to resolve for myself these nagging internal questions, I would have to abandon some of my own deeply held views, including any assumptions I had about the nature of business and charity as well as my left-of-center politics. Fortunately, as I later realized, I was not alone in so doing.

First to be abandoned, therefore, was the rigidity of the boundaries between the charity clinic and the marketplace because, despite my lingering fears to the contrary, the lines truly are blurry. As Peter Dobkin Hall noted in *Inventing the Nonprofit Sector* (1992), "For what, after all, is really meant when people speak of *nonprofits*? For some, the term implies altruistic and charitable activity, but many nonprofits do neither. For others, the term implies voluntarism; but many nonprofits are not voluntary organizations, nor do private agencies have a monopoly on voluntary action." He then observed:

> Although it makes sense to group institutions according to the products they provide, the services they deliver, or their forms of organization, the terms *nonprofit* and *nonprofit sector* have little to do with either, because any of the goods and services produced by nonprofits can be and are also supplied by businesses and government agencies. Nor can nonprofits claim a distinctive way of raising revenue. Although much is said about their dependence on donations, sales of services, government grants and contracts, bonding and investment income account for nearly 80 percent of nonprofit revenues. Even tax exemption is not distinctive to nonprofits: governmental activities have always been tax exempt; at various times, the exemption has been extended to for-profit enterprises as well; finally, in some times and places nonprofits have been denied the exemption.[7]

And so, while in the first chapter of this book I examine the sale of birth control supplies by charity clinics, in the last chapter I describe the ties that developed between charity clinics and commercial manufacturers through large-scale clinical investigation programs inside local clinics. The last chapter also describes the ideological overlap; charity clinics increasingly used commercial techniques to reach impoverished communities and adopted the language of consumer choice to make appealing the services they offered to potential clientele. In short, the lines between business and charity work are not so easily drawn, despite the birth control propaganda and the subsequent birth control historiography that often suggested otherwise.

The next assumption to be abandoned was the presumed benevolence of charity organizations. Certainly, scholars and activists alike have long noted the problems endemic to charity endeavors. For example, those engaged in charity often defined such things as the "worthy poor" and "deserving mothers." They also sometimes functioned as part of larger colonial projects.[8] But I always found myself wanting more, a sharper critique that dug more deeply at the problems that the engagement in charity might entail. Consequently, when I read Miranda Joseph's argument in *Against the Romance of Community* (2002)—that, despite the "persistent scholarly critique" made by feminists and poststructuralists of the 1980s and 1990s of the "disciplining and exclusionary" tactics of identity-based political movements, "a celebratory discourse of community relentlessly returns"—I was relieved once again.[9] Not only did I agree with this particular assessment, but I also could not help but notice the similarity between the persistent celebration of community with the persistent celebration of charity or nonprofit work. In other words, what is it about the desire to engage in nonprofit work, as opposed to profit, that in the grand scheme of things somehow makes it more noble, whatever its flaws?

Thus, the third assumption to be abandoned was the market's inherent selfishness. As Martha Ertman and Joan Williams wrote in their introduction to *Rethinking Commodification: Case Readings in Law and Culture* (2005):

> The conventional assumption is of hostile worlds: that the world is bifurcated into an economic arena dominated by rational self-interest and self-interest alone ("the market"), and a sharply different arena of intimacy and altruism that must be protected from the kind of instrumental behavior that is appropriate in market contexts.

But such a bifurcation, Ertman and Williams argued, is a flawed one, and only by moving beyond what they described as the "Hamlet question of 'to commodify or not to commodify,'" can we then consider the more useful question, where do we go next?[10] Or, as the historian in me is compelled to ask: how does this help explain from whence our current birth control laws and birth control technologies came?

Consequently, if this means at times appreciating the power of business, in this case in its most essential construction, then we must do so because it explains a crucial thread in the path of birth control to relegalization in the twentieth century. In other words, part of the market's liberatory power lies in the fact that when birth control was still illegal, the market looked to make abundant what the government looked to make scarce. And when combined with a charity movement that seemed, ironically enough, to want to limit the availability of birth control as well, there is something to be said for the market's desire to sell, and to sell a lot. Indeed, and as has been argued—see Andrea Tone's forceful argument about the importance of commercialization in the path to legalization—the growing legalization of birth control in the 1930s was as much a product of its commercialization by entrepreneurs as it was of the work of political, social, and medical reformers.[11] Thus it is all these perspectives that inform the *first* theme of this book: neither the worlds of business and charity nor the values attached to them are as distinct as we might imagine; and in terms of power, moments of oppression and resistance against oppression can be found within each. And only by appreciating the complexity of this overlap can we unpack in new ways the history of Planned Parenthood and that of its local birth control clinics.[12]

This book also contains, then, the results of my desire to trace the origin and evolution of local Planned Parenthood affiliates (those in Illinois), and especially the origin and evolution of the institution around which such local movements across the nation were usually based: the birth control clinic. Although there has been an effort in recent years to move beyond the activities of the national levels of the birth control movement by documenting life at the local level, what is strange is the consistency of the moment at which most of these recent studies stop: sometime in the 1930s or early 1940s. In some ways this makes sense because with the Depression came a dramatic period of growth that I refer to as the "first clinic wave." But with the onset of World War II, this expansion would come to a halt, bringing to an end not only the first burst of activity but also the excitement around what was once a new institution. However, it is for precisely these reasons we must move our story forward. Although the 1940s and 1950s marked a period of lull, these years also put into place a new set of variables that would lay the foundation for the movement's "second wave" of growth in the 1960s and early 1970s—a period characterized by another massive round of clinic establishment and the crumbling of some of the very bedrocks upon which the clinic was first built. A sustained analysis of the clinic institution over time uncovers, therefore, some dramatic transformations and fills in a striking scholarly omission.[13]

In addition, a sustained analysis of the local birth control clinic helps us better understand Planned Parenthood and its larger history. Where better to investigate such matters than from the perspective of the institution around which the organization was largely based? It is no small coincidence that, when thinking of Planned Parenthood, images of the clinic are among the first to come to mind. It follows that a useful way to frame this particular narrative is around the local clinic. For it was through the local clinic that the organization worked to control both the language of birth control and its provision; it was also through the local clinic that the predominantly female legions of local organizers found tangible expression of their less tangible beliefs, both establishing the organization's practical know-how to outside observers and earning the trust of the women they hoped to serve—a trust and an authority not easily, nor even always, achieved. Indeed, if there were two things the birth control organization learned through the course of its existence, it was that without authority, Planned Parenthood had no patients, and without patients, Planned Parenthood had no authority. And at the center of this never-ending whirl was the local birth control clinic.

Consequently, if we look at the clinic over time (from the 1910s into the early 1970s) and in terms of the many different relationships local clinics had—with their clientele and the national birth control offices, with the medical profession and the commercial birth control world, and even simply with each other—what we see is how this institution was less than simple and its success belied a less than unified movement. As clinic organizers themselves quickly discovered, their desire to engage in the provision of birth control became multilayered debates over whom the clinic should serve, who should do the serving, and even what birth control methods the clinic should provide. These debates were no small matters, for at their very heart lay fundamental questions about who was to engage in sex, who was to have authority over birth control, and even how to define the term "birth control" itself. Nor, for that matter, was the definition of the term "clinic" agreed upon by all. Throughout this sixty-year period, the local birth control clinic vacillated between so-called quackery and medical respectability, legality and illegality, all the while negotiating what had become its three main goals: the direct delivery of birth control services, the model to others engaging in birth control services, and the site at which to conduct research in the science of reproduction.

Thus it is the malleability of the term "birth control" and the form and function of the local birth control clinic that constitute the *second* and *third* main themes of this book. In part, such a flexibility helps explain the birth control clinic movement's many successes, in that it was able to adapt with chameleon-like ease to the many different circumstances it occupied. Yet with each clinic success came new dilemmas to be resolved, prompting new strategies and new discourses to be employed. For this reason, equally malleable was the term "birth control" itself. Not only did its changing definition underpin changing clinic operations, but its changing definition also lay at the heart of battles over reproductive rights more generally, often playing themselves out in unexpected arenas. In short, what follows is a narrative stormier perhaps than has been previously suggested. Certainly, there were many battles waged throughout the twentieth century *between* those for reproductive rights and those against. But there were just as many battles *within* the birth control clinic movement itself, internal battles that regularly threatened to tear the movement apart, and at the center of which lay those conflicting definitions of the term "birth control" and conflicting opinions about the form and function of the local birth control clinic.

The Birth of the Clinic and Its Curious Life Thereafter

When the birth control clinic institution of the first wave emerged in Illinois, New York, and elsewhere, it was in many ways a product of Progressive-era reform. It also differed greatly from Sanger's early work in the 1910s. Initially, when Sanger first began distributing her "Family Limitation" pamphlet and then opened her first clinic in 1916 (only to be shut down by the police after nine days), she promoted a radical vision of birth control services influenced by the Greenwich Village bohemians with whom she associated. As historian Linda Gordon noted:

> They used birth control to make a revolutionary demand, not a reform proposal. They did not want just to limit or schedule pregnancies but to change the world. They believed that birth control could alleviate much human misery and fundamentally alter social and political power relations, thereby creating greater sexual and class equality. In this they shared the voluntary motherhood analysis—that involuntary motherhood was a major prop of women's subjugation—and added a radical version of a new-Malthusian analysis that overlarge families weakened the working class in its struggle with the capitalist class. They also demanded sexual freedom.[14]

Thus with unabashed frankness Sanger talked about sex, about revolution, and about a variety of birth control providers and a variety of birth control techniques. Further, despite Gordon's claim that these sexual revolutionaries were "anticommercial" (an assertion with which I agree), Sanger even found use for the commercial world, occasionally mentioning specific bootleg entrepreneurs and describing the various methods that could be found at the local drugstore.[15] Bohemian radicals (like the early Sanger) and bootleg birth control entrepreneurs occupied a similar space, in that as political revolutionaries and patent medicine peddlers both existed on the ragged edges of respectability and legality.[16]

By the 1920s, however, Sanger promoted something else. As a doctor-run facility, which provided the most "scientific" method then known (the diaphragm), this new clinic institution resonated with the still lingering themes of the Progressive era: science and efficiency, experts and expertise. As a place intended to provide services to new immigrants and the poor, especially those of the industrial city, it resembled other Progressive-era work such as settlement houses, milk stations, and well-baby clinics.[17] In addition, the very idea of a clinic itself had become increasingly popular. As Paul Starr and other scholars of medicine have shown, throughout the early twentieth century the establishment of clinics had become an important part of Progressive-era public health reform, a trend that persisted into the 1930s when the economic hardships of the Depression made their presence even more necessary.[18]

That this new institution tapped into communities of women who were deeply interested in the needs of mothers and children suggests how the clinic was also tied to another cornerstone of the Progressive movement: infant and maternal welfare reform. It was in fact the forging of links between the clinic and these communities of women that in many cases helped ensure the clinic's initial survival and shaped the nature of its services. For example, although in some ways this new institution was decidedly medical in its inception (with doctor authority and an atmosphere of science and expertise), it was also decidedly nonmedical, a reflection of the many feminine and feminist touches that the often lay reformers brought inside. The emphasis on the diaphragm further reflected this amalgam: although it was doctor prescribed, it was also woman controlled. What clinic organizers had also done, therefore, was to pick up anew the tradition of what historian Regina Markell Morantz-Sanchez once called "sympathy and science," a culture of science and feminism that characterized the women's hospitals of the previous century.[19]

Yet also central to early clinic work was the charity birth control movement's embrace of conservative views of sexuality, which found tangible expression in the strict admission policy banning the unmarried from obtaining contraceptive services. In some ways, this was a product of the circles of doctors and middle-class female reformers from which the movement now drew physical and financial support, circles that did not necessarily share the sexual radicalism of Sanger's early days.[20] But this position was also an important strategy. Already walking on thin ice when it came to matters of sexuality, the movement realized that if it wanted to win the backing of the medical establishment, religious groups, and political leaders, it had to prove its work was not about promoting intercourse among the unwed but rather about strengthening the bonds of those already joined in matrimony. Consequently, it was the conservative position on sexual practices that figured heavily in the movement's arguments against the marketplace, whose openness about sexuality in the 1920s had by the 1930s come under full attack.[21]

It is crucial to appreciate this last point because while much has been made of the birth control movement's alliances *with* doctors and eugenicists in the 1920s and 1930s in its path to legitimacy, setting itself *apart* from the commercial marketplace was just as important.[22] Without a doubt, some of the efforts of the movement were intended to protect consumers from the many dangerous and ineffective products that had by the 1930s flooded the still illegal market. But this approach made sense for other reasons as well because for many middle-class reformers the commercial world represented danger and incompetence, lust and immorality, particularly for the poor, young, and unwed.[23] The writings of Jane Addams serve as a vivid reminder of these lingering white middle-class fears. In "lieu of innocent pleasure," she passionately wrote in 1909, the commercial dancehall "sold" nothing more than a few minutes of "allurement and intoxication," words which tellingly conjure images not only of profit and drink but also the height of physical arousal.[24] Thus the line the birth control movement hoped to draw was a fine one: one could object to the marketplace but still support birth control, as charity clinics and private physicians would preserve the sanctity of marriage by refusing to serve the unwed, or so the argument followed.

Notably, these strategies would in turn shape what was by the 1920s and 1930s becoming the charity movement's very narrow definition of birth control. Contrary, therefore, to what one historian said when he waxed poetic about the 1914 coining and subsequent use of the term "birth control"—that it was "so easily understood" and its "meaning so clear"—I would argue the reverse.[25] Precisely because its meanings were so potentially abundant, the charity clinic movement would have to work hard to contain it strictly. In part this meant distancing the term from the practice of abortion, as historian Leslie Reagan demonstrated.[26] But it also meant distancing it from other things: namely, commercially available birth control and sex among the unwed. As a result, the definition the charity movement now put forward went something like this: birth control was not only preventative in function, but it was also only used by the wed and only obtained through private doctors' offices or doctor-run charity clinics. And this method, the movement argued, was the diaphragm, which it now endowed with tremendous symbolic power.

However, by the 1970s—after the lull of the 1940s and 1950s and the second wave of clinic growth in the 1960s—everything had changed. Gone, for example, was the emphasis on the doctor-prescribed diaphragm, for which the rise of the pill was largely, though not entirely, responsible. Gone too was the heated rhetoric against commercial providers, for now Planned Parenthood had deep ties with the pharmaceutical manufacturing industry and even looked more favorably upon commercial sources of contraceptives.

Also gone were the charity movement's old complaints of sexual impropriety and the immorality of abortion, because now Planned Parenthood clinics were increasingly serving the unwed and helping women with the termination of their pregnancies.[27] Many of the old bedrocks upon which the birth control clinic movement was first based had dramatically given way. The question thus begs: what happened to bring about such an enormous transformation?

Part of the explanation might be found in the numerous court decisions enacted into law between the late 1910s and the early 1970s. After years of ever-tightening regulations about birth control, by the late 1910s they began to loosen, just when the birth control clinic movement was beginning to take shape.[28] Some of it began with local decisions. In New York, for example, while Judge Crane's 1918 decision shut down Sanger's first radical (and doctorless) clinic, it did make possible a legal loophole in which doctors could make contraceptives available in their private practices.[29] In 1923, court cases in Illinois established a similar exception.[30] In 1936, such local decisions took on national scope in *U.S. v. One Package*, which established the right of private physicians to prescribe contraceptives for reasons of health to their married patients.[31] These early years saw other important cases as well. Though condoms were rarely a part of early clinic work, the *Youngs Rubber* case in 1930 constituted a major victory for the commercial marketplace. So long as rubber prophylactics were sold through proper channels (such as the drugstore) and as preventatives of disease (rather than pregnancy), the ruling held that the sale of condoms was well within the law.[32] With the passage of years came even more loosening of legal restrictions. In 1965, *Griswold v. Connecticut* declared that contraceptives were not simply a right of physicians to prescribe but also a right of married couples to use, which meant the need for doctors' moral supervision had given way to rights of personal privacy.[33] Seven years later *Eisenstadt v. Baird* (1972) extended this right to the unwed.[34] Finally, *Roe v. Wade* and *Doe v. Bolton*—which in 1973 legalized the practice of abortion—constituted yet another important shift in the nation's birth control policies.[35] Striking in all of this, however, is that most of these decisions came *after*, not *before*, the practices that were already beginning inside the local charity birth control clinic. Therefore, the explanation for the charity movement's expanding definition of birth control and its radically shifting strategies need to be found elsewhere.

Indeed, many of the reasons behind these dramatic transformations can be found in the shifting terrains of business, medicine, and society, because the world in which the clinic was established in the 1920s was by the 1950s much changed. To begin with, there was the Second World War, a period in American history that, for all its tumult and tragedy, simultaneously heralded newfound opportunities in the workplace for women and minorities, particularly African Americans. Yet in the years that followed there came in response a clamping down, a concerted effort to quell deviance and disorder through propping up as an ideal the white middle-class nuclear family.[36] It was this ideal that, when combined with the fears of overpopulation as well as the second wave of African American migration to northern industrial cities, fueled concerns about what many saw as the new source of America's social disorder: the residents of color who dwelled in the nation's urban slums. Equally significant were such developments as these: First, the emergence of a squeaky clean new image for the pharmaceutical manufacturing industry.[37] Second, the postwar solidification of what historian Lizabeth Cohen described as "a consumers' republic."[38] And third, the rise not just of new methods of scientific research but also, and perhaps even more important, a new milieu—which brought together in unprecedented amounts the resources of the state, universities, and commercial enterprises in search of scientific breakthroughs.[39]

The effect of all of this was dramatic, simultaneously rendering obsolete some of the old rationales upon which the institution of the local birth control clinic was first founded and replacing them with new ones upon which to draw. No longer did Planned Parenthood need to distance itself from contraceptive manufacturers; now the medical profession had adopted closer ties with the pharmaceutical manufacturing industry. Embracing all that pharmaceutical companies had to offer also meant a golden opportunity to participate in the new milieu of scientific research, which brought status, prestige, and good old-fashioned money and supplies. Furthermore, to rely upon the language and practice of business had become useful to Planned Parenthood as well. Although charity remained a powerful tool, the organization increasingly replaced quiet respectability with bold commercialism and medical authority with an ethos of consumer choice. Nor, for that matter, did Planned Parenthood need to distance itself from the practice of sex among the unwed, because the dynamics had changed on that front as well. Whereas before, the provision of birth control to the unmarried constituted a threat to America's social fabric, by the 1960s it increasingly became the key to the nation's salvation. In other words, as concerns about overpopulation collided with visions of the unwanted baby and the massive demographic shifts of the postwar era, the use of birth control by the unwed—particularly by the poor women of color in the urban industrial slums—became less a vice and more a virtue, to borrow loosely the phrasing once used by historian James Reed.[40]

Equally dramatic was how these broader shifts affected the makeup of those who procured Planned Parenthood's services. The situation in Chicago serves as a striking example. During the 1920s, roughly half the local affiliate's clientele consisted of white middle-class women; the other half consisted largely of impoverished women, mostly new immigrants and a number of African Americans (somewhere between 10 and 20 percent).[41]

By the 1960s this had changed, and African Americans constituted more than two-thirds of the new patients the Chicago office now served, a presence that could be felt in the Planned Parenthood organization more generally, with nonwhites comprising approximately 50 percent of the total clientele.[42] Certainly, the transformation in healthcare—in particular the rise of private health insurance programs that enabled the growing middle-class to secure more easily the services of a private physician to accommodate their birth control needs—is one element of this shift.[43] But race is also important because it reveals both the ebb and flow of demographic currents and the complicated dynamics of social mobility. As new immigrants found themselves integrated into the mainstream of white America, African Americans, in contrast, found themselves once again left behind, with the task of achieving racial equality still their burden to bear.[44] As a result, the growing participation of blacks in the Chicago family planning movement constitutes yet another important transformation in the Planned Parenthood organization, though it would by the 1960s provoke battles among African Americans themselves about the proliferation of birth control clinics within their own communities.

Given the magnitude of these different shifts, therefore, if not also the speed at which they transpired, it should come as no surprise that not all within Planned Parenthood were in agreement; the organization's rationale of charity, moreover, would be in some ways ironic. For in this new era of birth control it would be Planned Parenthood's engagement in charity—the argument it used in the 1930s to stake its claim against the profit-driven exploitation of the marketplace—that would put precisely those women it hoped to assist in a new kind of risk. Put another way, in this new partnership with pharmaceutical companies and participation in this brave new world of biomedical research, the charity clinic patient had now become the potential scientific research subject, thus putting into jeopardy precisely those women whom the clinic's mission of charity was supposed compassionately and protectively to assist. In the end, then, for all the benefits these different changes may have wrought, they would simultaneously produce ever intensifying organizational debates as to what was to be the definition of birth control and the role of the local birth control clinic.

Not Just a Building, Not Always a Stable Movement

For all the larger patterns to be discerned in the local birth control clinic, variations always abounded. Exactly who the clinic patients were often differed greatly from clinic to clinic, and the presence of women from a variety of economic, racial, ethnic, and religious backgrounds determined each facility's unique atmosphere. In addition, although the local clinic operated within a larger model and organizational structure, it remained deeply tied to the needs of the community and was also restrained by the resources organizers had available to them. This meant that admission policies often varied considerably, as did the services the clinic could provide. As the national office would quickly learn, getting all the clinics to do the same thing was an impossible task and often the source of much frustration within the many bureaucratic layers of Planned Parenthood.

Complicating matters even further is that the clinic itself was never just a physical space. As the words used to describe early clinic work suggest, the noun "clinic" was more often understood as an act. For example, when in 1923 the Parents' Committee of Chicago (which by 1924 became the Illinois Birth Control League) announced the opening of its first facility in Chicago, the organization explained how Dr. Rachelle Yarros had "been engaged to conduct it"—terminology that suggests less a finite place and more a protracted moment spent by individuals engaging in work, leadership, even education.[45] Indeed, that the clinic was about teaching was never lost on those within the movement. Furthermore, that the clinic was also often not even located in its own building challenges our understanding of how medical institutions (or any other institution for that matter) might work. Unlike hospitals, for example, which are often self-contained facilities built precisely for the provision of healthcare, clinics in contrast generally operated as sessions.[46] As a result, most functioned within other institutions (such as hospitals, social service agencies, private medical offices, or even sometimes private apartments) and often for only limited periods of time. A flier put out sometime in the 1940s by the local Planned Parenthood affiliate in Champaign, Illinois, illustrates this well:

COME TO PLANNED PARENTHOOD TO LEARN
ABOUT BIRTH CONTROL
THE CLINIC IS IN THE PUBLIC HEALTH INSTITUTION
505 South 5th Street, Champaign
The 1st and 3rd Wednesdays of each
month at 9 A.M.
The 2nd and 4th Tues. Evenings
at 7 P.M.[47]

Hence for much of its first sixty years, the clinic was hardly a full-time agency but rather operated where it could, when it could. It was, in fact, this seemingly guerrilla-style flexibility that made clinic establishment as easy as it was.

For this reason, what also deserves closer scrutiny is the seeming stability of the charity clinic movement itself. Though in many ways it was characterized by steady growth (albeit punctuated by the lull of the 1940s and 1950s), local instability remained a persistent theme. Over the years, not only did clinics within a single affiliate open and close with great regularity, as was the case in Chicago, but even more dramatically, entire affiliates themselves would fade in and out of existence within a single community. Such was the situation in Springfield, Illinois, which saw the rise of two different local birth control organizations in which members of the second generation were often unaware that an earlier organization had preceded their own.[48] Such considerations should not minimize the strength of these local organizations as an institution, however. Precisely because new clinics kept popping their heads through the hard soil attests to a persistent (albeit sometimes latent) vitality. By fulfilling the needs of those who worked within as well as those who procured its services from without, the clinic seemed always to find fertile ground in which to grow, if not in one community then in another. It was through this rich resource of community clinics that Planned Parenthood found its strength; and it was also through this resource that Planned Parenthood found its authority—which in turn helps explain why the debates over its form and function mattered so much.

Structure and Sources

The story I tell here is broken down into four chronological chapters. Before their contents can be described, four important clarifications need to be made. First, although Illinois serves loosely as my cornerstone for the history of local birth control clinics in relation to the marketplace, I have tried (as much as I have been able) to keep the events of the entire Planned Parenthood organization within range of my analytical radar, occasionally zeroing in on affiliates elsewhere in the nation (in this case San Antonio, Texas) when events there directly impacted the clinic movement as a whole. But anybody familiar with the size of Planned Parenthood knows that a fully national perspective that still accounts for local variation is virtually an impossible task. Such a limitation, moreover, bleeds into my treatment of the various early national birth control organizations and the complexity of their relationships to local birth control clinics. Although at least one historian has rightly noted the many distinctions between these early national offices and how territorially the lines between them were drawn, I have chosen in chapters 1 and 2 to lump them all together (local and national offices alike) as the "charity movement" more generally, which would by the 1940s coalesce into the more singularly configured Planned Parenthood Federation of America, which then served as the umbrella organization to the many local Planned Parenthood affiliates.[49] Only with chapters 3 and 4 do I again pay close attention to the various distinctions and often heated debates between the organization's many bureaucratic layers. I do so, however, not without an appreciation of all that this glosses over. Second, despite the centrality of Illinois to my analysis, this study is also not intended to read as an exhaustive account of the

Illinois movement. Instead, the local events I describe (usually about Chicago, though sometimes about Champaign and Danville) serve more as points of analytic departure into the other ideas I wish to discuss. My sincerest apologies in advance to all those Illinois affiliates that received short shrift and especially those that had no mention at all.

Third, while I hint at the major historiographic themes in the introduction, I have also chosen to allow these debates to unfold more fully through the course of the chapters. My hope in so doing is to draw in a broader educated readership (beyond, in other words, the world of academics) who, I believe, would want to understand not just the story itself but also the nuances of the process behind it. Thus to mete out the analysis in smaller chunks makes it easier to follow as well as more clear why we have long thought one way when in some cases I'm trying to argue for another. I can only hope my efforts were successful. The fourth clarification concerns the end decade of this study: the early 1970s. Certainly the story of Planned Parenthood does not end there, but as far as this book is concerned these years make for good benchmarks nonetheless. While 1972 marks the legalization of contraceptives for the unwed (by way of *Eisenstadt v. Baird*), 1973 marks the legalization of abortion (via *Roe v. Wade* and *Doe v. Bolton*). The early 1970s also mark the revelations of the Tuskegee Syphilis Study and the emergence thereafter of new federally mandated rules designed to provide protections for those who served as subjects of scientific research.[50] In short, the years of the 1970s designate both the legal validation of what was already increasingly taking place inside the local charity clinic as well as the laying of foundations for future battles to come, for which Planned Parenthood would have to develop new mechanisms to cope. For these reasons, I look forward to reading all the new stories that will no doubt soon be written.

These limits noted, the chapters are arranged as follows. Chapters 1 and 2 trace developments in the 1910s through the 1930s, analyzing in particular the relationship between the commercial marketplace and the charity birth control clinic movement from the clinic's emergence through the first wave. Here we see the potential, real, and ideological overlap that existed between these two worlds—so much so that even commercial birth control clinics were beginning to emerge as part of what I call the irregular birth control clinic movement—prompting the charity clinic movement to work hard to set itself apart, which it did by adopting the following strategies. Asserting the virtues of charity and the evils of business, it eschewed loud commercialism and embraced instead quiet respectability; it then touted the merits of the doctor-prescribed diaphragm and the legitimacy of the bona fide charity birth control clinic as the embodiment of such ideals. Notably, such strategies were in many ways successful because the laws against contraceptives began to loosen and the charity clinic movement had by the end of the 1930s won the support of the American Medical Association.[51]

However, while the first two chapters are a rethinking of more familiar terrains, the next two move our story into relatively uncharted territories. Chapter 3, for example, turns to the intermediary period of lull during the 1940s and 1950s that, despite the dearth of new clinic establishment, witnessed other important developments. These included new battles between the national Planned Parenthood office (which looked to standardize its vision and consolidate its control) and local affiliates (who had other ideas). These developments also included new dilemmas about the prescription of the diaphragm; apparently it was a method many clinic patients didn't like, prompting them to abandon both the method and the message promoted by the charity movement and *return* to the marketplace for their birth control needs. In response, Planned Parenthood tried to address women's dissatisfaction, but because it clung fast to medical authority and charitable paternalism, its efforts were limited at best. Finally, this chapter also describes the emergence of a new conceptualization of family, which in turn yielded the concept of the "unplanned family" and all of its "unwanted children." As the new symbol of social disorder in America, this concept of the unplanned family produced a powerful new rationale that would in the decades to follow help fuel the clinic movement's second wave of growth, transform the organization's rationale of charity that lay behind clinic work, and dismantle its rigid definition of birth control.

Chapter 4 then turns to the late 1950s through the early 1970s. Here we see this second wave of clinic growth, the introduction of the pill, the influx of blacks in the Chicago family planning movement, and the rise of widespread clinical research inside the local Planned Parenthood clinic. Significantly, we also see the fundamental reevaluation of the bedrocks upon which the institution was first based, both in terms of the definition of birth control and what was to be the role of the local birth control clinic. In other words, all that the clinic had disavowed in the first wave of growth was now embraced in the second: contraceptives for the unwed, over-the-counter methods, the termination of pregnancy, close ties with pharmaceutical companies, and even the use of loud commercial techniques to promote its new family planning message. Successful as all this was, it was not without its costs, and this chapter also reveals how battles raged anew within the Planned Parenthood organization about what was to be the definition of birth control and the function of the birth control clinic. In the conclusion, I use the organization's newly incorporated abortion services to investigate briefly the trajectory of the book's three main themes—the malleable relationship between business and charity, the malleable definition of birth control, and the guerilla-style flexibility of the form and function of the local birth control clinic—as they manifested themselves in more recent decades, though not without an appreciation of the similarities they regularly bear with the lessons of the past.

The bulk of my primary documents comes from the charity clinic movement's early newsletter (the *Birth Control Review*) and especially the rich organizational material of the local and national Planned Parenthood offices, which in this case can be found in archives in Illinois and Massachusetts. In addition to revealing the inner bureaucratic workings of this massive organization, these records offered surprisingly rich accounts of daily clinic life at the local level, accounts that often differed from the more public rhetoric of the organization's many educational materials. Yet even the propaganda occupies a central role in this study, for it suggests what Planned Parenthood hoped to achieve, even if its efforts were not always successful nor the outcomes as it had intended. Also useful among the organization's records were the collections of local affiliate newsletters and newspaper clippings, the latter of which detailed outside reactions to key moments in the work of Planned Parenthood. Finally, these records provided hard-to-come-by material about the role of pharmaceutical companies in clinic affairs. As I quickly learned at the start of my research, access to the archives of pharmaceutical companies is often met with great resistance, which meant I needed to look elsewhere. Fortunately, because my research concerned persons who had direct contact with the birth control organization, Planned Parenthood had what I was looking for.

Other sources were important as well. The American Medical Association's Historical Health Fraud and Alternative Medicine Collection (mentioned at the start of this introduction) yielded a veritable treasure trove about the larger commercial world in which the early clinics operated and contained especially useful material on the inner workings of those clinic facilities that lay beyond the charity movement's scope. Investigation into a variety of popular press publications (including, but not limited to, women's magazines, black periodicals, Catholic journals, and business reviews) also provided much needed perspective from beyond clinic walls. In addition, the many published reports of birth control use—which regularly made their way into medical and public health journals—provided a good opportunity to learn more about clinic clientele, thereby deepening what I was able to glean from Planned Parenthood's internal records.

In recounting the sources I used, however, it would be remiss of me not to mention all that I borrowed from the work of other scholars. Three historians in particular come to mind. The first of course is Linda Gordon, whose influential *Woman's Body, Woman's Right* (1976) serves in many ways as the cornerstone to this study, but also as what I often want to argue against. Not only am I deeply indebted to the framework she brilliantly provided more than thirty years ago, but (and as I have also come to realize) she is apparently as difficult to avoid as is Margaret Sanger when it comes to writing about the history of twentieth-century birth control. So it goes with those who have made such important historical and historiographic contributions. The second historian to whom I am indebted is Andrea Tone; in all my research, she was always one step ahead of me in what I thought I was the first to uncover. For example, when I stumbled across the vitality of the 1930s contraceptive marketplace in the archives of the American Medical Association, she had already written about it in her 1996 article, "Contraceptive Consumers." When I then noticed the complexity of the relationship of the American Birth Control League to this commercial world, she was already writing about this too in her 2001 book, *Devices and Desires*, leaving me once again with the daunting task of differentiating my work from hers. Consequently, were it not for all that she had already written, my analysis would be much thinner and the book you are now holding would have far less to offer. I'm just grateful she didn't set her sights on the clinic. This brings me to the third historian to whom I am indebted, Cathy Moran Hajo, because she did write about the clinic.

Cathy and I first met at a conference a number of years ago and it has always been a great joy to have someone else around with whom I can engage in dense clinic conversation. However, I long lived in fear of how her work would outstrip my own. As an editor of the Margaret Sanger Papers Project, hers is a knowledge of Sanger and the various national birth control organizations vastly superior to my own. As the author of a book that analyzed the activities of more than six hundred early local clinics, *Birth Control on Main Street: Organizing Clinics in the United States, 1916–1939*, hers is a knowledge of the early clinic vastly superior to mine as well. It was with great trepidation, therefore, that I finally read the dissertation from which her book developed while I was still in the process of trying to figure out this book. But my fears were only partially born out because while in many ways she wrote the story I would liked to have written, she wrote what I apparently cannot write. It was a revelation strangely liberating, though, because were it not for her careful statistical analysis of hundreds of local charity clinics, which she then blended with her vast knowledge of the various national charity organizations, I would not have been able to spend my days contemplating more theoretical matters, namely, how this massive world of charity birth control negotiated the equally massive world of commercial birth control. So together, I think, we make a fine pair. And I was delighted to hear that she agrees.

Yet the sources that still stand the most prominently in my mind are the oral histories of five Planned Parenthood clinic workers who, with utmost graciousness, told me of their experiences from days long past. It is with great sadness that I must explain how little their specific stories enter into what about you are about to read. But what these women told me remains important because their insights helped frame this narrative in fundamental ways. As I waded through the organization's many materials, their words always stayed in the back of my mind, reminding me neither to believe all that policy stipulated nor accept what public rhetoric suggested life inside the clinic was really like. Indeed, providing birth control was part science, part art, a labor of love and a labor of frustration. And these clinic workers did the best they knew, even if it meant disagreeing with the advice outsiders so often had to offer. For these reasons and more, I am deeply grateful for all they told me. That they opened their doors and their hearts in an effort to answer my many unenlightened questions meant a great deal. That one of them sent me home with a bag of homegrown tomatoes meant even more. My only hope now is that although these women may have good cause to disagree with the interpretations I have chosen to lay over their clinic work, they may find at least a few grains of truth in the pages that follow.

Chapter One

The Birth of the Clinic

When Andrea Tone wrote *Devices and Desires* (2001), she breathed new life into what had become an old story about birth control, particularly in its illegal days. "Scholars," she wrote, "have often characterized the period between criminalization in the 1870s and Margaret Sanger's movement in the second decade of the twentieth century as birth control's bleakest chapter, a time when only a privileged few could afford the services of sympathetic doctors or of a dwindling number of merchants who would ignore the law for the right price." Yet, as was the case when Leslie Reagan looked into the history of illegal abortion, what Tone noticed was something quite different: although "not openly endorsed," there remained nonetheless a thriving black market of contraceptives for those interested in limiting childbearing.[1] The first birth control rebels, we might therefore conclude, were not the better known political radicals of the early twentieth century, but rather the bootleg entrepreneurs who had since the 1870s been breaking the law all along.

To appreciate the presence of these bootleg entrepreneurs is imperative; to take them seriously is imperative as well. As Tone described, the world of bootleg birth control was far more vibrant and complex than had been previously imagined, populated with individuals who defied Comstock laws long before Sanger began her work. Furthermore, their existence helps explain the long gap between 1873—when the Comstock Act (which banned fertility control techniques by making it illegal to send through the mail information about and devices for contraception and abortion) was first put into place—and the early twentieth century when Sanger began to defy this and other anti-birth-control laws herself. In other words, the world of birth control was not the vacuum that Sanger often liked to describe. Rather, a foundation (albeit underground) of fertility control advice and techniques was still firmly in place.

Equally important to appreciate is the intersection between these two rebel worlds of the charity clinic and the underground bootlegger, in particular the ways in which they fed off each other. To begin with, the early birth control clinic itself was in many ways a part of this bootleg world, in that it often operated in a realm of questionable legality. In addition, where was it to get its supplies if not from bootleg entrepreneurs themselves? They also influenced each other, to striking effect. In the 1910s, for example, political birth control radicals like Sanger were brash and loud while bootleg entrepreneurs tended to be quiet and discreet, least-wise they kept their message away from white middle-class publications. By the 1920s and 1930s, however, the behaviors and strategies of charity clinics and underground entrepreneurs began to switch. Emboldened by the successes of the early charity birth control clinic movement, bootleg birth control entrepreneurs grew ever more daring, moving noisily into the commercial mainstream. In response, the charity birth control clinic movement reversed its tactics. Now looking to cultivate an aura of respectability, it eschewed its loud rhetoric of old and embraced instead an air of quiet modesty. Thus within a few short decades, the strategies of both sides, responding to one another in dialectical fashion, had come full circle. For this reason, although we have long grown accustomed to viewing the commercial provision of birth control as somehow inherently distinct and separate from its more charitable distribution by way of the clinic, we should not. Instead, these worlds overlapped and their strategies intersected far more than has been previously suggested.

Our task here, then, is to recombine the two worlds of the charity clinic and the bootleg entrepreneur so that we might imagine a landscape differently than has been previously described—a landscape in which there existed a great variety of birth control methods, a great variety of birth control providers, a great variety of ways to make the availability of birth control known, and a great variety of motivations behind the desire to make the means to limit childbearing available in the first place. Our task is also to imagine what worked to pull these two worlds apart, ultimately giving rise to the dichotomy about this early period with which we are so familiar today. What we will see as a result is how in these early days when birth control was illegal, there existed a potentially broad definition of this newly invented "birth control" term, one that the institutionalized vision of charity clinic services would by the 1920s and 1930s seek to contain. It is this multilayered story that commands the attention of our first two chapters.

Radical Ideas in a Bootleg World

For all that has been said about the radical pamphlet "Family Limitation" that Sanger first published in 1914—in which she carefully described five different ways to limit childbearing—one piece of advice remains persistently absent in the scholarly conversations that describe it: her many references to the marketplace. Yet the "drugstore," the "reliable pharmacy," and even the names of several manufacturers were mentioned repeatedly by Sanger as good places to go to satisfy one's birth control needs.[2] Several years later, the same advice could be had in the radical clinic she briefly ran on Brooklyn's immigrant-populated Amboy Street. As Elizabeth Stuyvesant explained in a

1917 issue of the *Birth Control Review*, in addition to "desks, chairs, scrubbing brushes and soap," her friend Sanger had also purchased "a set of the articles" so that she might demonstrate to the clinic's needy clientele "just what they should ask for" on their next trip to the local drugstore.[3]

Given the prominence of marketplace options in Sanger's advice to women, scholars' failure to discuss it is curious. But it is an omission that speaks both to history and historiography. The illegality of birth control of course is in part to blame; if it was against the law, it could surely not have existed in any substantial way. As historian Janet Farrell Brodie wrote, and as Tone would later quote when she proved this characterization wrong, the Comstock laws of the 1870s drove "reproductive control, if not totally back underground, at least into a netherworld of back-fence gossip and back-alley abortions."[4] Hence Brodie argued that because of the law the picture was a bleak one. Yet, as Tone explained, not only was such a characterization misleading, it was also not born of law alone; Sanger was herself behind this inaccurate characterization as well.[5] Consequently, although Sanger's early advice suggests she knew otherwise, she would go on to paint a similarly bleak portrait—a portrait in which I could not help but notice she carefully erased all of her early marketplace connections. Here, then, is where the plot thickens because although the shift in Sanger's rhetoric was in many ways born of her desire to win over the American Medical Association (AMA), our buying of her claims speak to other things: in particular, what historian Nan Enstad in her brilliantly argued *Ladies of Labor, Girls of Adventure* (1999) described as the "analytical binary between consumerism and politics," which she declared to be a false one.[6]

Indeed, recognizing the overlap between these two things—the desire to buy and the desire to politick—has been difficult for historians, and nowhere does this appear more vividly than in our many stories of the young working women of the early twentieth century. As Enstad explained, on the one hand, much has been said about their lives as workers and as unionists who in turn "produced some of the most dramatic strikes of the century." On the other hand, there is the story of their leisure, a world of commercial goods and pleasures in which these working girls eagerly participated as well. Yet because of the ways in which these stories have been written, Enstad wrote, "it is hard to believe these books are about the same women," leading us to miss the ways in which these young wage earning women "used consumer culture to do political work."[7] To that end, then, and with respect to birth control, if we were to ask ourselves a similar question: what use could Sanger—the outspoken critic of capitalism that she was in her early days—have had for the commercial world? We could reply: a great deal because despite the radicalism of Sanger's critique and the militancy of her politics, when she first sought immediate solutions, she turned to the marketplace.

And why shouldn't she? If we go by what Tone found, Sanger could have added to her list of several manufacturers the names of many hundreds more.[8] That Sanger also repeatedly suggested drugstore sources makes just as much sense as well. They could be found in cities and towns across the nation; Chicago, for example, boasted of no less than 1,800 different locations scattered throughout distinct neighborhoods. Each also occupied an important niche, both economic and cultural, within the local communities they served, not least among them the various immigrant communities.[9] It should come as little surprise therefore that Sanger made mention, as did her colleague Emma Goldman, of this marketplace option in her efforts to reach immigrant communities.[10]

In fact, the work of two bootleg entrepreneurs who peddled their wares in the Midwest reveals the ties that could exist—indeed, already did exist—between these bootleg providers and their immigrant clientele. As Tone described, Antoinette Hon was herself a Polish immigrant newly arrived to America, and in 1905 she and her husband set up shop in South Bend, Indiana, to engage in the sale of various patent medicine preparations, not the least of which were several products that were contraceptive in nature. Further revealing are the ways in which she advertised her wares. As Tone explained, while Hon relied in part upon her status as a woman to appeal to her female clientele, she also drew upon their shared immigrant backgrounds to spread the word. As a result, advertisements for her feminine hygiene preparations could be found in such publications as *Zgoda*, a foreign-language newspaper that served Chicago's growing Polish community.[11] Yet Hon was hardly alone in using such methods. The Chicago-based Septigyn Company sought to win over an immigrant clientele as well, and while Hon looked to the Poles, Septigyn turned to the Czechs.

This in turn reveals yet another way our two rebel worlds could intersect. When Septigyn sought to win the patronage of the city's growing community of Czechoslovakians, it used fliers as part of its efforts, fliers that were written both in English and the native tongue of its prospective clientele.[12] And this, as Linda Gordon demonstrated, was precisely what Sanger did; the mass distribution of handbills, printed in a variety of different languages, constituted one of the main ways she educated women about birth control and advertised her clinic services.[13] In other words, although Sanger had perhaps learned such strategies through her Industrial Workers of the World (IWW) activism, such strategies were hardly confined to political or public service types alone; entrepreneurs used them as well. For these reasons, it is imperative we blend together what we know about the early politically radical Sanger (by way especially of Gordon's hugely influential Marxist-feminist account) with what we know about those bootleg entrepreneurs (by way of Tone's more business-friendly interpretation). For only then does the breadth of birth control possibilities emerge.

To begin with, in this early twentieth-century world, birth control was hardly the purview of doctors; nor did people expect it to be.[14] Sanger herself was a nurse who promoted the authority of other nurses as well as that of druggists and even perhaps of midwives.[15] Other individuals, such as Sarah Chase and Gustavas Farr, entered into the birth control trade with degrees in homeopathy.[16] As historians of medicine have long shown, this turn-of-the-twentieth-century world was replete with a great variety of medical providers whose authority persisted despite organized medicine's campaign against them.[17] Not surprisingly, they too would enter into the birth control trade. But then there were those who engaged in occupations seemingly unrelated, as we might imagine today, to their future birth control careers. George Brinckerhoff, for example, was once a grocer before he went on to establish the Eugenic Manufacturing Company. And the indomitable Julius Schmidt, the crippled immigrant from Germany, turned his day-job skills as a sausage stuffer into a business he developed at night: the manufacture of condoms, a story that Tone still takes great delight in recounting.[18] In other words, ordinary laborers and entrepreneurs could be just as knowledgeable about birth control as anybody else.

Nor, for that matter, were all these early twentieth-century providers intent upon promoting one single method, much less confining their work to the provision of contraceptives alone. While the German-born Joseph Backrach sold condoms for men, womb veils for women, and rubber ticklers to aid in sexual stimulation, others sold an equally diverse array of products. For example, the entrepreneur William Halleck sold rubber-stem pessaries, douching syringes, and abortifacients, while rubber manufacturers more generally made a variety of condoms, IUDs, and douching syringes.[19] Nor was the sale of contraceptives and abortifacients necessarily distinct trades, as Halleck's business suggests. Even the nineteenth-century career of Madame Restell makes this plain. Although she is more commonly known for her work as an abortionist, she also engaged in the provision of pregnancy preventatives.[20] Consequently, when measured against this backdrop, Sanger's "Family Limitation" pamphlet—with its recommendation of condoms, douches, pessaries, sponges, and even (more guardedly) abortion when all else failed—bears much in common with the goods and services provided by others.

Finally, no less expansive were the reasons to engage in the provision of birth control in the first place. While the early Sanger pushed it as a political matter, others saw in it just another way to earn a good living, a motivation that was particularly important to those individuals for whom other professional avenues were often closed. As Tone explained, the business of birth control was a magnet for women, for immigrants, and for those of limited means, making it a particularly appealing option for aspiring small-time entrepreneurs.[21] It would be unfair to suggest, however, that the pursuit of an income alone was all that drove these entrepreneurs on. They too could have been motivated by politics and even by a feminist sensibility. The career of Edward Bliss Foote—a graduate of Pennsylvania Medical College and birth control entrepreneur who would go on to have many run-ins with Anthony Comstock—is suggestive. Although he retired a wealthy man, his 1864 pamphlet for lay readers (*Medical Common Sense*) reveals other motivations for his work in contraception. As Foote wrote in reference to his one-size-fits-all diaphragm, "It places conception entirely under the control of the wife to whom it naturally belongs." To which he added, "for it is for her to say at what time and under what circumstances she will become the mother and the moral, religious, and physical instructress of offspring."[22] Contrary, therefore, to what the charity birth control movement would by the 1920s and 1930s like to have us believe, what we see here is how differing motivations could overlap, indeed did overlap, prompting us to take a cue from several historians of black business enterprises and to wonder if the analytical binary between politicking and *selling* could be false as well.[23]

Of course, this is not to say that there can be found no lines of distinction between them, because there was at least one: the ways in which they violated the Comstock laws. The early Sanger, for example, sought publicity and visibility, sought directly to challenge the Comstock laws in order to abolish them. Further illustrative of the boldness of her tactics is her "Family Limitation" pamphlet. Not only did it specifically describe various birth control techniques, but it also used simple line drawings to depict birth control methods commercially available as well as parts of women's reproductive anatomy. Readers were thus educated visually in precisely what to look for at the local drugstore and given a lesson in the workings of the female body.[24] In contrast, most of the early birth control entrepreneurs, though certainly not all (as was the case with Antoinette Hon and Septigyn), tended to operate quietly. However, they did so not necessarily out of a sense of shame or prudery, but rather because discreetness enabled them more successfully to elude Comstock's net. Bootleg birth control entrepreneurs relied on aliases to conceal their identities, stored their stock in a variety of locations, and camouflaged their products' contraceptive uses.[25] Thus the utility of Sanger's pamphlet, which made various birth control products and their uses plain. Here again, though, this should not minimize the radicalism of the work of these bootleggers. Not only was their defiance of the law often as great as that of the more political types, but their defiance of the law was also in many ways "direct action," to borrow the phrase used by Gordon to describe Sanger's early activities. In other words, these bootleg entrepreneurs saw in birth control both a need and a demand, and they, like Sanger, looked to provide for it directly.[26]

Nor is this to suggest that entrepreneurs operated without risk or that everybody, rich and poor alike, had easy access to the goods they offered. Merchants were indeed arrested and, if convicted, subject by the provisions of the 1873 Comstock Act to a hefty fine, hard-labor imprisonment, and the payment of court costs. Similarly, that many thousands of individuals wrote letters to Sanger looking for birth control advice suggests too that Comstockery, either the law itself or the larger culture that sustained it, posed no insignificant constraints.[27] But to borrow Tone's description, the law had its "limits," which meant that relatively few birth control entrepreneurs were ever caught, and when they were, they were either slapped lightly on the wrist or set free without any conviction at all, whereupon they resumed immediately the peddling of their wares, a decision the consuming public ensured was a wise one.[28]

My point therefore is this: if we wish to understand this early twentieth-century world of birth control, we must begin by describing the world of the clinic and the world of the bootleg provider in one breath because despite the restrictions posed by Comstockery, the nineteenth-century marketplace doggedly persisted into the twentieth century, keeping alive an important groundwork upon which political radicals could then seize. For this reason, we must reframe our perspective because only then can we begin to imagine the possibilities embedded in the provision of birth control. Indeed, when in the 1910s the term "birth control" first emerged, it *could* mean a great many different of things: it could mean methods for women, it could mean methods for men; it could mean methods to prevent pregnancies, it could mean those that terminated them; it could mean methods provided by doctors or nurses, it could mean those from homeopaths, patent medicine peddlers, and immigrant entrepreneurs; it could mean a way radically to change society, or it could mean simply a good way to earn a living. It *could* mean, in other words, so many different things. And only when we begin to imagine this can we begin to see more clearly the significance of the new vision of birth control that was by the 1920s set to emerge, the new vision embedded in the charity birth control clinic.

A Charity Is Born

There were many stories Sanger liked to tell about her conversion to the birth control cause, among them was her version of how she came upon the birth control clinic idea. It was on her 1915 trip to Holland where she had the opportunity to witness firsthand clinic operations sponsored by the Dutch Neo-Malthusian League. There she learned about Dr. Aletta Jacobs, who in 1882 established the first birth control clinic for the poor in Amsterdam, which had grown into a clinic movement that spread throughout the country. There Sanger also learned about the Mesinga diaphragm, a device she herself learned how to fit under the direction of Dr. Johannes Rutgers. Deeply impressed with what she saw, Sanger would later write how the "results of my visit to Holland were to change the whole course of the birth control movement."[29] Influential as her experiences no doubt were, what they do not explain is the birth control clinic's rapid embrace by reform-minded middle-class citizens in America. It wasn't so much that Sanger turned to these citizens; in fact she was often deeply hostile toward them. Rather, it was often they who turned to birth control, simultaneously bringing with them a shared desire to engage in charity work and a shared familiarity, as I have elsewhere argued, with the larger clinic movement born of the Progressive era. The seed of Sanger's Dutch clinic, in other words, fell on fertile American soil.[30]

Chicago illustrates this point well. In what has now become a classic story of the early days of the birth control clinic movement, Sanger's reaction to the city's tightly knit community of welfare reformers was one of hostility and disgust. "Chicago," Sanger later wrote of her experiences in 1916, "was so well organized by social workers, through the influence of Jane Addams of Hull House, that it was extremely difficult for me to reach [the women of the stock-yard] districts without sanction of a woman prominent in social work."[31] Sanger's derision, moreover, hardly applied to reformers in Chicago alone. In 1914, the editors for the radical magazine *Woman Rebel* decried "milk stations" and "baby benefits" as mere palliatives—the hypocritical window dressings of "The Church, State and big business"—which they believed only soothed and perpetuated women's misery, unlike birth control, which would empower them.[32] Yet the Chicago birth control clinic movement would become active nonetheless, deeply embedded in the city's vast network of maternal welfare reformers. Thus, despite Sanger's early animosity toward middle-class welfare reformers, it was in their arms that the charity birth control clinic movement was born.

The significance of this moment cannot be overstated; nor has it been overlooked. Following the paths laid by Ellen Chesler, Linda Gordon, Carole McCann, and James Reed, who documented the birth control clinic movement at the national levels, in recent years a wealth of new literature has emerged that describes the early rise of birth control organizations at the local level: in Arkansas, Ohio, Massachusetts, Minnesota, New York, North Carolina, Puerto Rico, Rhode Island, Tennessee, and Texas. Time and again, the story that emerges is the presence of middle-class women who were interested in charity work. Time and again, what also emerges is the complexity of their motivations to engage in such work.[33]

As the historians just named have described, the reasons why these women joined the charity birth control cause were many. In part they were driven by compassion. The first two decades of the twentieth century found Americans coping with the dramatic social and economic changes wrought by a period of massive urbanization, immigration, and industrialization. Of particular concern was the health of those who lived in the dirty and overcrowded cities. With higher-than-average infant and maternal mortality rates, the poor suffered the most. Through sanitation campaigns as well as settlement houses, milk stations, visiting nurses programs, and well-baby clinics, among other public health initiatives, maternal welfare reformers worked to improve the health of the nation's poor and immigrant communities. By the 1930s, this desire to engage in charitable services was propelled even more by the economic disaster posed by the Great Depression. Thus a genuine sympathy drove welfare reformers on, and they increasingly saw birth control as an essential component of public health reform.

Compassion, however, comingled with the desire to limit the number of children certain women bore. The 1920s fever pitch of nativism, wrought by the influx of immigrants from southern and southeastern Europe in previous decades, fueled support for the establishment of birth control clinics in the nation's poor and immigrant neighborhoods. The migration of African Americans to northern industrial cities likely fueled the fires as well. Moreover, persistently poor race relations in the South contributed to the movement's popularity in that region of the country as well. In addition, the ties that the early birth control movement cultivated with the eugenics movement were great, which has prompted in turn much scholarly debate: Was it compassion and sympathy that drove these individuals on? Or was it racism, nativism, and a desire for social control? Yet therein lies the significance of what this new body of scholarship about local birth control movements is beginning to reveal: the compassionate desire to help women and children often comingled to varying degrees with the impulse to limit the number of children that poor, black, and immigrant women bore. In short, the movement was as complex as it was vast; so too were the motivations behind it, products of the diversity of local circumstances and individual attitudes within given locales. As Cathy Moran Hajo put it in her analysis of the early birth control clinic movement, "one gets the sense that the movement was a hydra, whose many heads shouted different arguments, some contradicting others."[34]

However, for all the significance of these findings, the time has come to take the analysis forward by investigating what else this new relationship between charity and birth control yielded. While much has been made of the medicalization of birth control during this early phase of clinic development (with its emphasis on doctors, diaphragms, and science), much less has been said (in a sustained measure, at any rate) about what might be called its *charitification*. For this reason, the questions we should now ask are these: What exactly does it mean to have the provision of birth control increasingly framed within the context of charity? What in turn were its limits? To ask such questions is crucial because the effect of charitification was great: It influenced legal strategies and fundraising campaigns, the nature of enemies and the nature of friends. It also affected the type and location of birth control services and the attitude toward the women whom this new charity movement looked to serve. Charity thus served a powerful tool in gaining the physical and financial support necessary to establish and then run local birth control clinics, though the use of charity was not without its negative effects. Providing birth control in charity clinics also had serious limits, which meant that dabbling in the world of business remained important. Consequently, an examination of this shift in the birth control movement—from a radical movement to empower the working class to a charity movement run by the middle class—is now in order. Here again Chicago is a useful place to begin.

July 30, 1923, was a momentous day for the Parents' Committee of Chicago because it was on this day that the organization submitted to the Department of Health its application for a permit to engage in charity clinic operations. This day was long in coming. The Parents' Committee was first formed roughly seven years earlier in the wake of Sanger's 1916 visit. It immediately set to work, inspired, as one account would later explain, in part by its members' "belief in free speech" but also by their outrage that poor women were denied access to the means to control their fertility.[35] First among its many tasks was to determine the legality of birth control in the state of Illinois, and what the organization learned was encouraging. "So far as I am able to find," the attorney general wrote on February 24, 1917, in response to the group's inquiry about the matter, "there is no statute in this State, that would prevent physicians from giving such advice for the purpose of the prevention of conception." Nor was there, he added, anything "relating to the matter in the statute on the practice of medicine" or even "in the rules or regulations of the State Board of Health on this subject." He did go on to warn them of the "very severe penalties" they would incur if they engaged in the provision of abortion. But giving contraceptives to married women by their doctors fell well within the law.[36]

For the Parents' Committee this was good news, and although it would take six more years, the groundwork for its first charity clinic would be laid: The committee had met with the commissioner of public health, Dr. Herman N. Bundesen, who agreed to put aside his personal reservations against birth control and issue the required charity permit.[37] The committee had secured the services of Dr. Rachelle Yarros, a woman who was one of its founding members, to serve as the physician in charge of this local birth control operation. The committee had also decided not only on a name for its new facility (the Parents' Clinic) but also where this new facility would be—in a private apartment building on 1347 North Lincoln Street, deep in the heart of a poor, immigrant neighborhood on the city's northwest side.[38] All that remained was getting the charity permit itself.

However, this proved more difficult than the Parents' Committee anticipated because Commissioner Bundesen in the meantime changed his mind.

Technical deficiencies with the group's application were among the first things he cited. But when the Parents' Committee fixed these problems and reapplied, Bundesen refused again, citing first the law, then immorality, and finally the Bible directly. He solidified his position with a final p.s. in a letter of September 19, 1923, to Helen Carpenter, the president of the Parents' Committee: "Check No. 4 (Parents' Clinic) for $12.00 is enclosed herewith."[39] The Parents' Committee was not so easily daunted. With Harold L. Ickes and George Packard serving as its legal counsel, the group filed suit to force Bundesen to make good on what he promised to do, generating in turn a messy tug-of-war that pit the law against bureaucracy. Increasingly frustrated by what appeared to be an unwinnable case, the committee decided to pursue another route. "Reluctantly," as Helen Carpenter explained in 1925, we "abandoned the idea of a free clinic" and opened instead a facility that did "not require a license": the *fee-based* medical clinic. Although litigation had failed to produce what the group had originally sought, it did solidify the rights of doctors to provide contraceptives out of their private medical practices. As a result, the newly named Medical Center was born, and the services it offered came directly out of Yarros's private medical office.[40] Two years earlier Sanger had done the same in New York City.[41]

Although interesting to tell as a story, we need to pause to consider not only the practical obstacles that switching to a model of private medical practice raised but its ideological murkiness as well. To begin with, the clinic's new location was a problem. Located at 308 North Michigan Avenue, Yarros's office was right in the middle of the city's fashionable downtown, hardly the best place to attract the city's immigrant poor, a problem Helen Carpenter quickly noted. The "people who need us most," she commented, "are not accustomed to coming to Michigan Avenue for medical advice." New clinic locations, she explained, would have to be found.[42] Equally significant are the ideological implications of this tactic of providing birth control services to the poor by means of a private medical practice. While Gordon rightfully pointed out its significance in terms of doctors' unique power and professional autonomy (when describing the use of this strategy in New York City), what it also means is that the charity clinics in both of these cities were engaging in marketplace practices—goods and services were being offered in exchange for a fee.[43]

Indeed, strictly speaking, the charity birth control clinic could not help but dabble in the world of business and commerce. For example, in an effort to ensure a steady supply of Mesinga diaphragms for her New York clinic operations, Sanger solicited the help of her second husband, Noah Slee, to help establish the Holland-Rantos Company in order to manufacture the necessary clinic supplies. As Tone explained, to import them illegally from overseas was "time-consuming, impractical, and risky." Of course, Sanger looked to minimize her involvement but her intent was clear: she needed diaphragms, she needed somebody local to manufacture them for her, and she was going to make sure somebody did.[44] But then there were other ways to participate in this commercial world. The Illinois Birth Control League (formally the Parents' Committee) engaged in the sale of contraceptive supplies to patients—who were then charged by a sliding scale (anywhere from $7.50 at the downtown clinic to a maximum of $2.50 at all of its other clinic locations). It also sold contraceptives directly to local doctors who then made these products available to their patients in private practice.[45] Of course, the activities of New York and Chicago were in many ways unique, but they were not alone in such blurring of boundaries between charity and fee-for-service clinics; sliding fee scales were regularly used by clinics across the nation.[46]

In turn, the benefits of such businesslike practices were several. To charge patients something (even if it was a nominal fee) was often seen as important motivator for the clinic client herself. "Experience shows," noted Alice C. Boughton in a 1934 issue of the *Birth Control Review*, "that it is wise, when possible, to collect something, however small, to cover at least in part the cost of supplies, even if the cost in overhead is as much as the total sum involved." As she explained, "Clinic records seem to indicate that the woman who pays *something* for her supplies is more likely to follow directions than one who gets service and supplies entirely free."[47] Or, as the president of the Rhode Island Birth Control League noted, the "clinic was established for charitable purposes, but from the standpoint of modern social ethics it is advisable to have the patients feel that they are paying for a valuable service."[48] Thus the argument went something like this: not only would women feel less shame in taking charity but it might also prompt them to be more diligent in their birth control use.

In terms of the birth control clinic more generally, the selling of supplies also helped sustain charity clinic operations. The money it took in was constantly channeled back into the clinic—to cover the salaries of its paid workers (often physicians), the cost of rent (when rent was required), or the purchase of more supplies (when supplies ran out)—not unlike any other business operation.[49] Of course making a profit was not a goal; nor was the money the clinic took in ever close to fully financing clinic operations— though, in truth, the Illinois Birth Control League did quite well.[50]

Nor, interestingly enough, did the immigrant poor constitute the bulk of the Illinois Birth Control League's clientele. To the contrary, of the 1,340 women it served in 1929, 768 were listed as "American" (meaning white, native born); another 420 consisted of 170 "American colored," 74 Polish, 71 Italian, 45 Russian, 28 Mexican, 19 Bohemian, 13 Austrian clients; the remaining 152 were composed of a "scattering of Slovakian, Lithuanian, Hungarian, Armenian, Persian, [and] Croatian" clients. White nonimmigrant American women, in other words, constituted a sizable number of the women using the Chicago charity clinics. Moreover, many of the women in this category were not even poor. As a result, the Illinois Birth Control League's busiest birth control clinic was not housed in the city's poorer neighborhoods but rather in the city's fashionable downtown (though now at 203 North Wabash Avenue), a location that also served as the organization's main headquarters. Notably, the $7.50 fee these wealthier women paid was a hefty one, but this served a vital purpose. Much as was the case in New York City, it helped ensure a solid financial basis for the local office and, perhaps even more important, sustained those clinics that served poorer communities.[51] As Hajo pointed out, Chicago and New York were unique in the number of middle-class women they served. But the practices of the clinics in those cities suggest the possibility, indeed the reality, of the ways in which clinics might be in competition with private physicians for paying patients, a point that will become more salient in the chapter to follow.[52]

Such blurring of boundaries between free and fee-for-service practices notwithstanding, charity remained a vital framework for the model of the birth control clinic, offering powerful practical solutions to some difficult problems that the early clinics had to resolve. Chicago's problem of less than suitable clinic locations to reach the black and immigrant poor was quickly solved with the assistance of the city's many philanthropic organizations. Of the six clinics the Illinois Birth Control League opened by 1928, one found its home in the Henry Booth House, another in the South Side Community Center, two more in the Jewish People's Institute and Hull House's Mary Crane Nursery. Also alleviated was the matter of lagging caseloads. As Helen Carpenter of the Illinois Birth Control League wrote, the "first three months of our work were a little discouraging," and although newspaper publicity from the battle with Bundesen boosted attendance slightly, patients, she explained, still "come slowly."[53] But by 1930 things appeared to have turned around. As the league proudly reported on the pages of the *Birth Control Review*, not only had it served more than 1,300 women in the previous year, but its totals also drew increasingly from the foreign born, a shift the league credited to "the various social organizations [that] have been of the greatest assistance."[54] The Associated Charities of Chicago even helped out by paying the fees of the women it referred.[55] Notably, Chicago (as well as New York City) was unique in the depth of its ties to such agencies, particularly in the prevalence of birth control clinics operating through settlement houses.[56] But clinics across the nation cultivated ties to charities of their own; it was just a matter of how and to what degree.[57]

Charity also served as a powerful propaganda tool. In part, it pulled on the heartstrings of those whose support local birth control groups looked to solicit. For example, despite the fact that the Illinois Birth Control League regularly served wealthier women, it was the stories of poor, pitiful women that more commonly appeared in its public announcements. "Many of the cases are very pitiful," explained one report appearing in a 1925 issue of the *Birth Control Review*. It then provided the following examples:

> Case No. 59—Referred by United Charities and Municipal Tuberculosis Sanitarium. The man is 54 years of age, street cleaner, Colored-Protestant. The woman is 40 years of age, married at 20 and in twenty years has had sixteen pregnancies. Of the fourteen children, whose ages range from seventeen years to eighteen months, seven died in infancy.

> Case No. 318—Referred by United Charities. The man is 28 years old, laborer. The woman is 20 years old, German-Catholic, married at 19. Both feeble-minded. One child feeble-minded.[58]

More such stories made their way into the Illinois Birth Control League's application for membership in Chicago's local community chest, the Welfare Council.[59] Of course, that the local birth control office described such cases when applying to a charitable organization certainly seems appropriate. But the more birth control is pitched that way, the more it becomes that way. Charity also pulled on people's purse strings, though often in less than charitable ways. As one commentator remarked in a 1936 issue of *American Mercury*, "Of proper consideration . . . is the amount of money which might be saved by more widespread use of birth control machinery."[60] Or, as Gordon later argued, "Birth controllers seized upon the relief crisis [of the 1930s] with gusto" because "birth control would cut public costs and thus taxes," an argument that held considerable appeal.[61] Perhaps most illustrative of the centrality of charity to the propaganda of the birth control movement was the slogan adopted by a birth control group in Waco, Texas, that read: "A charity to end charity."[62]

This is not to say that all charities supported clinic work. The Illinois Birth Control League's repeated efforts to join the Welfare Council in Chicago—the massive umbrella organization that drew together all those engaged in charitable work—demonstrates this point well. Time and again the league applied, and time and again it was denied; the primary obstacle being the council's powerful Catholic constituency.[63] It is little wonder that, in the face of such long-standing opposition, the Illinois Birth Control League took great delight in announcing the large presence of Catholic women at its various clinic locations. "It is interesting to note," remarked Dr. Yarros, "that almost a third of our patients are Catholics, and when the center is located in a Catholic neighborhood the proportion rises much higher."[64] But such opposition from local charities was not confined to Chicago. Birth control clinic groups across the country regularly faced resistance; and while often it was the result of Catholic opposition, that was not always the case. Jimmy Elaine Wilkinson Meyer, for example, recounted similar difficulties in Cincinnati, Albany, and St. Louis, while Denise Hulett explained how the birth control group in Waco, Texas, had trouble getting support from the local community chest.[65]

Finally, to frame the provision of birth control as an act of charity was also not without another important effect: the creation of the "case," a term increasingly used within the birth control clinic movement to describe those women who procured clinic services. Scholars Stanley Wenocur and Michael Reisch, authors of *From Charity to Enterprise: The Development of American Social Work in a Market Economy* (1989), offer insight into the roots of this terminology. In part, it was a product of the language of physicians, who often used the word "case" to describe their patients. By the early twentieth century, the practice was picked up by social workers, who, in their quest for professionalization, looked to the medical profession as a good model to follow. As Wenocur and Reisch explained, social workers "argued that the function of the caseworker was rehabilitation, and that since diagnosis and treatment went hand-in-hand, a good caseworker should emulate the skills of a good doctor." Hence the term "case" and in turn the "caseworker." Given that both doctors and social workers were entering into the birth control clinic movement in increasing numbers throughout the 1920s and 1930s, the language they used followed. But just how egalitarian this relationship between specialist and patient should be remained the subject of much debate.[66]

As a result, as birth control services moved into the hands of charity organizations, deeply rooted notions of paternalism could not help but influence the movement's perceptions of the women it looked to help, those women whom they now regularly referred to as "cases." Sanger's own shifting rhetoric illustrates this vividly. While the early radical Sanger emphasized the skill, agency, and the ability of the poor not only to use birth control but also to teach others (as is evident in early editions of "Family Limitation"), by the 1920s a decidedly different tone emerged. "Printed matter," she wrote in her call for the organization of local clinics, "will carry the message to those who have been educated. But the woman who has been denied such advantages must be told by word of mouth and shown by demonstration what to do and how to do it."[67] The poor, in other words, needed especially to be taught. Remarks made by Yarros reveal this attitude as well. "Our experience," Yarros wrote in 1928, "shows that the poor, ignorant and foreign-born are just as eager for this information," and when instructed, they "followed carefully and successfully."[68] Granted, her words were in part an effort to counter the elitist criticism that the poor were simply too stupid to learn, but there remains a patronizing air to what she had to say: the poor may be simple, but they certainly can be taught, and we of course are the ones who can do it. As Eleanor Rowland Wembridge said of the women who attended the Cleveland clinic, "At these clinics the dull could be taught Birth Control, as patiently and persistently as they have been taught everything else."[69]

Thus the power of charity within this new birth control clinic movement is evident; so too its limits—all things that would eventually haunt the clinic movement in the decades to follow. But for the time being, many women (rich and poor alike) were deeply grateful for the services this new institution offered, whatever its practical and ideological flaws. As one Illinois woman wrote, "Where I am living now I have access to a Birth Control clinic where the best scientific methods are used and I feel much more secure about the future than I ever did before."[70] Another Illinois woman said in a letter to Sanger, "I am one of the many women you have helped, for which I can never thank you enough." To which she added, "I would almost do anything for you in my gratitude, yet there seems to be nothing I can do at present time, except tell other unhappy mothers about your wonderful work."[71] As the preceding letter suggests, the most visible sign of patients' appreciation could be found in their generous word-of-mouth publicity. Consequently, although local birth control organizations throughout the nation cultivated a more formal network of referring agencies by way of charity groups and medical institutions, often the most common way women learned about their clinics was through the recommendations from women themselves.[72] In Chicago the number of new clients referred by ordinary women stood at roughly 50 percent, the significance of which was not lost on the local organization. "This is most encouraging," the local office proudly announced on the pages of the *Birth Control Review*, "since our advice is evidently giving satisfaction."[73]

But it is on that note that we should perhaps pause in our story about the strengths and limits of charity and turn more directly to life inside the local clinic. For only there is it possible to see all there was to like about this new institution—and all there was not.

Birth Control the Clinic Way

Although prescriptive, manuals of clinic procedure offer a good place to begin describing what a trip to a local birth control clinic was like in the 1920s and 1930s. A woman enters a local clinic. She is greeted, asked a series of questions about her personal and medical background, and then told that the doctor will soon be ready to see her. She proceeds into a separate office, or simply steps behind a privacy screen, where she is to undress partially and await the doctor. Upon the physician's arrival, she is asked to lie on the examining table and put her feet in the rubber stirrups, spreading her legs wide open, so that the gynecological exam might begin. A general examination of her private parts—with fingers and a speculum—might be the first place the doctor starts. But then the physician would turn to the primary task at hand: the prescription of birth control. And so, as the woman continues to lie on her back with her feet still in the stirrups, the doctor determines which size diaphragm is best by measuring "the depth of the vagina, the tone of the perineum, and the condition of the pelvic organs," as Dr. Hannah Stone (of Sanger's New York clinic) advised. The woman then learns how to use the device herself, inserting and removing it several times until she has mastered the process well enough to do it at home. There would end, then, this new birth control prescribing ritual, and after dressing, paying whatever fees the clinic may have charged, and being told to return at a later date for a follow-up examination, she would gather up her new diaphragm, her new tube of contraceptive jelly, and head out the door, confident in the knowledge that she had learned what the charity movement now called birth control "the clinic way."[74]

That the early birth control movement emphasized the diaphragm is something historians have already described. But to remind ourselves of this scene is crucial nonetheless because it highlights the dramatic shift that had taken place. For in light of all that was laid out in the previous section of this chapter, what we notice is a vision of birth control radically different from what the larger marketplace, even the early Sanger, had to offer. The clinic could, for example, have provided condoms; it could have provided douches. It could have also recommended the supplies of drugstores, the goods of patent medicine peddlers, as well as the authority of nurses, mid-wives, and immigrant entrepreneurs. It could have even determined the proper diaphragm size by relying upon each woman's childbearing history, which is what Sanger did in her first clinic, her radical clinic on New York's immigrant-populated Amboy Street.[75] It did not. Rather, what this new birth control institution promoted was a new kind of ritual, one that rested squarely upon three important things: the doctor, the diaphragm, and the vaginal examination.

Yet equally important to appreciate is the clinic's persistent malleability, which enabled it to accommodate a variety of local circumstances. Consequently, although the birth control clinic was in many ways becoming more institutional, it still carried with it a guerilla-style flexibility that enabled it to flourish quickly, easily, and in any number of different settings. This in turn yielded many moments of uniqueness within the larger clinic mold: in terms of staff, clientele, and even institutional setting. Further contributing to the clinic's lack of uniformity was the complex amalgam of sympathy and science upon which the institution was based—because it was an amalgam not consistently applied. Thus to appreciate all these features of clinic life—the rigidity of its ritual practices and its simultaneous flexibility—are central to our understanding of the clinic. Not only do these features help explain the early rise of the birth control clinic, but they also help explain what the clinic would become in the decades to follow. For the moment, however, let us continue with our investigation of the clinic's early days.

In January 1938 there appeared an article in Bernard McFadden's *Physical Culture* magazine, "I Went to a Birth Control Clinic," offering a nice window through which to peer. Classic in its account, the article bears many of the hallmarks of such stories: the distraught wife, the brutish husband, and the salvation to be had by way of the clinic. Fictional, sentimental, exaggerated, it is surely intended to evoke an emotional response.[76] This does not mean it is without merit; if we combine it with the clinic movement's voluminous prescriptive literature and the many accounts that describe practical clinic life, the story simultaneously provides a useful way to appreciate the promise of this new institution as well as the limits of the quixotic ideal its proponents propagated.

Fearful and distraught, with a referral from a social worker friend Martha Martin makes her way to a birth control clinic, and as she arrives so do we. "I went up the steps of a two-story, red brick house," she writes, and it "did not even look like an office building, and certainly not like a hospital or a clinic," she adds with "some relief." Still nervous, she enters anyway. First to greet her is a kindly female receptionist, a woman who proceeds to ask her a series of questions about her personal and medical background, and who, when her questions are over, tells Martha to take a seat in the adjacent room. Martha does as she is told and is surprised to discover six women are already there, women, as Martha tells us, who come from a variety of economic backgrounds. Several, we learn, are "undernourished," "shabbily dressed" and wear "tired, unhappy faces." Others, however, are "nicely groomed." But, as Martha explains, despite their economic differences, she and her fellow clinic patients are drawn together by the similarity of their "need," their uniquely female need for birth control.[77]

As she and her fellow patients continue their conversation, another woman enters the room, a nurse dressed in "crisp white" who speaks to the group as "one woman to another," explaining what the doctor would do. Martha's anxiety lessens, only to have it return when her time to meet with the staff physician arrives. "I was nervous on the examining table," Martha explains in what is a rather vague description of the diaphragm fitting ritual. But Doctor Rosemary "was very gentle." She even "patted my shoulders" when it was all over and said that I could "come to [the clinic] at any time in the future for additional supplies, or for advice." Deeply moved by all that she has experienced, as she prepares to leave Martha finds herself unable to contain her deepest emotions. It "means a lot to a woman to be treated so kindly and sympathetically," she says to the woman at the front desk. "I was afraid—but the entire atmosphere here—everything—everybody—so reassuring and kind." With "tears in [her] eyes," she then turns and flees the clinic.[78]

Martha's account reveals a great deal. Her description, for example, of the exterior of the clinic is a telling one. Clinics had a way of popping up in any number of differing settings. Some were in welfare agencies, some were in community centers, and some were in private doctors' offices or larger hospital facilities. But others, as Martha's story describes, made their way into more domestic settings, such as the private house or the apartment building. In fact, the chain of Illinois Birth Control League clinics in Chicago alone illustrates this variety well.[79] Yet Martha's relief about this more domestic setting is equally suggestive because it serves as an important reminder that not all women were interested in going to a medical facility to secure their birth control supplies. As can be gathered from Dr. Norman Himes, *Medical History of Birth Control* (1936), cultural differences among immigrants may have been one factor. As Himes wrote, a "European peasant woman would no more contemplate the desirability of consulting a physician to limit her family than the majority of the populace even in our day will consult a physician for a common cold," a striking observation given how different things are today.[80] It was something with which Chicago welfare reformers of the early twentieth century were already familiar. Unable to convince immigrant women to take their sick children to hospitals, which many foreign-born people viewed as places one went to die, they opened instead outdoor baby tents, which proved enormously popular.[81] It could also be the case that native-born, white women (like our fictional Martha) were not all that keen on going to medical facilities either. As one *Birth Control Review* contributor remarked, "women do not want to go to a hospital for contraceptive advice."[82] In short, they hadn't done so before, so why start now?

Martha's description of the interior of the clinic is equally suggestive because she invites us to imagine a space that had all the privacy and comforts of home. Manuals of procedure regularly encouraged organizers to decorate the waiting and interview area in "any pleasant informal and noninstitutional manner" with "cheerful color, plants and books." They also recommended a separate space for clinic interviews where women could discuss personal matters without fears of being overheard.[83] Furthermore, a separate examining room, or at least a space divided by a curtain, was especially important and was intended to assuage the fears of women who, in order to get birth control, found themselves lying partially undressed and in a compromising position in front of an unfamiliar doctor, a position that contradicted social codes of sexual propriety and modesty.[84] For this reason, how clinic workers arranged the examining room space mattered the most. While privacy and a female doctor alleviated some of the stresses of the diaphragm fitting, other features—such as the examination table, stirrups, specula, and rubber gloves—could still provoke anxiety among patients. Clinics that were well equipped, as those in Chicago reportedly were, were therefore advised to keep at least some of these things hidden from the patient's view. As the charity movement's Dr. Robert L. Dickinson chastised in his 1938 manual of clinic procedure, there is "nothing more callous and careless . . . than the free and general exposure of instruments. No woman can imagine a painless or considerate treatment possible in full view of that ponderous engine called a Graves' speculum, lying with its valves spread wide among lesser horrors like long scissors and scissor-shaped hooks." He added that "bloody swabs" and other potentially distressing items should also be tucked away.[85]

That the clinic was staffed by women, compassionate women, also comes through in Martha's account. Given the intimacies of the gynecological exam, it was particularly important that the clinic doctor be a woman; although men sometimes served as the clinic doctor, female physicians were a common sight.[86] "The qualities of the physicians have much to do with the success of the center," wrote Mary M. White (executive secretary of a birth control league clinic in Massachusetts). As she explained, while "technique" was important, so too were "personality and understanding."[87] The use of female physicians also eased concerns of the patients' spouses. As another manual of procedure remarked, "the husbands of underprivileged women are usually more willing to have their wives examined by women than men doctors."[88] But it was not just about making the patients and their spouses feel more comfortable; women doctors were indeed drawn to clinic work. In part their status within the medical community may have fueled their participation in clinic programs. With few avenues for professional advancement and difficulties in building up practices because of their sex, female physicians may have viewed the clinic as a place to put their expertise to work.[89] As women, they also had a uniquely female initiative. As Dickinson himself humbly noted in his manual of clinic procedure, women physicians "tend to be more socially minded, and in this matter have shown more courage than their male confréres." He also added that female doctors were "more impressed with [their patients'] need."[90] In other words, it was in particular a female sympathy that often guided the efforts of women doctors, a sympathy historian Molly Ladd-Taylor described as a shared "capacity for motherhood."[91]

Such sensibilities likely held true for the rest of the staff, as the legion of nurses, social workers, and lay volunteers—areas of work often dominated by women—were vital to clinic operations as well, another feature of clinic life that comes through in Martha's account. While doctors were responsible for conducting the pelvic exam and fitting patients with the diaphragm, the rest of the staff did everything else. They interviewed patients, answered the phone, made appointments, and sometimes did follow-up work with patients, either by mail or through home visits. They also set up the facility before each clinic session began and cleaned and put away all the supplies once it was over.[92] Theirs was a presence, in fact, that had as much influence on clinic operations as did that of the staff physician. Consequently, it made sense when Dr. Stone of Sanger's New York clinic wrote in a 1927 issue of the *Birth Control Review*, "Of all the equipment, the most important is a staff with 'a breath of inspiration,' a truly sympathetic attitude, and a sincere interest in the work."[93]

Furthermore, to have on hand staff members who spoke several languages proved especially valuable when looking to serve immigrant communities. The clinics operated by the Illinois Birth Control League in Chicago were particularly successful in that regard. Dr. Olga Ginzburg, who received her medical training in Russia, was able to instruct Germans, Poles, and Russians in their native tongues. Another clinic worker, Miss Francesca Mollenaro, put her language skills to use in the league's South Side clinic, which served a large number of Mexican and Italian women. That the Chicago office specifically singled out Ginzberg's and Mollenaro's contributions in its annual report suggests their importance to the success of clinic operations in immigrant communities.[94]

However, what Martha's story especially drives home is the presence of women as clientele. Certainly a few men occasionally came by. As one New York nurse explained, they sometimes showed up in order "to hold the baby," "interpret," or to pick up their wife's "supplies." For all practical purposes, though, the clinic was a world of women, many of whom had children in tow. For this reason, great care was taken to have such things as a baby basket available or toys for older children. First-floor locations were also regularly recommended so that they might more easily accommodate the inevitable baby carriage.[95] In light of all this (atmosphere, staff, and clientele), it is little wonder that historian Ellen Chesler later described the clinic romantically as "a community of women."[96] Or that the New York nurse waxed poetic that her facility was a site for "family reunions for sisters, sisters-in-law, cousins, and aunts."[97]

Yet for as much as the clinic was to convey a "warm, friendly atmosphere," organizers also strove to achieve a scientific medical environment, which Martha's account also illustrated vividly.[98] For the most part, those clinics associated with medical institutions tended to convey a more professional atmosphere, having the advantages of what one instructional guide described as "proper medical standards and adequate medical supervision." In contrast, those facilities found in private houses and apartments were in general more informal. Nevertheless, the national birth control offices still expected clinics "to conform to accepted hospital standards" and to cultivate a "dignified and professional atmosphere."[99] Clinic duties performed by the staff promoted a scientific environment by replicating professional medical hierarchies, which placed doctors at the top of the totem pole of expertise. As one clinic manual explained, while the use of nurses and other staff members was "desirable" to perform the clinic's many jobs, unlike physicians they were "not indispensable."[100]

Notably, this pursuit of medical professionalism was not simply a strategy intended to win the support of physicians. Sometimes it was done with the patient in mind. As Mary White from the Massachusetts clinic wrote, the "impression made upon the patient at the time of her first visit is of vital importance. To come to an office where a dignified and professional atmosphere is carefully maintained, impresses upon her the seriousness of the visit and banishes fear." It was also for the benefit of "hospitals, physicians and social agencies." As White urged, "we must prove [to them] that we are not asking them to endorse bungling amateurs, but an organization with the stringent professional standards which they themselves demand."[101] In addition, to have doctors in the clinic was also a source of great pride. Clinic organizers even began to view European facilities, which were often run by nurses or midwives, with growing skepticism. Not even the Holland facilities where Sanger took her training escaped such criticism. As Dr. Stone remarked, the Dutch Neo-Malthusian League clinics can "hardly be called clinics in the meaning we apply to the word," and although she went on to explain that European centers were likely providing women with quality services, she believed the doctor-run American institution held greater promise.[102]

Finally, the benefits of the individually fitted diaphragm are clear as well. Its safety, effectiveness, function as a female-controlled method, and (eventual) respectability by way of its association with doctors and scientific medicine were among the many reasons why the device held such great appeal among clinic organizers.[103] But there were other reasons as well. For example, the pelvic examination itself proved highly valuable. In addition to enabling a better diaphragm fit, it also served as an effective moment to detect health problems, which was particularly important for poor women who may not have had access to this kind of medical care.[104] Demand for the diaphragm, moreover, often came from women themselves. "It is not convenient to use douches," wrote a woman from North Dakota to one birth control proponent, "and I don't think they are absolute safe."[105] A "friend of mine," said another to Sanger, "told me of a doctor that would give me a dangerous gold internal appliance which was a sure preventative." Much to her dismay, not only did this twenty-four-year-old mother of two experience internal hemorrhaging, but three months later she also discovered she was pregnant.[106] Still another explained to Sanger how she tried calendar methods (along with contraceptives) to no avail. "I am simply one of those women who have *no safe period*," she lamented.[107] In other words, women themselves expressed a desire to use something different and better.

What Martha's account illustrates vividly, therefore, is the nature of the birth control clinic and its widespread appeal, but in so doing she has a habit of glossing over those things that might not fit into the quixotic ideal presented by clinic supporters. To begin with, the romanticized notion of female camaraderie, one that transcended economic, ethnic, and racial differences, deserves scrutiny. The daily interactions between the middle-class women who worked in the clinic and the poor women they looked to serve suggest that camaraderie was more often a fanciful dream rather than a concrete reality. Clinic staff was often frustrated with its clientele. As one New York nurse complained, some women "put off" using their referrals and showed up "to[o] late, pregnant," a situation the nurse viewed as "tragic" yet ultimately a product of these women's irresponsibility. Still others, the nurse reported, said the patients "were too stupid to learn" how to use the diaphragm.[108] In addition, the historian Cathy Moran Hajo noted this problem: although the middle-class women who ran clinic operations believed they could cultivate an alliance between themselves and their working-class female patients, it was an alliance that required them to pit these working-class women against their working-class husbands. "The underlying philosophy at the clinic," noted Hajo, "sought to separate working-class women from solidarity with their men, in favor of an unequal sisterhood with the clinic activists."[109] Certainly, some clinics may have been more successful in cultivating good relationships with their clientele; specific individuals may have been more successful as well.[110] But economic, racial, and ethnic differences remained a chasm not easily bridged.

Nor should we accept so readily Martha's romanticized notion of a shared camaraderie among the patients themselves. Records for Chicago simply do not bear this out. As one 1928 report noted in reference to its downtown clinic, "The type of patient at this office is quite different from the other Medical Centers." It described how this facility served mostly white, middle-class, Protestant women, while the other clinics served the poor, immigrants, and African Americans, each according to the neighborhood in which it operated. The report then made a list that detailed the patients each of the Chicago charity clinics served:

Medical Center #1 (203 North Wabash, downtown): predominantly white, middle-class, Protestants.

Medical Center #2 (1347 North Lincoln Avenue; northwest side of downtown): working-class, Catholic immigrants from Germany, Poland, Lithuania, and Slovakia.

Medical Center #3 (701 West 14th Place; just southwest of downtown): African-Americans and immigrants; largely Catholic.

Medical Center #4 (3201 South Wabash Avenue; the "black belt" district): largely African-American.

Medical Center #5 (3500 Douglas Boulevard): mainly Jewish women.

Medical Center #6 (Hull-House; also southwest of downtown): Mexicans and Italians; largely Catholic.[111]

It is a striking list to look at. In part because it reveals another unique characteristic within the larger clinic mold, in that each clinic took on the character of the neighborhood in which it operated; but it also reveals a

more blunt reality: not only would you be hard-pressed to find a poor immigrant woman attending the Illinois Birth Control League's downtown clinic,
but you would be equally hard-pressed to find a wealthy white woman attending one of its facilities on the city's South Side, deep in the heart of the black
belt district.[112] Female camaraderie went only so far, as is further evidenced
by the common practice of segregated clinic sessions.[113] And so, although
in Martha's imaginary waiting room women of different backgrounds could
sit side-by-side with one another and share their personal woes (though the
differences she describes were economic rather than racial or ethnic), real
clinic life suggests a different story.

In addition, there were other features of clinic life that the patients found
equally undesirable. Many of the women detested the gynecological examination, which required an intimacy with which most were unaccustomed.
But even the initial interview itself could be overwhelmingly invasive. As
Hajo brilliantly illustrated when, in rapid-fire succession, she went through
the list of questions interviewers were supposed to ask:

> Who referred you to the clinic? What does your husband do for a living? Is he
> working at present? How much money does he make? Do you work, and if so
> how much money do you make? When was your last menstrual period? How
> many times have you been pregnant? How many children have you borne?
> How many are still alive? Are they normal? Have you had any abortions? Were
> the abortions induced or spontaneous? Were you born in this country? Was
> your husband? What is your ethnic background? Your husband's? What reli-
> gion do you practice? Have you tried birth control methods before? If so, did
> they work? How often do you have sex? Do you enjoy it? If not, why not?[114]

So put off was one woman by this bombardment of questions that she composed a two-page, typewritten letter expressing her outrage, which would
later be found by the historian Jimmy Meyer in the records for the Cleveland, Ohio, clinic. "In the first place, I object to your third degree," she
vented. "You ask questions which you have no business knowing, no business
asking. Probably you feel justified in knowing everything about a person you
have on charity. But I question even that."[115] The clinic, as she (and probably others) saw it, was asking for a lot—invading their bodies and their privacy—and she was not going to stand for it.

Thus, the clinic had its strengths and its limits; nevertheless, this new
model of birth control services would be enough to win people over. Not
only did it win support from beyond its doors, but it also won support to
keep it going from *within*—from the women who labored inside and, perhaps even more important, those who procured the services it provided.
Indeed, without patients there was no clinic, a lesson clinic organizers
quickly learned when sometimes faced with empty reception areas, which
they then worked hard to fill. Further illustrative of the charity movement's

success was the magnitude of the "first clinic wave." By 1940, Illinois, for example, could boast of sixteen birth control facilities. While most were concentrated in the Chicago area, four additional facilities (each sponsored by its own separate local league) now operated downstate. These included: Springfield (the state capital), Champaign (a university town), Danville (an industrial city on the eastern border), and Centralia (a mining town in the southern part of the state). Nationally, the growth was equally dramatic. As Hajo noted, by 1940 more than five hundred clinics were in existence throughout the nation.[116]

Notably, the spread of local clinics even convinced Sanger's rival, Mary Ware Dennett, of their value. Dennett, as historians have described, was another of these early birth control reformers. Dennett also established her own organization in New York City, the Voluntary Parenthood League, in which she adopted a program of action radically different from that of Sanger. At first the differences between their strategies went like this. While initially the early radical Sanger openly challenged Comstock laws and broke them, Dennett worked through the legal system in order to remove the label of "obscenity" from birth control, arguing that prohibiting the dissemination of information about birth control was a violation of free speech. By the 1930s, Sanger shifted tactics. While Dennett still argued for free speech and the removal of the obscenity designation, Sanger now opted for more conservative measures by way of a doctors-only bill that would make birth control legal as long as it came through physicians. Seeing this still as a violation of free speech, Dennett strenuously opposed this doctors-only strategy.[117]

Interestingly enough, though, as Dennett and Sanger argued about the best way to challenge Comstock laws, Dennett (like Sanger) found herself inundated with requests from ordinary individuals for practical and immediate assistance about how to limit childbearing. Unable to ignore their plight, she too eventually began to recommend these newly established local birth control clinics. And so, although still much opposed to Sanger's decision to put birth control into the hands of physicians, Dennett recognized the utility of an institution that gave individuals direct and immediate assistance. "The best suggestion which I can make," she wrote in 1930 to a man in Wheaton, Illinois, "is that you get in touch with the Illinois Birth Control League," which would supply you with the "contraceptive information" you desire.[118] She gave similar advice to women in Michigan, New York, and California.[119] Consequently, great as Dennett's ideological differences with Sanger may have been, when faced with individual demands she was unable to resist providing women (and sometimes men) with concrete advice about how to limit childbearing, even if it meant giving in to Sanger's vision of a doctor-run clinic.

Thus the success of the charity-clinic movement was dramatic; its success, however, simultaneously ushered in a narrow definition of birth control and a narrow understanding of how best to make it available. Out were patent medicine peddlers, homeopaths, nurses, and druggists who could make available a variety of birth control methods directly to consumers. And in were doctors, diaphragms, and the now mandatory pelvic examination. For all the promise, then, of this new institution and its guerilla-style flexibility, what it brought to Americans were ever more rigid definitions, definitions the charity movement then expected everybody to share. As the following chapter reveals, not everybody did.

Chapter Two

Rising Above

"The cause of birth control has reached that stage of development where charlatans, quacks and commercial interests are trying to turn it to profit and ride in upon the wave of popularity," warned the American Birth Control League's executive director, Marguerite Benson, in a 1935 issue of the *Birth Control Review*.[1] Indeed, fueled by Depression-era hardships as well as the charity movement's efforts to promote birth control and help with the establishment of local charity clinics, the 1930s witnessed a massive expansion of birth control methods, birth control providers, and the rise even of irregular birth control clinics—those facilities not associated with the charity movement but run instead by nurses, chiropractors, and entrepreneurs.[2] Americans therefore, particularly those in larger cities, found themselves with newfound access to a remarkably large and openly available selection of goods and services to assist them in limiting childbearing, despite the Comstock laws that continued to ban birth control.

But, as Benson's words also suggest, this was not something about which the charity movement was pleased because, when taken together, the radicalism of old had now become commercially mainstream. While the radical Sanger of the 1910s had originally promoted a variety of birth control techniques, a variety of birth control providers, and frankness in sex, this new commercialization of contraceptives and providers now did much the same, with an even greater openness than before. Given that this new world of birth control products and services was vast and overlapping—with its many participants, goods, and messages difficult to differentiate—the position the charity movement thus found itself in was a tricky one. Consequently, if it was to win the backing of the conservative American Medical Association, institutionalize its chain of doctor-supervised clinics, and successfully lobby against Comstock laws, it would somehow have to set itself apart, which it did by working to establish once and for all what birth control was and what birth control was *not*.

This too is a process scholars have already begun to describe. As Leslie Reagan demonstrated, in its efforts to establish its legitimacy, the charity movement distanced its understanding of the term "birth control" from the practice of abortion.[3] True birth control, in other words, was only contraceptive in nature. But this did not mean that all pregnancy preventatives were met with an eager embrace. As Amy Sarch argued, commercially available feminine hygiene preparations—such as vaginal powders, douches, jellies, and crèmes that women could buy over the counter—were also *not* met with enthusiastic interest by the charity movement, for these were tainted by the vulgarity of the sexual female body and the illicitness of marketplace.[4]

In addition, Andrea Tone implicitly suggested yet another feature of what birth control was *not.* The charity movement sought, as Tone described, to wrap itself in a cloak of corporate science and ally itself only with so-called ethical manufacturers (those who made contraceptives available only to the medical profession, and not to the laity). I will in turn argue explicitly that, according to the charity movement, birth control was also *not* to be seen as a commodity of the marketplace—a product openly available to consumers that anybody could buy, make, or sell. Instead, it was concealed and hidden, a product of corporate science over which only doctors, scientists, and ethical manufacturers were to exercise control.[5] Yet if we are to appreciate fully the breadth of the charity movement's campaign to establish its legitimacy by containing the meaning of birth control and its provision, still needed in this story are two additional themes. The first is the complexity of what had by the 1930s become a massive commercialization of birth control. The second, the crucial thread in the birth control movement's efforts to rise above that commercialization: its mission of charity.

This chapter begins, therefore, by weaving together the many stories mentioned earlier, the stories often told in isolation, as a way to remind ourselves of the many different methods, providers, and ways to make birth control available in the first place. In other words, the many different meanings to which the terms "birth control" and the "birth control clinic" could still be attached. But because the charity movement also sought to distinguish itself from this massive commercialization of birth control, this chapter turns to the charity movement's attempts to rise above it. Consequently, while an emphasis on science, medicine, ethical business practices, and sex within marriage were certainly important strategies in the efforts of the charity movement to rise above commercial birth control, it was the moral weight of charity that served as the glue to hold these many strategies together. For it was the (quiet and demure) moral weight of charity—in contrast to the (bold and brash) profit-driven motives of the marketplace—that the charity movement used to ennoble both the almighty diaphragm and the bona fide birth control clinic.

Embedded within this campaign therefore are three striking ironies, which in turn force us to reevaluate our understanding of the charity movement's efforts to legitimate itself during this crucial period of professionalization. First, while the movement was indeed looking to democratize birth control through clinics catering to the poor, it was simultaneously working to limit what women of all classes used by promoting the diaphragm above all other methods. Second, while the movement was also regularly calling for the establishment of birth control clinics throughout the nation, it did not suffer lightly the presence of those that failed to conform to what would become its strict new rules. Third, while it had long criticized Comstock laws for limiting the availability of birth control, now the reverse argument was in effect: because of Comstockery, there was far too much availability. In other words, because of its illegality, birth control had spawned a massive commercial industry—an industry that, in the eyes of the charity movement, was not only dangerously unregulated but also far too open, accessible, and directly available to consumers. Consequently, when one pro-Sanger journalist saw fit in 1934 to note that the charity movement and its supporters "are obliged at one and the same time to advocate more and less birth control," she could not have been more accurate in her assessment.[6] Were she to have said the same about clinics, she would have been right once again.

A Veritable Sea of Birth Control

Perhaps the best place to begin this section is by describing the Historical Health Fraud and Alternative Medicine Collection, the contents of which had turned my analytical world upside down. For those unfamiliar with this particular manuscript collection of the American Medical Association Archives, it is, as Reagan's study of illegal abortion demonstrated, a goldmine of primary sources for historians of medicine because it houses the internal records of an agency that by 1925 was known as the Bureau of Investigation. First begun informally in 1906 by the AMA, the bureau's purpose dovetailed neatly with the aims of the Progressive era, in that it looked to provide protections for consumers in the massive though still largely unregulated marketplace, in this case the production of patent medicine. Consequently, just when the federal government was enacting the Food and Drug Act (1906), the Bureau of Investigation began operations of its own, serving as a clearing house of information—an agency to which people could write in order to learn more about a particular product they hoped to buy or to complain about something they had already purchased. The bureau was also proactive in its activities. It regularly published a column in the AMA's monthly professional publication, the *Journal of the American Medical Association*, in order to warn physicians of the useless products it had found, and it even occasionally used spies to investigate what it believed were shady operations.

Patent medicine was not the only thing that concerned the AMA however; nor was the desire to protect consumers its only goal. Also important was the protection of the medical association itself and its vision of medical practice in America. As a result, other practitioners—such as homeopaths, osteopaths, and midwives—regularly endured the bureau's scrutiny as well, as did "illegitimate" medical practices, which in this case meant contraception and abortion. Ironically enough therefore, particularly given the bureau's larger purpose, this collection has preserved for us a remarkable window into the larger world of medicine, one the AMA hoped to suppress.[7]

What made this collection so useful to me, however, was not simply the information housed within it but the skepticism it embodied as well. Although by the 1930s the AMA was slowly coming around where charity birth control clinics were concerned, its suspicion of birth control more generally remained decidedly palpable. In turn, the AMA's doubt had on me a curious effect. On the one hand, I grew ever more suspicious of all the birth control providers in existence by the 1930s, charity clinics included. On the other hand, I found myself believing every word, including every word found in commercial feminine hygiene advertisements and also every word in the literature put out by the irregular birth control clinic movement—all of it rhetoric that, if I abided by what the charity birth control movement would have me believe, I was supposed unquestioningly to deride. In viewing the Historical Health Fraud and Alternative Medicine Collection, therefore, I found myself seeing this world for the first time from the perspective of an ordinary 1930s consumer: someone who might have supported birth control or opposed it; someone, however, who was still unbound by the lines of distinction the charity movement would try to impose around the meaning of birth control and how best to make it available. What then did I see?

To begin with, by the 1930s women as well as men were neither as utterly ignorant about birth control nor as entirely ashamed to talk about it as the charity movement would have us believe. To the contrary, women and men sought out and obtained assistance from a variety of sources. They consulted pharmacists, department store saleswomen, door-to-door peddlers, magazine advertisements, commercial circulars, radio shows, physicians, and even the AMA to help them narrow down the choices that lay before them.[8] The questions they asked could be quite specific. "I am interested in the quality and effectiveness of Lanteen and Certaine Jelly," wrote Mrs. Henrietta Rusin of Chicago to the AMA. "Will you please give me the results of your findings regarding these products?"[9] They then shared what they learned with family and friends, as the derisive phrase "back-fence" birth control suggests.[10] Even the letters people wrote to the charity movement offices reveal a growing savvy and a sense of entitlement in obtaining birth control information. In previous years, remarked one contributor to a 1933 issue of the *Birth Control Review*, requests for advice were "personal and emotional," laden with "reasons to justify an exception being made in their individual cases." "Today," she tellingly added, the letters are more "matter-of-fact," as if information "can be had by any one, on request."[11]

Also contrary to what the charity movement would have us believe, although income did influence what people used, the organization tended to overplay the diaphragm's desirability, particularly among those who could afford it. For example, according to one 1930s study, white-collar workers relied heavily on the condom, which, according to one advertisement, sold for 73 cents a dozen. In contrast, those on relief tended to rely upon the more economical douche, which need only be purchased once and in 1937 could be had for anywhere between 49 cents (for the Sears and Roebuck "Low Priced" model) and $2.89 (its deluxe "Miracle Douche"). The poor also practiced withdrawal regularly, which of course cost nothing at all. Diaphragm use, in contrast, was consistently low among all classes, and its sales accounted for less than 1 percent of the total contraceptive market.[12]

Further contrary to what the charity movement would have us believe, many of the consumers who used methods other than the diaphragm were often satisfied with the results. "I heard about something the druggist was selling," explained Florence W., a Jewish woman born in 1905. "You insert it, it looked like a suppository. I asked him to make up some for me and he did." To which she added, "He did very well with it because all my friends bought it too." About condoms, Italian-American Dorothy, born in 1915, had this to say: "Most of [my friends'] husbands used condoms. That's the safest."[13] Even abortion, the method Sanger regularly described as "the most dangerous remedy of all," was not necessarily always the horror the charity movement would have us believe. As we know from Reagan's study, by the 1930s safe ones could increasingly be had by trained practitioners.[14]

Consequently, with so many choices available the competition was fierce, and in an effort to win the public's patronage and trust, providers all drew upon a common language of science, medicine, and sensitivity to gendered concerns. In many ways the messages put out by the commercial industry resembled those put out by organizations engaged in charity. While the charity movement argued that birth control was a matter of doctors and science, so too did many of the advertisements. As one feminine hygiene advertisement read, Dr. Clotilde Delaunay, a "leading gynecologist of Paris," reassures a "bride of a few months" by saying: "When it comes to a crisis—involving life itself—the ablest physicians always turn to 'Lysol.'"[15] While the charity movement also argued that birth control was a matter primarily of female authority and concern, commercial advertisements reflected much the same. As another ad for Lysol proclaimed, ladies could take comfort knowing that the company had asked "an eminent woman physician" to prepare its educational booklet. "It answers the questions you would like to ask [her] in person," the company reassuringly asserted.[16] And while the charity movement regularly promoted birth control as the key to female health and happiness, so too did the materials distributed by others. As one pamphlet put out by one of the irregular birth control clinics in Chicago announced, the "use of jelly and the diaphragm is the greatest aid a woman can have in maintaining her charm and beauty." It went on to describe how freedom from the "fear of pregnancy" would dispel the "continual worry" that so often caused "feminine nervous ailments and fading youth"—words that bear striking resemblance to those put out by the charity movement.[17] Interestingly enough, however, despite the similarity of the rhetoric, when it came from the mouths of advertisers, the charity movement would dismiss it as deceptive euphemisms. Or, as Sanger called it, the work of "Clever copywriters"—a characterization that historians would subsequently perpetuate.[18]

But then there were all the messages the charity movement did not want to promote. While it wanted to advance only the diaphragm, clearly the commercial world promoted all types of contraceptives—diaphragms, condoms, douches, and the myriad of other vaginal preparations—often selling them side-by-side.[19] While the charity movement wanted to assert the authority of doctors, the commercial industry regularly promoted the authority of other medical practitioners, in particular nurses. As a result, department stores regularly clad their salesclerks in white coats and caps, hoping to lend an air of nursing professionalism to the advice they had to offer.[20] Door-to-door peddlers adopted this strategy as well, drawing perhaps upon the tradition of visiting public health nurses.[21] Certainly, such deceptiveness is hardly to be commended. But charity clinics were hardly immune from such practices, often dressing their lay personnel in nursing whites.[22] Nurses even appeared in condom advertisements, though for a different effect. In ads geared toward women, the image of the nurse or female physician conveyed medical expertise tempered by motherliness; in ads for men, the picture of the young, pretty, blonde nurse in a display for Ramses condoms suggested science tempered by sexiness.[23]

But this promotion of a wide range of methods and the authority of nurses were not the only messages and strategies the charity movement looked to avoid. It also backed off from the more overtly feminist arguments, from which at least one manufacturer did not. "Why wasn't I born a man?" came the question from a rather determined looking woman in an ad for the Zonite Products Corporation. To which the description below it read, this might "sound like a complaint, but [it is] really a protest—a protest against those burdens of life which are wholly woman's."[24] The charity movement also wanted the specifics of birth control to be discussed quietly and discreetly. In contrast, the marketplace was, as the evidence suggests, open and loud.

As a result, with so many options available, Depression-era Americans must certainly have found themselves wading through a complex maze of birth control products and providers. With such names as American Bureau of Hygiene, Hygienic Company of America, Dilex Institute of Feminine Hygiene, Feminine Institute, Servex Laboratories, and Naturol Laboratories, to name but a scant few, companies must have all started to sound the same.[25] So too the methods they sold. In fact, when one manufacturer, Rufus Riddlesbarger (about whom you will soon read more), decided to color-code his line of products—Lanteen Blue indicating the antiseptic jelly; Lanteen Lilac, the diaphragm and jelly; Lanteen Russet, the sponge and jelly; plus a few more with equally colorful designations—it is clear he was anticipating the confusion consumers might face and looked therefore not only to create brand recognition but also to help consumers sort through the maze of choices even within his own line of merchandise.[26] But even the national birth control organizations associated with the charity movement—the American Birth Control League, the Birth Control Clinical Research Bureau, and the National Committee on Maternal Health—must also have all started to sound the same, even blurring into the names of the manufacturers. Further contributing to the fuzziness of boundaries between charity birth control organizations and commercial manufacturers was what was happening in such places as the health and hygiene sections of at least one mail-order catalog. In addition to offering a variety of contraceptive products, the 1937 Sears catalog sold books by Sanger and by Hannah and Abraham Stone (prominent figures within the national charity movement) alongside manuals about birth control and sex written by others not necessarily associated with the charity birth control movement.[27]

However, it wasn't just supporters of birth control who might find themselves confused; opponents were likely confused as well. And given that to opponents the cause of birth control amounted to nothing more than profiteering, quackery, and immorality, it really did not matter if it was about charity or about profit—all birth control providers were sinners. Resistance, for example, within the medical community was great, and getting the backing of doctors no easy task. Some doctors expressed concern about sex among the unwed, as at least one letter to the Bureau of Investigation suggests. "Is there no law," complained Dr. Edith Flower Wheeler in 1933 about mass-mailed leaflets for Lucorol (a vaginal crème), "to prevent circularizing this kind of literature among unmarried people?"[28] Another common complaint among doctors was that the charity clinic movement was simply an extension of the commercial world. Because contraceptive companies often took advantage of the charity movement's frequent public-speaking tours, such an assumption was not without merit. Always alert for free publicity, sales representatives kept track of these lectures, which were often announced in local newspapers, and made sure local suppliers were stocked with their goods. Once the lecture was over and the ground ripe with interest, detail men then leafleted physicians about the merits of their particular products.[29] In 1929, such strategies provoked no small furor between the charity movement and a local medical society, which questioned the birth control organization's intentions. In fact, so great did the controversy become that Dr. Murray N. Hadley (of the Indianapolis Medical Society) implored Dr. Morris Fishbein (of the AMA) to clarify whether one of the American Birth Control League's speakers (Dr. James Cooper) was a "properly accredited and scientific speaker" and not simply a "paid representative of a commercial house selling pessaries and contraceptive jellies."[30]

Not surprisingly, Catholic opponents played upon similar scenarios of greed and sex among the unwed. Editors of the Catholic magazine *Commonweal*, for example, drew upon images of profit-driven manufacturers in order to discredit anyone who supported birth control. "So does the Protestant principle of private and individual opinion," the magazine asked in April 1931, "finally surrender a supremely important moral problem into the hands of a clique of birth control advocates—incidentally to the huge profit of commercial interests, the makers and sellers of contraceptives." The magazine also exploited fears of sexual license among the young and unwed who might more easily obtain contraceptives through local drugstores.[31] In addition, many Catholics remained unconvinced by the charity movement's attempts to distance itself from premarital sex or abortion. An article appearing in a 1934 issue of *Catholic World* demonstrates this well. The author shocked her readers by describing a visit with a woman doctor, whom she claimed "was on an executive committee with a leader of the birth control movement." When this doctor "noticed her engagement ring," the author wrote, she bluntly encouraged her to engage in sex before the honeymoon and even offered "information" and "devices." The author then described the doctor's attitude toward abortion. Though the doctor claimed she did not believe in abortions, she still "recommended such cases to an acquaintance of hers."[32] To many readers, this account must have fit right in with what they thought was really going on—charity clinics vehemently opposed abortion at the front door while offering referrals for the procedure out the back.

Thus the perspective of 1930s consumers (be they supporters of birth control or opponents) is an important one. We see in part how theirs was a world in which the charity clinic movement was not necessarily the only authority, but rather one among many individuals, organizations, and commercial interests vying for peoples' patronage and trust, and whose messages regularly diverged and overlapped. We also see that there were a great many different birth control methods available, which could be obtained through a variety of settings—sometimes charitable in nature but more often commercial. Finally, we see how the dilemma I mentioned at the start of this chapter arose for the charity movement: the radicalism of old had become commercially mainstream, and unless the charity movement could somehow manage to set itself apart, it was a shift that could jeopardize its efforts to win over the AMA, institutionalize its chain of physician-supervised clinics, and put an end to the legal rule of Comstock. For the charity movement, these were grave matters indeed. Worse still was that these issues were not confined to birth control methods; they also made their way into birth control clinics. And it is to this story that our chapter now turns.

Other Kinds of Birth Control Clinics

Sometime in 1930, a woman known only as "R.H.S." attended a birth control clinic located at 190 North State Street, deep in the heart of Chicago's downtown business district. Upon entering the "pleasant and clean" office, she spoke with the receptionist, who asked her a series questions about her marital status, number of children, and previous birth control practices. R.H.S. then met with a female doctor who fit to her "exact measure" a diaphragm, gave her careful instructions on its use, and supplied her with a tube of contraceptive jelly.[33] Given everything that was described in the previous chapter, it would be easy to assume that R.H.S. attended any one of the growing numbers of charity clinics now in existence, in Chicago and elsewhere in the nation. She did not. Rather, R.H.S. went to a place called the Medical Bureau of Birth Control Information, a clinic operated by Lanteen Laboratories, a major contraceptive manufacturer in the burgeoning Depression-era marketplace. The Medical Bureau of Birth Control Information, in other words, was no charity institution but rather a commercial enterprise.

As the presence of this facility suggests, by the 1930s the establishment of diaphragm-dispensing clinics had become a popular idea. The facility R.H.S. attended, for example, was first established in the late 1920s and was part of a network of facilities in the Great Lakes Region that, in addition to Chicago, had locations in Milwaukee and Detroit. In fact, it was a "glorious 'chain'" of facilities, to borrow the words Sanger used to describe her own clinic aspirations, that neatly dotted the perimeter of Lake Michigan. And the man behind the operation was Rufus Riddlesbarger, president of Lanteen Laboratories and the entrepreneur who color-coded his many commercial contraceptive products.[34]

But then there were the birth control facilities operated by others. Indeed, the flurry of clinic activity in Chicago is striking. As one look at the local telephone directory under the heading "birth control" reveals: Bureau of Birth Control Information (1511 East Fifty-Third Street), Illinois League of Birth Control Clinics (203 North Wabash), Medical Bureau of Birth Control Information (190 North State Street), and Woman's Bureau of Birth Control Information (32 West Randolph).[35] Equally striking are their locations. As any geographically inclined Chicagoan would be quick to point out, the clinics' close proximity in the phonebook was matched only by their close proximity in the city itself; with one exception, these facilities operated not only within several blocks of each other but also within several blocks of the main office and busiest clinic of the Illinois Birth Control League itself. In other words, and in the city of Chicago at least, competition among clinics was perhaps more vigorous than we might have previously imagined.

This does of course raise the question of just how common the phenomenon actually was. Determining the existence of other such irregular facilities has been difficult and is made more difficult by the seeming uniqueness of the "birth control" heading in the local telephone directory of Chicago. Phone books for other major metropolitan areas (such as Los Angeles, New York, and Washington, DC) had no comparable designations, and why Chicago did while other cities did not is not entirely clear. But there can be found shreds of evidence suggesting the presence of at least a few more such facilities elsewhere in the nation. There is rumor of a clinic in New York City, which can be gleaned from one letter written between birth control proponents in 1933; and there is a rumor of a facility in Los Angeles, as evidenced by one of the individual listings in the city's telephone directory, several years earlier.[36] However, scant or pervasive as these clinics may have been, they would be enough to provoke a response from the charity clinic movement.

Also worth noting are two additional considerations. First, much as was the case with those early bootleg entrepreneurs, we must take seriously these irregular birth control clinics (those sponsored by nurses, chiropractors, and commercial entrepreneurs) because to do otherwise would be to perpetuate what the charity movement would have us believe: that such clinics were nothing more than the work of quacks or scoundrels whose only purpose was to profit off of their patrons' desperation, a characterization historians have subsequently repeated.[37] Using the word "irregular" to describe them is important too.[38] Among historians of medicine, this is a term used to define such practitioners as chiropractors or homeopaths, whom the regular medical profession (the AMA for example) regarded less than favorably. Admittedly, my use of the term "irregular" covers a much broader range of providers, but I do so with good reason. In part, grouping these many individuals together shows the similarity of their status with respect to organized medicine, as the AMA had about as much love for the entrepreneur or the self-reliant nurse as it did the irregular practitioner. But to group them together, under this term especially, captures also organized medicine's long-standing campaign against this world of irregular providers, a campaign in which the charity movement, in its efforts to win the backing of the AMA, was now becoming an avid participant.[39]

So what was it, then, that seemed to distinguish these irregular facilities from those that were more regular (hence more medical) in nature? First and foremost were the types of practitioners who worked in them. Regular doctors supposedly ran the regular clinics of the charity movement, but in these irregular facilities this was not always the case.[40] Nurses, for example, were common in these clinics, and not just nurses whose job was to assist the doctor (as organized medicine hoped to define their position), but nurses who conducted the entire examination and prescription process themselves, and who only consulted the doctor when they felt it was necessary.[41] Chiropractors could also be found within irregular clinics, as was the case with the

Woman's Bureau, whose operations were directed by a practitioner by the name of Dr. Dennis Blood.[42]

Then, too, there was the matter of publicity, an issue that rippled into questions of propriety and discussions about service to the unwed. Charity clinics were supposed to announce their facilities quietly, if not also tactfully, in part to avoid breaking the law but also to ensure that news of such services would not "fall into the hands of high school children and unmarried girls, thereby doing unlimited harm," as the vice president of Chicago's Illinois Birth Control League wrote.[43] Such discreetness, however, was not necessarily the case where irregular facilities were concerned. Advertisements for the Lanteen-sponsored Medical Bureaus appeared seemingly everywhere: on the radio, in form letters (mailed out both to potential female clients as well as to potential professional referrers, doctors themselves), in drugstores (across the nation), and even inside the boxes of sanitary napkins.[44] But the Woman's Bureau operated overtly too. Not only did those associated with the clinic leaflet pedestrians at downtown street corners, they also left stacks of fliers inside downtown office buildings that plainly illustrated a diaphragm resting snugly against a cervix and the insertion of spermicidal jelly from a tube cleverly bearing the clinic's name.[45]

All of this, in turn, reveals a great deal about the various views about sex. While charity clinics were supposed to promote a "wholesome attitude" about it and leave such discussions to the staff physician, irregular clinics seemed to think otherwise.[46] There is even evidence to suggest that at least one practitioner inside the commercially sponsored Chicago Medical Bureau had few reservations about serving the unwed. Further revealing are her readily expressed opinions about the importance of female sexual fulfillment, views that resonated with those of Sanger in her earlier, more radical, days.[47]

But in determining the many differences between irregular clinics and regular ones, there remains one more important distinction: the existence of commercial connections if not also businesslike practices. While the regular clinics of the league were charitable operations, irregular clinics—as was especially the case with the commercially sponsored Medical Bureaus—often were not. Customers were therefore expected to pay for what they got.[48] Moreover, when it came to the method itself, the company's clinics prescribed only what the company manufactured.[49] In short, the chain of clinics (like the rest of the company Riddlesbarger ran) was a business, and Riddlesbarger ran it with a businessman's flair, as the following exchange between him and Sanger illustrates. "You may be assured," Riddlesbarger wrote in explanation of the possibility that he would expand to the East Coast, "that we would not consider opening a branch in New York City without first consulting with you." "Such [an operation]," he added with an air of entrepreneurial congeniality, "would be opened only on arrangement of friendly cooperation with your clinic." Although he believed there was a "need for a clinic there," he would not hone in on what he regarded as Sanger's territory.[50]

It would be a mistake, however, to overdraw these distinctions between the irregular and the regular clinic because this would oversimplify the complexity of birth control clinic operations. Regular clinics could, in fact, sometimes behave quite irregularly. For example, that the *Birth Control Review* consistently reminded its readers that "no trained worker will attempt to give contraceptive advice to a client" suggests that some clinic workers occasionally did.[51] The same could also be said about the charity organization's exhortations about the need to promote "wholesome" attitudes about sexuality, as public words could differ from private practice.[52] Nor, as we saw in the previous chapter, were these charitable clinics averse to charging their wealthier patients fees for what they received, fees that were in line with the going market rate. Equally important are the various attitudes toward abortion. Although, officially, charity clinics were to avoid the procedure entirely, there is evidence to suggest that some occasionally broke the rules.[53] Thus, the regular clinics of the charity movement could easily be mistaken for their irregular counterparts. But this fuzziness could work both ways. I have elsewhere described a nurse (Adele Gordon) who ran the commercially sponsored Medical Bureau in Milwaukee; not only did she regularly read (and often heed the advice found in) the *Birth Control Review*, but she also saw her work as in keeping with that of Sanger herself. Furthermore, although some of her irregular colleagues may have espoused more liberal views about service to the unwed or the provision of abortion, this Milwaukee nurse expressly did not.[54] Irregular clinics, in other words, could sometimes behave quite regularly.

Where services were concerned, therefore, the boundaries between these various birth control clinics were decidedly blurry. The only thing blurrier was the names of the clinics themselves. A list drawn from both sides of this clinic movement makes this maddeningly clear:

Bureau of Birth Control Information
Bureau of Contraceptive Advice
Maternal Health Clinic
Medical Bureau of Birth Control Information
Medical Center
Mothers' Birth Control Clinic
Mother's Guidance Clinic
Mother's Health Clinic
Parents' Clinic
Woman's Bureau of Birth Control Information[55]

Telling the difference must have been difficult enough for practitioners; telling the difference must have been virtually impossible for consumers themselves.

It was precisely this muddiness that troubled the charity movement so because in many ways such clinics bore striking resemblance to Sanger's radical work in the 1910s. While irregular clinics graphically depicted contraceptive techniques as well as parts of the female anatomy, so too did Sanger's first educational pamphlet. While irregular clinics promoted a variety of practitioners, so too did the early Sanger. And while irregular clinics relied upon open leafleting and brash tactics to publicize their efforts, this was something Sanger did as well when she was still engaged in the direct-action radicalism of her IWW days. The only difference now was that these were precisely the strategies the charity clinic movement wanted to leave behind.

Almighty Diaphragms and Bona Fide Birth Control Clinics

If we recall the quote with which this chapter first began, the shrillness of the charity movement's attack is striking. "The cause of birth control has reached that stage of development," warned Benson in September 1935, "where charlatans, quacks and commercial interests are trying to turn it to profit and ride in upon the wave of popularity." She then concluded her many criticisms of the marketplace with the following rallying cry:

> The need for vigilance against misrepresentation is growing and it is the responsibility of those engaged in educating the public to *right thinking* on a subject controversial as it is. Let us be on guard, that the cause of birth control may be kept free of quackery and that the consumer may be protected as far as is humanly possible.[56]

Right thinking indeed. But what exactly did this mean? In part it meant adhering to the strict dichotomy that was now emerging within the charity camp, one that pit everything that was "good" about birth control against everything that was "bad." Or, everything that birth control was versus everything that birth control was *not*. Consequently, while the diaphragm signified all that was good about birth control—doctor prescribed, respectable, safe, effective, contraceptive in function, and used only by the wed—feminine hygiene products stood for everything that was bad. They were dangerous, unreliable, and pushed by unethical commercial vendors and unqualified medical providers (like irregulars or nurses); they were also recommended by misinformed family and friends and used by the poor (who could afford nothing better) and by the unwed. Because of the high failure rates of feminine hygiene products, moreover, their use potentially led to abortion, a connection drawn by the charity movement that was neither superficial nor coincidental. But the glue that held this complex dichotomy together was the belief that any provider who failed to adhere to these standards of "good" birth control was motivated, not out of the compassionate desire to help, but rather the greedy desire to sell. Hence the necessity of the doctor-run charity clinic.

Therein lay the horror of the rise of these irregular birth control facilities. As Benson went on bitterly to complain, the "League has received numerous reports of commercial fly-by-nights maintaining 'Birth Control Bureaus' or 'clinics,'" which unscrupulously prey on "innocent purchasers." The derisiveness of her words is matched only by the frequency of her use of quotation marks; these appeared regularly around terms designating irregular birth control facilities.[57] Consequently, the situation for the charity movement was a dire one, and if it was to rise above commercial birth control and irregular birth control clinics, it would have to teach people, not just the merits of the almighty diaphragm but also the legitimacy of the bona fide birth control clinic.

Of course, it would be wrong to assume that the movement's faith in the diaphragm and concerns about commercial vendors were without merit. The following scene vividly illustrates why. "A nurse came to my home about 2 months after the birth of my child," wrote a much distressed woman from Minneapolis, Minnesota, and "assured me that a pregnancy simply could not take place" when using the Surete kit, a product endorsed by an organization called the American Bureau of Hygiene. Although her husband was "very skeptical" about its reliability and put off by its cost, the woman prevailed upon him to let her try it. Despite "us[ing] it exactly as per directions," she explained, two months later this mother of a six-month-old found herself pregnant once again and desperate not only about her health but also her marriage. "It has almost broken up my home," the young wife lamented, "my husband is furious." Angry at being so deceived, she wrote a letter "to report . . . this failure," which she mailed off to the American Health Association, an organization like the American Bureau of Hygiene (which supposedly endorsed the product she purchased), whose affiliations or existence remain unclear.[58] That the letter eventually made its way to the American Medical Association suggests again the muddiness of medical boundaries.

Such incidents were common. Because the birth control industry operated outside the law until 1936, regulations to ensure both the efficacy and safety of the thousand of products available simply did not exist, leaving consumers vulnerable to the exaggerated and often false promises made by many manufacturers. As historians have described, douches and vaginal inserts often contained caustic chemicals or failed to live up to manufacturers' claims of effectiveness.[59] Moreover, assured by promises of gentleness and desperate to avoid pregnancy, women sometimes strengthened douching solutions—to disastrous effect. As Dorothy Dunbar Bromley noted in her 1934 birth control manual, one woman "disregarded directions and poured the germicide into the bottom of the douche-bag, without stirring it after she added the water. She was so badly burned that she later died."[60] Similarly, lack of quality-control requirements also resulted in inferior condoms, easily broken and with holes in them. As one *Fortune* journalist noted, without regulations manufacturers had little incentive to carry out tests of reliability, which only contributed to production costs.[61]

One possible solution was to regulate the market by establishing contraceptive standards and then publicizing the names of those products that met them. For Dr. Clarence Gamble—supporter of the charity movement but opponent of the need for medical supervision—this strategy seemed ideal. With the assistance of the National Committee on Maternal Health, in 1934 he formed the Standards Program to establish guidelines to determine the safety and effectiveness of various over-the-counter preparations. White lists would then be published and made available to physicians—with the ultimate goal of making "birth control so easy that people could doctor themselves effectively," according to historian James Reed. In addition, Gamble was not as enamored of the diaphragm as those around him were. For this reason, he promoted the use of a wide range of over-the-counter preparations—even feminine hygiene products (which could also include spermicidal preparations); he believed all methods deserved recognition as acceptable ways to reduce the risk of pregnancy.[62]

Others within the charity clinic movement saw things differently. Certainly they too understood the importance of contraceptive testing. As the self-described authority on birth control, the movement needed to know what worked and what did not so that women might obtain reliable advice from its clinics. In fact, one of the services the national charity movement would by the mid-1930s provide to local clinics was lists of methods it found to be safe and effective, and suppliers that it found "satisfactory," a reference likely to manufacturers who engaged in ethical practices by limiting the advertisement and sale of their products to physicians. As one clinic manual stated, the "supplies should be sent to the physician in charge of the center. . . . The fact should be stressed that the <u>responsibility of giving the advice rests with the physicians alone</u> and not with the social worker or nurse referring the patients."[63] Indeed, according to this line of logic, allowing women, or anybody else for that matter, to make decisions on their own would invite only disaster. As the fictional nurse in the imaginary waiting room in "I Went to a Birth Control Clinic" explained to Martha Martin and the women seated around her, "Many a woman has prescribed for herself and made purchases without knowing anything about her anatomy. Is it any wonder she has had disastrous results?"[64]

Safety and effectiveness were not the only issues about which the charity movement was concerned; the question of who had access to the best methods of birth control was also important. In many ways such diligent oversight was motivated by noble reasons of various persons in the movement. "Women in their desperation," wrote Bromley in her 1934 birth control manual, "believe anything and everything they read in advertisements, just as they believe whatever a friend tells them." She went on to attack commercially available feminine hygiene preparations, which she viewed as either ineffective or unsafe, or both.[65] Bromley then quoted Chicago's Dr. Yarros to present the diaphragm as the best way to limit childbearing: "If properly applied . . . the pessary is by far the best and most adequate method."[66]

Implicit in the charity movement's vision of birth control, therefore, was that if given a choice, women would want to use the diaphragm, and those who could afford it did. For example, when offering advice in the 1934 issue of the *Birth Control Review*, Alice C. Boughton explained how the "privileged" could "afford the services of a private physician" while the "young and the poor" were the most susceptible to the "irresponsible advertising of contraceptives and abortifacients."[67] Those with money, in other words, went to doctors and obtained the diaphragm while those without were forced to depend upon feminine hygiene products or terminate their pregnancies. Thus, sharp critiques of class inequities—holdovers from the charity movement's more radical roots—took on new meaning in its quest for legitimacy. In assuming this new kind of moral high ground, the movement often accused its rivals of preying particularly upon impoverished women whom it claimed were too poor to afford a doctor or too misinformed to know they could have something better, a situation the movement argued often resulted in abortion.

However, this question of accessibility quickly bled into concerns about sex among the unwed. Evidence of this can be seen in the quote from Boughton; when she spoke of the victimization of the poor, she also pointed to the susceptibility of the young, a reference no doubt to the unmarried. Similar language can be found in Bromley's discussion in a 1931 issue of the *Woman's Journal*. When she argued that not only were commercial sources of birth control "hardly for the best interests of either the individual or of society at large," she added that it was also "certainly . . . not for the best interests of the young."[68]

It was a concern, moreover, that came up regularly in the popular press. The argument went something like this: although advertisements for commercial goods—which appeared in magazines and drugstore display windows, for example—phrased their slogans to suggest that only married consumers would be interested in their products, critics doubted the sincerity of the sales pitches. "Presumably," sarcastically remarked *Fortune* magazine about drugstores, "contraceptives are not available to unmarried women."[69] Or, as the *Woman's Home Companion* pronounced: So "important" is the subject of birth control that we must hold it "on a high level of decency and dignity." For this reason, the article added, "We do not believe that *methods* of birth control should be discussed in public prints" because these would "fall into the hands of children and young people who will be harmed, not helped, by a premature interest." The pro-Sanger article then advised married women and men to obtain "full information" from physicians.[70]

Notably, all throughout these discussions references to greed and profit abound, as do remarks about charlatanism and quackery. Characterizations such as these ran rampant: "Quacks, bootleggers and unethical vendors," read the *Woman's Home Companion* piece.[71] "Charlatan," "fraud," and "abortionists' fortune," read another in *Colliers* magazine.[72] "The profiteer, the bootlegger, and the abortionist," read a piece by Sanger in *Forum* magazine.[73] But in being able to make such accusations, the charity movement would have to allow itself to believe an exaggerated image of benevolence on behalf of those entrepreneurs with whom it was okay to associate: those ethical birth control manufacturers who made their wares available only to the medical profession. "Now these firms had high ethical standards," wrote journalist Elizabeth H. Garrett in her pro-Sanger piece in a 1934 issue of the *New Republic*. "They were, in fact, non-commercial in character since their officers were for the most part men and women who had been active in the birth-control movement. . . . And because they sold only to the medical profession, their profits were necessarily limited."[74] At least one birth control manufacturer was quick to call her on this. Wanting to counter the notion that some of the early diaphragm manufacturers were noncommercial in character, George Stubbs (who was apparently one of them) was compelled to reply. "I am afraid that she here permits her natural sympathy for the older babies to color her judgment. Certainly I had a difficult enough time explaining to doctors the reason for the exorbitant price of products that cost only a few cents to make."[75]

Nonetheless, the argument stuck and also made its way into the attacks against the irregular birth control clinic movement. Indeed, the charity movement's campaign against abortion and the commercial sale of feminine hygiene products dovetailed neatly with its campaign against those other kinds of birth control clinics. Significantly, it was a campaign that received assistance from the AMA's Bureau of Investigation. In fact, by 1930 both the charity movement and the AMA were investigating these clinic operations and then sharing with each other what they learned, suggesting the deepening though still decidedly ambiguous ties between them. While both were concerned about the irregular birth control clinic movement more generally, it was the commercially sponsored Medical Bureau in Chicago that bore the brunt of their scrutiny; they collected all references to its president, Rufus Riddlesbarger, and even took steps to find out what was going on behind closed doors. Consequently, while the charity movement's Dr. Dickinson visited the facility himself on at least one occasion, the AMA sent in a woman from its own office to find out what was going on. In other words, the woman known only as R.H.S. was no ordinary Medical Bureau patient but rather a spy.[76]

The handful of reports submitted by R.H.S. were damning, revealing not only that the clinic may have served the unwed but also that it offered frank and detailed advice about birth control methods and even about sex. "Even though I told her I was not married," R.H.S. explained, Dr. Buzza "was more than willing to fit me."[77] Dr. Buzza then told her how best to enjoy sex. Open discussion between husbands and wives about intimate relations is "key to [a] successful marriage," Buzza explained. Mutual sexual satisfaction was important as well. "Don't be prudish about your relations," Buzza advised her patient, as it is "perfectly all right for husband to do anything that makes life more interesting for wife and vice versa." In order to liven up sex, the doctor also recommended nudity, privacy, and "proper positions," which the report did not describe.[78]

Characterizing such advice as "raw," the AMA was in turn quick to defend its own tactics and especially the respectability of its office spy, knowing that the use of a single woman to carry out such investigations might provoke comparable criticisms of impropriety. "In justification," responded the AMA to the editor of a Colorado medical journal who had inquired about the commercial facility, "the young woman in question" was not only married but also "the mother of a child."[79] Many in the charity movement were likely in shocked agreement about the advice Buzza had to offer. As was mentioned earlier, at least one contributor to the *Birth Control Review* took pains to point out that clinic workers should promote a "wholesome attitude" about sex and not harbor what she described as "warped" views.[80]

Equally critical was Dickinson's report, which he wrote after his visit to the Chicago Medical Bureau that same year. As he waited to speak with Riddlesbarger, Dickinson carefully observed clinic operations and listened in as the receptionist made appointments with three patients. Like the AMA, he was shocked by the clinic's openness. While charity clinics were to leave the details of contraceptive devices to physicians, the Medical Bureau's receptionist casually showed the "various appliances" to at least one woman who stood at the front desk. Remarks from the other two patients proved even more distressing. "I could not help hearing them say that they were 'overdue,'" Dickinson wrote, and noticed how they "were given appointments" nonetheless. The inference was clear: these women wanted abortions and because the Medical Bureau did not immediately turn them away, as charity clinics were expected to do, he concluded that the commercial facility was giving women what they wanted.[81]

The Medical Bureau's relationship to the booming abortion industry is elusive yet suggestive. Reminiscent of charity movement rhetoric, at least one of the Bureau's pamphlets reminded women of the "Evils of Abortion," which they were not to confuse with birth control. In addition, Riddlesbarger himself publicly denounced the practice in the *Chicago Daily Tribune*.[82] Yet, as Dickinson's observations suggest, the clinic may have occasionally helped women with the termination of their pregnancies, or at least put them in touch with someone who would. Indeed, the seventh-floor Medical Bureau was only one flight of stairs up from the sixth-floor Gabler-Martin abortion clinic, the bustling illegal operation at 190 North State Street whose activities Leslie Reagan described. And although the Gabler-Martin clinic provided its services quietly, it drew upon deep networks within the medical community and among women themselves.[83] It is unlikely, then, that Riddlesbarger, whom we know cultivated ties with at least one other physician in the building, would have remained oblivious to such an operation.[84] At least some members of Riddlesbarger's staff probably knew of its existence as well. Whether any referrals were given remains unclear, but I would not be surprised if some on occasion were.

The Medical Bureau was not the only irregular birth control clinic being watched; to a lesser degree, the Woman's Bureau of Birth Control Information endured scrutiny as well. The clinic's use of nurses and later a chiropractor did not sit well with the AMA, who increasingly viewed birth control as a medical matter that fell under the purview of regular doctors. One letter of complaint about the clinic even appealed to the AMA's sense of professional integrity. Nurses, rather than physicians, were providing medical advice, complained Dr. George Nichols, and he felt confident that the AMA would "take pains to see that this concern is put out of business immediately."[85]

The charity movement could not have agreed more. Fiercely protective of the birth control clinic institution (which it saw as its own creation), it launched a major offensive against this irregular birth control clinic movement. It did so in part by lashing out against it verbally, taking pains to draw out any commercial motivations, whether they existed or not. Evidence of this can be seen in Benson's blasting 1935 indictment on the pages of the *Birth Control Review*. Birth control manuals further promoted such sentiments. As Drs. Rita Irwin and Clementina Paolone wrote in their 1937 guide, *Practical Birth Control*, "We cannot emphasize too much that such 'clinics,' are primarily interested not in the welfare of their patients, but in making money."[86] The charity movement then took steps to distinguish its clinics officially. At the prodding of Dickinson, in 1935 it began to issue certificates of authenticity to "bona fide" birth control clinics—those clinics, in other words, that met its minimum standards of approval.[87]

Central to these standards were four important rules. First, the clinic was required to have a physician in charge, one who had graduated from a "recognized" medical school. Hence no chiropractors, osteopaths, or nurses need apply. Second, the clinic was to "have a representative medical advisory board" composed of a minimum of three doctors, which in practice often meant securing the support of the local medical society. Third, the clinic was to be "a non-profit organization" and "in no way . . . affiliated with or subsidized by any commercial manufacturer of contraceptives," which meant the clinics run by Riddlesbarger were also eliminated. Fourth (though this was only a recommendation), clinics were to serve only the indigent.[88] Singled out directly, therefore, were the practices of irregular birth control clinics, thereby proving the charity movement's allegiance to the AMA. Notably, also singled out directly were those clinics already situated in the charity movement's camp, but whose activities might blur into the world of the irregular clinic. Among these were charity clinics like those in Chicago and New York City who took in a middle-class clientele, much to the consternation of the medical profession, who saw this as competition for paying patients. As Cathy Moran Hajo noted, "Opposed to any form of medicine that took away patient dollars, doctors characterized the clinics that treated paying patients as 'rackets' that sought to profit from birth control."[89] Thus this last recommendation was a way to assuage organized medicine's fear of competition from charity clinics. Having achieved all of these standards, local clinics were then encouraged to hang their newly minted certificates of authenticity on their reception area walls so that patients would know they made the right choice for their birth control needs. As Benson explained, with this "the reputable, scientific clinic is differentiated from the commercial."[90]

Consumers were not the only ones who needed to be educated; doctors needed to be educated as well. "A patient brought the enclosed literature to my office," wrote a Michigan doctor to the AMA about Riddlesbarger's Medical Bureau, "and questioned me as to the truth of the information given."[91] Aware that such scenes were likely common, the AMA worked to make sure physicians gave the appropriate answer to their patients: the clinic in question was not a "scientific organization" but "merely a commercial outfit organized for the exploitation of its products."[92] Of course some doctors already viewed the Medical Bureau with great suspicion. "I have never sent a patient to this quackery. I wonder what sort of game they are trying to play," scribbled one angry Illinois doctor on the margins of a form letter Riddlesbarger sent out.[93] But the AMA could not be sure all physicians shared such sentiments, knowing that many increasingly turned to pharmaceutical literature and detail men for advice. As one physician noted in a book review of Palmer and Greenberg's *Facts and Frauds in Woman's Hygiene* (1936), "At times [doctors] succumb too readily to the literature of pharmaceutical houses and to the detail men who overwhelm them with their free flow of pseudo-scientific language."[94] Consequently, when the AMA decided to punish those who associated with Riddlesbarger's facility—by publishing the names of the doctors with ties to the irregular clinic in its "Bureau of Investigation" column in the *Journal of the American Medical Association*—it was clear that it wanted to make sure all physicians got the message.[95]

Here again, though, it would be unfair to suggest that the AMA's and the charity movement's concerns were without merit. Much as was the case with the birth control marketplace more generally, there were probably those who wished to take advantage of the situation, either by setting up shoddy clinic operations or by pretending that clinical work was a part of their mission, even when it was not. In fact, so visible had the concept of the "clinic" become that it appeared regularly in advertisements for commercially available birth control.[96] Furthermore, Riddlesbarger was not always aboveboard in his advertising techniques. As Andrea Tone noted, a fictional doctor graced the cover of one of his most popular birth control pamphlets. In addition, at least one patient had cause to complain about the improperly fitted diaphragm she received at his Chicago Medical Bureau.[97]

Problematic as these incidents may be, we must still exercise caution in our indictments against irregular clinics. It would be wrong to assume that all doctors, even those who worked in charity clinics, knew how to fit diaphragms properly; this was clearly not the case, as several studies at the time revealed.[98] It would also be wrong to assume that nobody ever complained about charity clinic services; this was also not true, as evidenced by the letter described earlier that was sent to the clinic in Cleveland, Ohio. Moreover, the charity movement's concern was not simply about the quality of clinic services, but also who it was that was providing them. For example, and as I have elsewhere described, the irregular clinic in Milwaukee (the one run by Nurse Gordon and backed by Riddlesbarger) not only provided reliable birth control assistance but also had the support of Sanger herself. But it too found itself under attack, first by the local medical society and then by the national charity birth control movement.[99]

And in the grand scheme of things, the charity movement's efforts paid off. Legal restrictions against birth control loosened even more in 1936 with the passage of *U.S. v. One Package*, which established the right of physicians to prescribe contraceptives to their married patients for reasons of health (thus Sanger's strategy of a "doctors-only" bill was successful). Support from the medical profession was growing as well; while charity clinics themselves were slow to jump on the certification bandwagon, the AMA finally came around. In June of 1937, it formally recognized "birth control as a legitimate part of medical practice." It also officially endorsed charity birth control clinics, so long as they were "under medical control."[100]

Notably, although irregular clinics continued to be monitored, it was hardly to the same degree as before. While Riddlesbarger's Chicago Medical Bureau was investigated by the AMA again in 1948, the chiropractor-run Woman's Bureau regularly felt the AMA's watchful eye through the early 1970s.[101] But in the eyes of the charity movement, the perceived threat of the irregular clinics seems to have diminished, though the reasons why are unclear. Perhaps it was because the charity movement now had the law and the AMA on its side. Perhaps also because irregular clinics were never all that widespread and failed to catch on. But, even if the charity movement's vigilance had waned in this regard, it still saw itself as the model of clinic services that others should follow. For this reason, the charity movement's message about the superiority of its clinics over those run by others still occasionally continued to make its way into the popular press.

Case in point: an article that appeared in a 1950 issue of the *American Mercury*. The contrast that author Grace Naismith drew between charity clinics (now Planned Parenthood) and those operated by others is striking. Carrying out an investigation of her own, she attended one of these other facilities. The clinic, Naismith wrote, was "dirty, cluttered and quite unpleasant." It was also staffed by an "unkempt" male doctor, who even offered to perform a "pre-marital operation" (likely a reference to the surgical breakage of a virgin's hymen), for which she would have to "fork over another ten" dollars. Shocked and confused, Naismith blurted, "But—but . . . I thought this was a clinic, a Planned Parenthood Federation clinic."[102] Apparently, her assumption was incorrect. Readers, therefore, were expected to draw the obvious conclusion: Planned Parenthood clinics were everything this disreputable facility was not—warm and inviting, safe and reassuring, and above all a decent place for women to go.

Thus the charity movement's desire to distinguish itself from other birth control providers remained a persistent desire; controlling the meaning of the term "birth control" remained a persistent desire as well. But these were goals not easily achieved, neither in the 1920s and 1930s nor in the decades that followed. As this first wave of clinic establishment reveals, the term "birth control" slid almost effortlessly between contraception, feminine hygiene, and abortion while providers themselves slipped in and out of categories of quackery and legitimacy, despite the charity movement's efforts to contain the meaning of birth control and who were legitimate providers. Moreover, that the commercial contraceptive industry continued to flourish even after the Supreme Court's 1936 decision to place birth control in the hands of doctors suggests that not everyone shared the charity movement's vision. Indeed, controlling the marketplace, controlling consumers, and controlling clinics sponsored by others and even those under its own auspices would remain a difficult, and often unachievable, task for the charity organization. Adaptability would be required.

Consequently, that Planned Parenthood would eventually reverse its ban against ties with pharmaceutical companies, embrace over-the-counter methods, more openly describe contraceptive techniques, and even open its doors to the unwed and provide abortions, suggests that, for all the value of its campaign in the 1930s to narrow the definitions of the term "birth control" and limit who were legitimate providers, later decades would require strategies far different. Among these were a new use for the power of charity, a new use for the power of business, a radically transformed birth control clinic, and a radically new definition of birth control, upon whose meaning the clinic institution fundamentally rested. And it is this complex process of transition that commands the attention of our last two chapters.

Chapter Three

Old Habits Are Hard to Break

When turning to the charity clinic movement's activities in the 1940s and 1950s, it is hard not to appreciate what Linda Gordon had to say about the period in the groundbreaking *Woman's Body, Woman's Right* (1976): these years constituted the third major shift in the birth control movement more generally, one that the organization's new name—which changed from the Birth Control Federation of America to the Planned Parenthood Federation of America in 1942—made plain. As Gordon explained, "The radical associations of the term 'birth control' seemed inescapable to many in the movement in the 1920s and 1930s. Opponents still called Sanger a free-lover, a revolutionary, [and] an unwed mother." Consequently, despite the charity birth control movement's efforts to contain the term "birth control" and transfer notions of sexual impropriety to commercial entrepreneurs, it couldn't quite shake the term's radical associations and the charity organization's radical past. Thus the significance of adopting a new term altogether. Gordon noted that a number of terms were proposed, but it was "Planned Parenthood" that won out. All contained, however, a similar message. As Gordon explained, they "took the focus away from women and placed it on families or children." The terms were also "designed to have as little sexual connotation as possible."[1]

Gordon's interpretation has had an enduring effect, and most accounts depict the rise of family planning as the organization's final effort to shed the vestiges of radicalism embedded in birth control, both entering into and creating a safer discourse revolving around children and family rather than feminism and sexuality.[2] The pronatalism embedded in the new rhetoric is unmistakable. As one 1943 educational flier announced, "The country needs and wants lots of babies, of course."[3] Here again, though, for all the accuracy of this particular argument, the time has come to give this period more careful scrutiny as well because—if we situate the newfound language of family planning within the context of practical clinic work, and Planned Parenthood's charitable underpinnings within the context of the commercial contraceptive marketplace—a richer story emerges, not just about the Planned Parenthood organization but also its local birth control clinics.

This chapter begins (and ends), therefore, with the *language* of family planning, exploring further its origins as well as its larger effects. Certainly, the rise of the new rhetoric was a product of the organization's quest for a more sanitized, conservative image. But closer investigation also reveals that

it was equally rooted in a new conceptualization of family life more generally, a product of America's postwar preoccupation with psychology, rationality, and the quest for control. Closer investigation also reveals what this
new rhetoric yielded: not just new ways to envision the family but also new
reasons why to practice birth control. In other words, the "planned family"
with all of its "wanted children" was the key to America's salvation. For only
through rational planning could its members be spared the suffering generated by a whole host of social ills, which first destroyed individuals, then
families, and ultimately society.

Equally suggestive are the methods through which this new message was
delivered. Although Planned Parenthood continued to remain quiet about
the specifics of contraception, its propaganda campaigns increasingly bore
the more overt commercial advertising techniques prevalent in the 1930s:
it mass produced educational pamphlets, theatrical skits, comic-book styled
educational melodramas, and even the occasional movie script in an effort
to advertise its new family planning message, all suggesting a slow abandonment of its emphasis on quiet respectability. The chapter ends with a discussion about what this new vision of family planning also inevitably yielded: the
unplanned family with all its unwanted children. As the new symbol of social
disorder in America, the unplanned family would have equally dramatic effect
by putting into place the conditions necessary to facilitate the clinic movement's second wave of growth, its broadened definition of the term "birth
control," and its new use for the rationale of charity in the decades to follow.

Yet in turning to the 1940s and 1950s, we also need to consider the *practical* obstacles the clinic movement simultaneously faced. This means appreciating in part the limits of the shift in language. While the rhetoric of the
organization may have grown more conservative, what happened inside the
local clinic often did not, as the prescription of the diaphragm remained the
institution's primary function, at the heart of which still lay the early feminist impulse to give women control over childbearing. Also worth appreciating is women's dissatisfaction with the diaphragm prescription regime.
While clinic organizers thought the diaphragm was the answer to women's
birth control needs, many of the women who attended the clinic did not.
As a result, when women were dissatisfied with what they received as *cases* or
as *patients*, they exercised their rights as *consumers* by returning to the methods they had formerly used, those various methods of the marketplace. And
so, for all the success stories local clinics may have rightfully been able to
boast, that so many women simultaneously chose to abandon the diaphragm
suggests something else: the charity movement's campaign of the 1930s to
teach women both the limitations of commercial products as well as their
immoral ramifications had in other ways failed miserably.

Equally important to investigate are the ways in which the clinic movement responded, first to this situation and then to others. With respect to

the diaphragm, despite the efforts to address women's dissatisfaction, the clinic's combination of charitable paternalism and medical authority complicated the solutions it proposed, which meant that while a variety of methods was urged, doctors (rather than the women themselves) were still to decide what method to use. Moreover, in the many calls made for the necessity of research into "simple" methods of birth control (methods, in other words, that were not as complex as the diaphragm), the justification remained chronically rooted in elitist assumptions about the inabilities of the poor; that they especially needed a simple method, even when middle-class women themselves were as unhappy with the diaphragm as were their less well-off sisters.

Further complicating matters is that throughout the 1940s and 1950s a contest of wills was emerging within this massive Planned Parenthood organization. On the one hand, there was the ever expanding national umbrella office, which, just when it was looking to standardize its vision of birth control by way of this new family planning motif, was simultaneously changing its mind about what this vision ought to be, even reevaluating the necessity of the local birth control clinic. And so, whereas before, clinic establishment and the direct delivery of contraceptive services were among the charity movement's primary goals, now the national office insisted that local organizations shift their efforts elsewhere. They were to spend less time establishing clinics and more time lobbying public heath agencies and hospitals in order to get them to incorporate family planning services into the programs they offered. Of course, in opposition to much of this stood the local Planned Parenthood affiliates themselves. They chafed under the national office's growing scrutiny, disagreed with many of the new directives coming from above, and often continued to do as they had done before, which was the establishment of local clinics so as to engage in the provision of the diaphragm. For everyone involved, therefore, old habits were indeed hard to break.

Planning Your Family

In the records for the Chicago affiliate (newly incorporated in 1947 as the Planned Parenthood Association–Chicago Area), there is a script for a play called *Sunday Afternoon*.[4] Written sometime in the late 1940s, the author of this educational melodrama was Jennette Dowling of the American Theatre Wing War Service, Inc., in New York City.[5] Its presence in the Chicago affiliate's records is something of a mystery. It is neither clear how the Chicago office obtained a copy of the play nor if the national Planned Parenthood organization promoted this theatrical skit. Nor is it apparent if anybody in Chicago, or elsewhere in the nation, ever put the play on. And, if they did, who or how many saw it. *Sunday Afternoon* remains significant nonetheless because its message reverberates loudly the organization's new family planning theme—a theme that made its way into the millions of educational materials Planned Parenthood distributed throughout this period and that also regularly appeared in the popular press.[6] For this reason, it offers another useful window through which to peer.

The story opens in Terry and Jim Davidson's small apartment. Looking to relax on this Sunday afternoon, Jim sits on the living room couch with the newspaper; after finding the section with the theater listings, he throws the rest in a pile at his feet. His wife Terry quietly enters the room. "Asleep?" Jim asks about their son, Davy. "Uhuh—at last," she replies. Though worn out and tired, Terry continues picking up pieces of Davy's clothing, which are strewn on the floor, all the while still holding the boy's plate, cup, and spoon, leftover apparently from his afternoon meal. Also leftover are several articles of the boy's soiled clothing, which are now slung over Terry's weary arm. Terry and Jim continue talking, Jim hoping to entice his wife into catching a movie at the local cinema. Polite conversation, however, quickly bleeds into bickering, until finally a full-scale fight erupts, only to be interrupted by a knock at the door.

In enters Helen, a friend of Terry and Jim who has come to watch Davy for the afternoon. Helen is a smart woman, married and with three children of her own, and quickly she realizes the nature of Terry and Jim's argument. She understands how although they still love each other, the stresses of marriage and parenting have taxed their personal well being, which has in turn made it difficult for them to enjoy each other and even their young son. Consequently, both are quite unhappy, so much so that Terry has even just mentioned the dreaded d-word: "divorce!" Fortunately for Terry and Jim, Helen also knows the solution, and as the play unfolds she will enlighten the unhappy couple about the joys of the planned family, an ideal in which each member contributed in order to achieve personal happiness, familial bliss, and ultimately a stable community.

That *Sunday Afternoon* and other such materials depicted daily life at its most intimate, and perhaps its most mundane, reveals not only the nature of this new household ideal but also the new reasons behind it. Rather than the wife's responsibility, everyone contributed in some way to the life of the family, not just the husband but the children too. *Sunday Afternoon* also reveals a new conceptualization of domestic discord, one that justified the need for family planning. It was not solely about catastrophic events, such as major illnesses or deaths of overburdened mothers, an image that so often characterized the propagandistic tales of the two decades preceding. Rather, it was increasingly about the daily interactions between husbands and wives, parents and children, and between the children themselves. In other words, family planning was about domestic harmony; and domestic harmony was about improving the daily web of familial relationships, a web that was underpinned by emotional stability, which the anxiety produced by uncertainty only threatened. Indeed, while emotional stability was the glue that held the planned family together, instability was what tore it apart, as instability led to such irrational behavior as divorce, juvenile delinquency, miscarriage, infertility, and a whole host of other social ills.

The influences behind this new family planning culture were many. Linda Gordon connected it to the culture of governmental planning as it emerged out of the New Deal and then World War II.[7] But it also could be found in the urban planning movement more generally, which by some accounts had its roots in the urban development movement of the turn-of-the-twentieth century whose primary goal was to create order and efficiency among the nation's rapidly growing cities. Notably, by WWII this urban planning movement had entered an era of new vigor, with the influx of massive monetary incentives from the federal government.[8]

This planning motif could also be found in a variety of other social, cultural, and economic arenas. For example, the analogy Planned Parenthood literature repeatedly drew between the planned family and home ownership resonated with the larger trend of postwar suburban planning, which also embodied the need to map everything out beforehand.[9] As William Levitt, among the most famous housing developers of the era, remarked: "We planned every foot of it—every store, filling station, school, house, apartment, church, color, tree, and shrub."[10] In addition, the 1948 publication of psychologist B. F. Skinner's *Walden Two*, a psychological utopia based upon expert and meticulous planning, suggests another thread in this cultural fabric.[11] The planning imperative even gave rise to another new (though now familiar) trend: personal financial planning.[12] Finally, a sense of preparedness in order to assuage anxiety also figured prominently in the "culture of the Cold War," to use the phrase coined by historian Stephen Whitfield.[13] Put another way, backyard bomb shelters not only provided protection in the event of nuclear attack but, and perhaps more important, also ensured peace of mind before a catastrophe even took place. Preparation thus meant control in the face of uncertainty, and in the postwar era control meant security and therefore happiness, or so the argument went.

At the same time, equally influential was the growing presence of psychology in American culture. Much as was the case with the city planning movement, World War II and the years that followed marked newfound strength and authority for this field as well.[14] As a result, by the 1940s everything had psychological roots, and such things as divorce, juvenile delinquency, unwed motherhood, and even infertility and miscarriage were defined as problems of the irrational and anxious mind, which first destroyed individuals, then families, and ultimately society.[15] But in psychology also lay the solution; the way to curb such destructive behavior was by helping mothers and fathers take control of their lives in order to ensure emotional security for themselves and, in turn, their children. Indeed, although Planned Parenthood literature still promoted doctors as the voice of authority on *how* to plan, the reasons *why* increasingly drew upon the language of popular psychology. Thus by stitching the perceived weaknesses of family and society into a patchwork quilt of psychological frailties, such propagandistic tales as *Sunday Afternoon* showed how the planned family could help prevent any tears in the fabric through rationality and control. And so our story of the planned family begins.

World War II and the years that followed were marked by a number of contradictions: unprecedented prosperity coincided with continued poverty, and middle-class optimism was interwoven with fears of social instability. For example, many Americans found themselves living more comfortably than ever before, a level of prosperity that was buoyed by the massive wartime and postwar production booms. For others, however, especially in the nation's rural areas and the growing but cash-strapped cities, poverty often remained acute. Money was not the only issue, however. Concerns about broken marriages appeared regularly in mainstream publications, and the topic of juvenile delinquency became an issue of growing anxiety and debate. The threat of unwed motherhood, often linked with "sexual delinquency," loomed large as well.[16] Planned Parenthood in turn participated in this contradictory fervor, and its educational literature regularly bore newspaper headline collages testifying to the urgency of all these problems. While banners such as "Marriage Like a Mine Field" evoked fears of broken homes, others like "Rising Prices Beat Earnings" and "City Will Solicit Aid for Children" drew upon concerns about money, be it personal financial woes or having to support through taxes the economic hardships of others. Still another headline, "Orgies in Youth Gangs Charged," reminded readers of the problems not only of juvenile delinquency but also adolescent promiscuity. Postwar life had become an "American Drama," to use the words of one such collage-bearing pamphlet, which, according to the educational rhetoric, the planned family could help make less turbulent.[17]

Central to achieving the planned family was rational preparation and control. "It takes forethought, preparation and a certain amount of strategy," announced the World War II pamphlet "The Soldier Takes a Wife."[18] Although such militaristic language waned with the war's end, a domesticated version of such strategic maneuvering persisted in educational materials well after the boys returned home. Rather than leave things to chance, parents now took charge of their marital destinies by determining when and how many children they wanted to have before they had them. "You've been lucky," Terry says to her friend Helen, whose children were born several years apart. To which Helen replies, "Lucky! No Terry—Joe and I planned it that way."[19] Other materials—which depicted metaphoric architectural floor plans and parents gazing upon the specifications of their blueprint baby—also suggest this push to get people to think ahead of time.[20] In fact, prescriptions for married life in general reflected this time warplike mentality, and Planned Parenthood regularly encouraged engaged couples to find out in advance, through marriage education classes, for example, what life after the exchange of vows might hold. As the fictional character Helen explains to her friends Terry and Jim, "Even when two people are born to be suited to each other, a perfect marriage doesn't just happen—without education."[21]

If education was so important, what then were couples supposed to learn? If we look at what the literature had to say, we find out that the planned family was about teamwork and began with both husband and wife pooling their efforts to create a healthy and happy household. Together, they assumed the responsibility not only of childraising but also in the decision-making process before pregnancy even took place. "Newly married couples dream of a house that will expand to fit their growing family. They also dream of their ideal family," proclaimed one Planned Parenthood flier.[22] Another encouraged husbands and wives "to talk it over *first* from every angle" how many children to have and when. It then showed images of the husband and wife visiting the doctor together and later basking in the glow of their happy families, thereby reinforcing the idea that couples, rather than the wife alone, made such decisions and enjoyed of course the results.[23]

In turn, such cooperative planning yielded emotional well being for everybody involved. For women this was especially important. By not having to worry whether she could afford the next child or whether she had the time or room to care for another baby, she would not have to endure anxious days or sleepless nights. As Joan Harper, married mother of three in Planned Parenthood's comic book-style pamphlet entitled "Escape from Fear" tearfully says to her husband late one night, "I don't know what other people do, Ken. Maybe they just go on having a baby every year and not caring about food or clothes or bills." With no reply from equally troubled husband, Joan then buries her anxious head into her pillow.[24] Certainly, such emphasis was not entirely new, as arguments for birth control had long described the emotional suffering mothers experienced as a result of constant childbearing. As one daughter in the 1920s wrote, "Poor mother! No wonder that she is a mental and physical wreck today when only in her early forties," which she explained was brought about by "twenty years" of childbearing.[25] But by the 1940s mental health arguments took on new fervor. So powerful had such arguments become that on occasion they completely overshadowed the more materially grounded demands for birth control that had characterized the propaganda campaigns of the two preceding decades. As the remarks made in 1946 by one speaker at Planned Parenthood's twenty-fifth anniversary conference suggest, mental rather than material, relational rather than physical rationales underpinned the need for family planning.[26]

That mothers now found themselves in a state of mental turmoil after only one child marked a dramatic shift from the stories of overburdened motherhood of the past. Whereas before, overwhelmed mothers were women who had many children (six, eight, ten, often more), now they could feel such stresses regardless of family size.[27] As Helen of *Sunday Afternoon* explains to her friend Terry, "Having a baby takes a lot more out of the woman than just going to the hospital and having it. That's only the beginning . . . just getting used to having a baby in the house at all—is a complete readjustment in itself."[28] In other words, fear of future babies was only part of it; getting over the anxiety of the one you just had, even if it was the first, was now equally important.

With this newfound emphasis on mental health came benefits for the husband. Although he did not have to endure the physical rigors of childbearing, the emotional stresses of parenthood could take their toll on the father as well. As a result, while tales of tragic motherhood characterized the older literature, by the 1940s tales of tragic fatherhood also started to appear, as the following story reveals. The melodrama begins with George and the history of his "cruel childhood." The eldest of twelve children, his mother died in childbirth when he was a teenager and his father abandoned the family soon thereafter, leaving George the sole breadwinner. At twenty-two, George married Mary and was delighted with the birth of their daughter. Then came a set of twins, followed by another girl. So distraught was George by the birth of his fourth child that he showed up at the maternity ward drunk, only to be thrown out. His wife Mary worried strenuously and turned to the doctor for help. "Another baby and George might go to pieces altogether," she explained. "A fifth child too soon and George might follow in his father's footsteps."[29] More such tales—in the form of letters from "A Soldier Father," a "Tubercular Father," and an "Army Air Force Private [whose] buddies need help too"—made their way into Planned Parenthood materials.[30] Even Ken, Joan Harper's husband in "Escape from Fear," finds himself trapped in a pit of existential darkness, spending his days and his nights in moody and melancholic distraction worrying about the possibility of another mouth to feed and the lack of physical intimacy with his wife because both worried about another pregnancy.

The husband's role in the family planning ideal is dramatic. Consider, for example, what the pamphlet "The Soldier Takes a Wife" has to say. "So much sweetness and light have been poured on the institution of motherhood that American men are likely to gain the impression that they are useful only at conception and in paying the bills afterwards." Fathers were also told just how much they could enjoy their children. "Men who with their wives invest time, care, money and affection in their children never fail to get it back in double interest," the WWII pamphlet explained. Perhaps even more significant is how the educational literature even on occasion chastised husbands for not doing their part, sometimes subtly blaming them for any suffering they endured if they did not help their wives plan. "Don't wait to have your children say, 'I can't see how Father got through the last war. Mother has to do all the planning.'"[31] In other words, if the planned family was to achieve emotional stability for all its members, the husband had to work at it too. In fact, the emotional stakes could be just as high for him as for his wife.

And of course the key to this emotional well being for both husbands and wives was the opportunity to express physical intimacy. As *Sunday Afternoon* demonstrated, those couples who lacked intimacy suffered great discontent. In the heat of Terry and Jim's argument before Helen arrives, Jim tries to reach out to his unhappy wife, but when he puts his hand on Terry's shoulder, she snaps, "Don't." Angry, Jim shouts back, "There! You see! It's been like this ever since Davy was born. You don't want me to touch you."[32] Similarly, Planned Parenthood's comic-book pamphlet painted an even more overt scene in the bedroom, right on the front cover. Sexily clad yet obviously distraught, the wife sits in bed, alone and with her head buried in her hands. Her bathrobed husband looms large in the foreground, frustrated, dejected, staring out in space, and smoking a cigarette. "Joan and Ken Harper's marriage was on the rocks," the caption read, "*because they loved each other!*"[33] In short, their desire to be intimate only provoked fears and then fights about the possibility of pregnancy, which in turn squelched their desire, their ability, to be intimate. All hope was not lost, however, because through family planning marital bliss could once again be achieved. While Terry and Jim recaptured old feelings of romance by going on a date, Joan and Ken sat lovingly in each other's arms while their children played around them.[34] Thus rekindling the spark was another key to happy, hence strong marriages, which meant that rational planning also made room for spontaneous moments of lightheartedness and fun.

While family planning was intended to improve the lives of husbands and wives, the culmination of such blissful unions was planned (or wanted children), who, much like their parents, were happy and emotionally secure. As one pamphlet explained, "His food and physical well being and safety are important, but his happiness and mental health are even more important in determining the kind of person he will grow to be."[35] Best exemplified by the childrearing manuals of Dr. Benjamin Spock, this shift toward caring for children's psychological needs has long been noted by historians.[36] In previous generations, good parenting meant providing food and shelter. Now, however, mothers and fathers needed to nurture their children's emotional development. In addition to being well clothed and well fed, therefore, the wanted child was well adjusted too. This idea of wanted children also had much to say about the love within a family, not just love that parents bestowed upon their children but also love that existed between husband and wife and even among the siblings themselves. As the fictional Helen explains in *Sunday Afternoon*, "no child was ever made happy living with parents who didn't love each other." Put another way, parents in love loved their children. Wanted children also loved (and were loved by) their brothers and sisters, as the educational melodrama depicted. Because she and her husband had planned, Helen's boy Richard was not jealous but instead "excited at the idea of a tiny baby in the house" and insisted on holding his newborn sister all the way home from the hospital.[37]

How were couples to achieve such blissful households? The answer was to use birth control, but now it also required two important rituals of waiting. The first took place between the exchange of nuptial vows and childbearing. Rather than get pregnant right away, couples were told to wait, to get to know each other as individuals first, so as to solidify the marital relationship before the rigors of parenthood complicated matters.[38] The second took place between pregnancies, with what one flier called a "'breather' between babies."[39] Thus emerges another new conceptualization of family life. Birth control advocates had long argued for spacing the birth of children, but because this message ran counter to the popular belief that having children close together promoted sibling bonding and camaraderie, it took on new fervor. So adamant were some advocates of the well-spaced planned family that they even began to chastise parents for holding on to outdated conceptualizations of family. As one marriage counselor remarked at a Planned Parenthood conference, the "sentimental concern to have children close together for their companionship to each other is based on a myth."[40] Remarks made by Helen in *Sunday Afternoon* suggest the problems that ill-spaced children could generate. Had she not spaced her offspring, she explains to Terry, she would have been "ganged up" by too many infants, imagery that also tapped into the fears of juvenile delinquency.[41]

All of this, then—the loving and in love parents, the affectionate siblings—meant family planning worked at the individual, familial, and community-wide level. While parents who planned found happiness for themselves as individuals and couples, they in turn raised wanted children who would then become better adults. As *Parents' Magazine* advised its readers, "Babies who are wanted and planned for happily have the best chance in life."[42] Communities comprised of such planned families also benefited. As C.-E. A. Winslow, professor emeritus of Yale's School of Public Health, noted in a 1948 issue of *Survey* magazine, "The stability of the household and the stability of society are as vitally affected by planning the family as is the health of the individual mother and child."[43]

It would be unfair to suggest, however, that it was Planned Parenthood alone that cultivated such ideas; popular demand contributed as well. The emphasis on husbands and fathers, for example, was in part a product of men's interest in family planning, much as it was for women. To assume as one historian did that Planned Parenthood "needed to appear to be more friendly to men's concerns because men controlled the agencies from which [it] sought support," shortchanges men's participation in family affairs.[44] Indeed, contrary to propagandistic exaggerations of men's lack of involvement, which showed the "unknowing husband" stumbling upon his wife sewing "tiny garments," men had long helped their wives, daughters, and sisters in such matters. For example, they helped them procure contraceptives and abortions.[45] They regularly contributed to the *Birth Control Review*. Widespread condom use further indicates men's interest in reproductive matters.[46]

Likewise, the desire to keep marriages from falling apart was not solely a measure to shore up conservative family values but often reflected a long-expressed desire (among women and men) for help when faced with marital strife. As one clinic patient explained to the attending nurse in the 1930s, my husband "told me he'd go out with someone else, and that made me mad."[47] Another lamented how her husband "goes with others."[48] Yet husbands themselves had long faced distressing predicaments. "I am a married man with two children, but I am not with my wife now," wrote one husband in the 1920s. "I don't want any more children any more than she does . . . [and] . . . I think that if I could get that information I could get her to come back to me."[49] In other words, men were also keenly interested in maintaining intimacy with their wives, and while there is much to be said about Peter Stearns and Mark Knapp's argument that sex for men was by the 1940s more about physical expression than emotional affection, such sentiments as the following must surely have persisted among at least some men.[50] As one man explained (in the 1920s): "Of course 'abstinence' would be the answer to my problem, but both my wife and I are of an affectionate nature, and we could hardly apply abstinence with any kind of success. I know from past experience."[51] Still another wrote quite desperately that he and his wife "have occupied separate bedrooms for five years and I crave her kisses and affection which under the conditions cannot be satisfied."[52]

Finally, the parental desire to spend time with their offspring and create a happy home life contributed to the emphasis on children's happiness. "My life was a constant hell of fear of pregnancy. I didn't enjoy my children because of the strain," wrote one woman in the 1940s. She then explained how her daughters were more fortunate because birth control freed them from such stress and as a result their homes were "happy, joyous, and comradely."[53] Men wanted to enjoy their children too. As the sociologist Ralph LaRossa demonstrated, despite the widespread belief that involved fatherhood is a modern invention, fathers earlier in the twentieth century expressed an interest in childrearing practices and actively participated in the very personal daily concerns and routines of parenthood. The letters they wrote about their infants to the Children's Bureau (the federal agency established during the Progressive era to improve the health and well being of women and children) suggest that they wanted advice about such things as feeding, sleeping, thumb sucking, and bed wetting. Letters that fathers wrote to Angelo Patri (who had a popular syndicated column and weekly radio show called "Our Children") as their children grew older indicate their continued interest in the "psychological health of school age children."[54]

What all this suggests therefore is that men and women wanted help with their marriages, wanted help raising happy children, in short wanted help with family planning. Where then, according to the rhetoric, did one go to find assistance regarding such matters? The answer can be found in Helen's advice to her friends Terry and Jim in *Sunday Afternoon*. For couples with money, they could see the local doctor. For couples without, there was the local clinic, though, as Helen admits, the nation needed more. "We need clinics," Helen explains, "places where the right kind of knowledge about marriage and child spacing can be given freely—because when the marriage is right—when children grow out of a home based on the very best marriage has to give—it's—it's the fulfillment of the birthright of every human being."[55] And so, although by the 1940s and 1950s the message of Planned Parenthood was in flux, in this case its clinics remained "the solution," to use Sanger's rallying cry of 1920.[56] On that note, *Sunday Afternoon* slowly drew to a close, with newfound happiness for the Davidson family. "Oh Jim," Terry says lovingly and with great relief to her husband, "we've got a chance now—a chance to be a family!"[57]

A Voice from Above, Dissent from Below

Meanwhile, sometime in the early 1940s a member of Illinois' newly established Champaign County Planned Parenthood wrote to the head office in New York describing the work she and her colleagues were carrying out in this midwestern college town. She first explained that in order to raise money for their clinic and reach prospective patients, they held rummage sales in the basement of a local black church in one of the poorer sections of town. The Champaign woman went on to describe the fliers they stuffed in the bags of each customer's rummage sale purchase. "It is <u>imperative,</u>" she insisted, "that altho[ugh] the idea of the Planned Family be emphasized, that the title [of the fliers] bear the words 'Birth Control.' They can be taught to plan their families, and that is part of the clinic's job, but the term Planned Family does not bring them to the clinic. More frequently than any other term, when they come into the clinic for the first time they say, 'I want to get me a birth control.'" She then enclosed a copy of the affiliate's flier, which bore the simple words "A Birth Control Clinic."[58]

Hers is a telling note. In part because it reveals the role Planned Parenthood clinics were to play in educating Americans about the new family planning ideal. From the late 1930s through the 1950s, Planned Parenthood literature and manuals of procedure show dramatic changes in clinic policy, changes that met the broader family planning mission. As a result, rather than simply give women the diaphragm, local clinics were to provide a range of contraceptives, including methods men could use, and to offer a variety of programs, such as infertility counseling and marriage education programs.

Yet, as this letter also suggests, what happened inside local Planned Parenthood clinics often differed little from previous decades, despite the changes in policy and rhetoric. As accounts of practical clinic work reveal, most patients continued to receive only the diaphragm, few clinics offered on-site marital or infertility services, and the teaching of family planning remained largely a female affair during which clinic doctors fitted women with the diaphragm, much as they had done in the decades preceding. Even getting people to use the language of family planning proved no simple matter. Consequently, much as Planned Parenthood tried to change the language people used and broaden the services local clinics provided, implementing these new visions was an entirely different story. And so, our story of practical clinic work returns.

After the massive proliferation of contraceptive facilities during the Depression years, clinic movement growth stabilized during the postwar era. Of the almost six hundred Planned Parenthood clinics that existed nationwide,[59] Illinois was home to at least eleven: seven in Chicago, one in Evanston (a Chicago suburb), and the remaining three scattered throughout the rest of the state.[60] Despite local fluctuations—such as the opening and closing of several clinics in Chicago and elsewhere in the state—by the end of the 1950s, the number of clinics nationwide changed little.[61]

But it was a stability that hid rocky waters; during this period the national Planned Parenthood organization tried to strengthen its authority over this loosely connected chain of affiliates, especially through newly instituted field visits and reports. It was an endeavor, however, that had a way of provoking as many problems with the local committees as it was supposed to resolve.[62] Of particular concern for the national office was how well local offices worked with the national umbrella organization. Often the ties were amicable. "The present relationships between California and the Federation are very good," described a 1942 summary of Planned Parenthood activity throughout the United States. Twelve other affiliates received similar praise. Not all did, however. New Jersey and Illinois (in particular the Chicago office) bore sharp criticism in the early 1940s, though it is not entirely clear why. "Illinois is very sensitive at the point of its prerogatives and is consequently very critical of the National organization," the report chided.[63] Even those who subscribed to the national office's authority still occasionally vented their frustrations over the federation's increasing demands. Hardly a unified movement therefore, such tensions suggest conflicting opinions within the Planned Parenthood organization about how best to promote family planning and how especially to carry out clinic work.[64]

Trouble first began with the kinds of contraceptives local clinics were giving their patients. "Clinics everywhere thought they had a method so generally applicable," wrote Dr. Robert Dickinson in his 1938 manual for birth control clinic procedure, "that the movement required merely multiplication of centers." "Follow-up," he added, "gives this comfortable belief a jolt."[65] Indeed, study after clinic study consistently revealed that women were unhappy with the diaphragm regimen. The numbers are striking. In her analysis of Cincinnati clinics, for example, Dr. Regine K. Stix found that of the 1,621 women who were prescribed the method, just over half (51.4 percent) had abandoned it, and an additional 2.6 percent never used it at all.[66] When Dr. Ruth A. Robishaw analyzed clinic services in Cleveland, she found similarly disappointing results: of the 3,264 women who were prescribed the method, 1,504 quit, most of them (1,353) doing so "deliberately."[67] Given all the benefits of the individually fitted diaphragm, the question is why were women so dissatisfied?

If we listen to what women themselves said about the diaphragm—responses, admittedly, that are framed by the questions researchers asked—we find all sorts of reasons. As Dr. Marie E. Kopp listed in her analysis of more than ten thousand patients at Sanger's New York clinic:

Patient personally objects.
Patient dislikes using method.
Patient objects to use of pessary.
Patient afraid it will injure her health.
Patient believes that her husband will object to [its] use.[68]

Improper fitting by doctors, moreover, contributed to women's complaints. Women "did not use the method after being given it," concluded one report of clinic services in Minneapolis, "because of discomfort incidental to the large size diaphragms used."[69]

The findings of Cathy Moran Hajo shed even more light on the situation. Clinic patients simply did not like the diaphragm. Many "found it cumbersome and distasteful." She explained:

It forced them to touch their sexual organs, it had to be cleaned and maintained between uses to prevent rubber deterioration. Spermicidal jelly could be greasy and stained clothing. In some rare instances it caused irritation to either the patient or her husband. But perhaps the biggest adjustment was that using the clinic method put women in charge of contraceptive decisions. Unlike withdrawal, condoms and periodic abstinence, the clinic method did not rely on the cooperation of the husband.

Hajo concluded, "While women often came to the clinic in order to get more control over their reproductive lives, they sometimes balked at the amount of work the method required" and "complained that it was 'too complicated' or 'sordid,' and viewed the many rules as annoyance and bother."[70]

It is little wonder, then, that so many women quit, often returning to their *old* birth control habits. As Stix noted in her 1939 analysis of Cincinnati clinics, "There was a marked tendency for couples who did not use the clinic prescription or who discontinued its use to turn to the same types of contraception they had used *before* they attended the clinic." These included none other than withdrawal as well as commercially available condoms and douches, methods the charity movement had once worked so hard to discredit.[71] And so, although contraceptives were technically legal only in the hands of physicians, their over-the-counter sale persisted, and more than a few consumers (including those who went to local birth control clinics) continued to demand their availability.

Given this reality, strikingly little has been written about the relationship between consumers and the contraceptive marketplace during the 1940s and 1950s—the period between, in other words, the *U.S. v. One Package* decision in 1936 and the introduction of the pill in 1960. But we do know a little. According to James Reed, now that the Federal Trade Commission (FTC) could regulate the contraceptive industry, the quality of condoms, for example, dramatically improved. As Reed explained, because condoms found to be defective were then destroyed, "Suddenly it became profitable to test condoms, and a permanent improvement in the quality of prophylactics on the market resulted."[72] Andrea Tone noticed this development. "By the late 1940s, the small-scale condom entrepreneurs who had made sheaths by hand in small shops had become a thing of the past." Now, she added, "In their stead stood corporate Goliaths, automatic assembly lines, and name-brand condoms meeting industry specifications set by Washington."[73] Thus, long gone were the days of the indomitable Julius Schmidt—who stuffed sausages by day and made condoms by night—because the manufacture of condoms was becoming big business.

So too was the feminine hygiene industry, which continued to produce its vast array of douches, vaginal suppositories, crèmes, jellies, and foams. But in this case, Tone noted, the government's efforts to regulate the trade were "mixed." The "FTC's authority was limited, confined to the elimination of false and misleading advertising." As a result, Tone explained, this "regulatory vacuum encouraged companies to resurrect euphemistic language to obfuscate the intended contraceptive use of their products."[74] Thus the over-the-counter sale of feminine hygiene products persisted, and women continued to demand their availability—even among those given the opportunity to use the more effective diaphragm through the local clinic. In short, they just didn't like the diaphragm and made the decision to use something else.

In contrast, many in the clinic movement viewed women's dissatisfaction with the diaphragm rather differently, a product likely of the clinic's culture of medical authority and middle-class elitism toward the poor women they served. As Jimmie Elaine Wilkinson Meyer noted in her historical account of the early Cleveland movement, characterizations like these abounded in one 1931 report of unintended pregnancies among clinic patients: "lazy and ignorant," "apparently too shiftless to care," "careless," "questionable mentally," "difficult," and "moderately difficult."[75] Or, as Hajo noted in her study, "Blaming the patient was easier than finding fault with the method, which the middle and upper-class activists saw as scientific, advanced, and effective."[76] At least one patient, moreover, internalized such views. Meyer quoted from one of the patient letters she found in the Cleveland clinic records: "I'd like you to know that I realize what a fool I've been," wrote one woman in explanation of her unintended pregnancy. "I have felt so ashamed of being pregnant again, I[']ve even avoided my mother," she confessed.[77]

To others within the charity movement, however, it was becoming increasingly apparent that the diaphragm—or at least clinics' singular emphasis on it—was part of the problem, regardless of the patient's class or educational level. As Stix's 1939 Cincinnati study also demonstrated, women of all classes quit the method, indicating that the reasons behind its unpopularity were more complicated than money and intelligence. Although impoverished living conditions often influenced how well women used the diaphragm, so-called levels of intelligence did not. In addition, that Stix also found a 37 percent drop-out rate among the wives of white-collar workers—a figure that is admittedly somewhat less than that of the wives of manual workers (47 percent) or welfare recipients (56 percent) but significant nonetheless—suggests that women of more comfortable backgrounds found the diaphragm unappealing as well.[78]

As a result, some within the clinic movement began to suggest that the prescription of a variety of methods inside the clinic was now in order. As Stix wrote, "clinic policies" needed to be "changed to permit the more flexible prescription of a variety of contraceptives, suiting each to the individual patient."[79] Dickinson agreed; when he made his disparaging remarks about the limits of diaphragm-only services, he went on in his clinic manual to describe a variety of methods—including condoms, douches, tampons, spermicidal preparations, sterilization, celibacy, and even the safe period before ovulation—as possible methods to use.[80]

This did not mean that patients were granted agency in the decision-making process. Instead, medical authority and charitable paternalism remained firmly in place. For example, although there was a growing appreciation for a variety of contraceptive methods and for individualized advice, this still meant the physician, rather than the patient, was supposed to choose the most appropriate method. As Dickinson's 1950 manual informed prospective patients, "When you see the doctor, he (or she) will select the method which is best for you to use."[81] Furthermore, the old habit of connecting class and intelligence with the ability to use birth control continued to influence these new policies. In his advice to physicians in his 1938 manual, Dickinson advised them to consider what he called "intelligence," "living conditions," and "character" when deciding what method to prescribe.[82] In short, while women deemed more intelligent and economically secure should be given the diaphragm, women who were not were to get something else, something presumably easier to use. It was a philosophy Clarence Gamble shared. As Laura Briggs noted in her study of the birth control movement in Puerto Rico, Gamble believed fervently in the "idea that other methods—even less effective ones—would be necessary, particularly for impoverished and colonized people."[83]

Notably, such conclusions also underpinned the push for research into simple methods of contraception. Certainly, Sanger had dreamed of a simple method in the form of a pill since as early as 1912, and women's dissatisfaction with the diaphragm more generally must surely have contributed as well.[84] But more often than not it was arguments such as the following one that carried the most weight in fueling contraceptive research. As Johanna Schoen explained in her study of birth control and public health in North Carolina and elsewhere, in 1937 "birth control nurse Doris Davidson bemoaned the problem to Elizabeth Barclay, field director of the American Birth Control League":

> We all know the ever present need for a simpler method for unintelligent, illiterate, lazy and poverty-stricken patients. Although the diaphragm method may provide greater safety in the hands of the intelligent patient, it often acts in just the opposite way in the hands of the unintelligent patient, no matter how carefully she may have been instructed. This type of patient (and I am referring to the low-intelligent strata found by the hundred[s] in North Carolina, South Carolina, Tennessee, and West Virginia) can learn a thing one moment and unlearn it the next with bewildering rapidity. Often by the time the poor creature has arrived back in her home, she is uncertain about technique and therefore hesitant in applying it. . . . If we are going to help this low-grade patient, do we not have to meet them on their own level?—give them something which is EASY for them to apply, and which they can readily understand?[85]

In other words, the uneducated poor especially needed something simple in the way of contraception.

And Nurse Davidson, of course, was hardly alone in her sentiments. As Briggs argued, from the late 1920s forward most scientists who engaged in contraceptive research regularly used such logic to justify their work, following the lead set by Dickinson, who argued "for the need for something simple to be used in colonial regions."[86] Even Sanger was of this opinion.

In a letter written to Katherine Dexter McCormick (the woman who would ultimately bankroll the development of the pill), she would have this to say, "I consider that the world and almost our civilization for the next twenty-five years, is going to depend upon a simple, cheap, safe, contraceptive to be used in poverty stricken slums, jungles, and among the most ignorant people."[87] Thus the rationale for simple methods was not because women, regardless of their class or intelligence, wanted something else, but rather because the illiterate poor were incapable of using something too difficult.

Despite all of this—the widespread dissatisfaction among patients and the federation's growing efforts to change clinic prescription policies—clinic prescription practices changed very little. A survey conducted by Planned Parenthood Federation of America (PPFA) in 1960, shortly before the dramatic shift to the pill, illustrates this vividly: of the 73 Planned Parenthood affiliates that responded to the national office's request for information, more than 90 percent prescribed the diaphragm virtually exclusively.[88] In fact, so prevalent was the prescription of the diaphragm in local Planned Parenthood clinics that by the late 1950s the organization had become almost synonymous with this particular method. As the federation's president, Dr. Alan Guttmacher, wryly remarked, the diaphragm ought "be emblazoned on the coat of arms of the U.S. Birth Control Movement."[89]

The reasons why local clinics remained so preoccupied with this particular method are elusive, but we can speculate. Perhaps the original reasons for prescribing the diaphragm may have continued to appeal to the legion of women who worked in local clinics or served on their administrative boards. Indeed, although male doctors increasingly made their way inside the local clinic—in part perhaps because of birth control's increased respectability but also because of the declining numbers of women in the medical profession—women remained the cornerstone of the clinic institution by carrying out its many other functions.[90] In addition, despite pervasive pessimism about the poor's ability to use the diaphragm, many clinic workers still likely believed in their ability to teach the method and that all women could learn, a paternalist attitude still, but at least a more generous one.

Furthermore, there were still plenty of women happy to get the diaphragm at the local clinic and who often viewed birth control as something that women in particular needed to control. Although many women discontinued the diaphragm regimen, many others continued. It all depends on how you interpret the numbers. Even when as many as 46.1 percent quit, which was the case at the clinic that Robishaw studied, this still meant 53.9 percent continued, which in the grand scheme of things were not bad results.[91] Moreover, that women or their partners could choose to use other methods that they could get elsewhere might also explain why many patients did not mind the clinic's emphasis on the diaphragm. As Planned Parenthood's national medical director, Dr. Mary Steichen Calderone, speculated in 1961, perhaps those "preferring [other] methods don't bother to come to the Centers."[92] Finally, despite men's interest and active participation in the efforts to limit fertility, it was women who remained tied to their biology and who in turn wanted something they could control. "I'm tired of having children for these men folks," explained one African American woman. "Menfolks ain't got no feeling for women having children 'cause they don't know what it means."[93] Indeed, many women still resisted the male-controlled condom because, in the rare instances clinic patients were offered this method, it was often met with "great disappointment," as was explained in one federation-sponsored workshop about clinic procedures.[94]

In other words, the clinic's long-cultivated reputation—as a place where women went to get the female-controlled diaphragm—continued to precede it, despite Planned Parenthood's larger family planning message. A strikingly familiar photo layout of clinic services that appeared in a 1947 issue of *Look* magazine illustrates this well: "Mrs. Jane Doe" first meets with a female nurse who gives her "woman-to-woman" advice; she then sits in an "instruction room" with four other women, where the nurse explains what "child-spacing" is; finally, she sees the "woman doctor" who "equips and instructs her." And although such "child-spacing demonstration[s]" were available for husbands, not a single man appeared in any one of the photos. Furthermore, the thinly veiled reference to what the patient encountered when she met with the doctor probably meant a diaphragm fitting.[95] The clinic, therefore, was still not the place where a man who was interested in family planning would go.

Consequently, for all the emphasis that PPFA placed on how the husband and wife worked together to plan their families, the message remained that women ought be responsible for getting and using birth control. For example, for all the discussion of men in the literature, the organization continued to direct virtually all its materials toward women; and rather than telling husbands to talk to their wives, the line of communication generally went the other direction, from wife to husband.[96] Even those pamphlets told from the husband's perspective (like the comic book-styled "Escape From Fear") still made birth control a woman's job, as the following shift in pronouns suggests. After learning about birth control from his doctor, the fictional Ken excitedly heads home to tell his wife the good news. "Once and for all *we're* going to find out," and then adds, "*you're* going down to that Planned Parenthood center first thing tomorrow."[97] Furthermore, despite all the discussion about the need to provide a variety of contraceptive techniques, none rested upon the argument that men wanted to, or even should, get directly involved by being in charge of contraception, suggesting again how the early feminist influences remained in place.

In addition, the national office contributed to clinics' failure to move beyond the diaphragm in other ways. Despite PPFA's rhetoric about the need to provide a variety of contraceptives in the local clinic, the organization often failed to provide enough concrete advice about how to go about doing this. While clinic manuals described in great detail the many different methods available, when it came to actual clinic procedures, they all dropped entirely from view, that is except for the diaphragm. Consequently, when explaining what supplies clinics needed to have on hand, manuals only mentioned diaphragms and jellies, which patients were to use together. No sponges, condoms, nor douching outfits appeared on the lists. Moreover, when explaining how to discuss birth control with patients, the sample "Instruction Talk" was devoted entirely to the diaphragm.[98] Even when the federation held workshops run by staff members of Sanger's New York clinic (as was the case in 1940 at which representatives from thirty-eight affiliates attended), it is clear that despite the discussion of other methods, the diaphragm was still promoted above all.[99]

However, even had the national office provided good advice about how to expand their services, there is no reason to assume local affiliates would have followed its directives. The federation's demands and constant intrusions into clinic matters often rankled local affiliates. The newly instituted matter of annual dues to the national office was one example. So angry were some affiliates over this new requirement that they even quit the organization because of it.[100] But there were other conflicts as well, as the situation in Danville, Illinois, reveals. When in December of 1955 PPFA's field office representative visited the central Illinois affiliate to check up on its affairs, Miriam Garwood made some shocking discoveries. First, she learned that although the Danville group had withdrawn its affiliation, it continued to use the Planned Parenthood name. Second, the Danville office fell well short of PPFA's recommended standards regarding clinic work: there was little privacy in the clinic (which was located in the basement of the local YWCA); there was no nurse in attendance (just lay volunteers); and the doctor was only called in when a patient had arrived, a practice that was actually quite common in the smaller clinics. That the Danville affiliate lacked a medical advisory board and had no board of directors also meant it had completely disregarded the required organizational standards as well. Worse still, there seemed to be little interest in complying with any of these requirements. As a result, Garwood's findings provoked considerable concern, and a flurry of visits ensued to see how they could improve Danville's clinic services while at same time getting the local committee back into the Planned Parenthood fold.[101]

But complaints went both ways. PPFA's required board work, for example, was decidedly unappealing for many local organizers. As Mrs. L. T. Allen, chair of Danville's now defunct board of directors, explained, she was "unwilling to assume any initiative in the reorganization of a Planned Parenthood Board" and the "clinic is her only interest."[102] Likewise, Dr. Tanner, the Danville clinic's physician, was particularly hostile toward the national organization's intrusions. According to Garwood's report, he was upset that his name appeared without his permission in a letter announcing Planned Parenthood services to new mothers, which he claimed put him at odds "immediately and forever after" with the other male obstetricians and gynecologists in the area, who perhaps viewed such services not only as disreputable but also, and perhaps more important, as a threat to their own private practices. Dr. Tanner also saw little use for the national office. "It would take a tall lot of talking to convince me that the national organization is good for anything except the literature they put out," he reputedly told Garwood.[103]

Thus the level of hostility between the Danville office and the federation serves as a vivid reminder that not all affiliates were interested in working through their differences with the national office. As Tanner's complaints suggest, it was not always clear just how much PPFA did for local organizations, sentiments that were shared by other affiliates. As one PPFA report complained, "There seems to be some resistance against reporting to National." For this reason, the federation ought "help Leagues understand the value of keeping the National office informed."[104] The federation also often voiced sharp criticism about local clinic operations, which likely did little to engender allegiance to the national organization. For example, this same report complained that local committees were "too casual" and took too little "pride" in their work. The "fact that clinics are not better attended in many areas is due primarily to the fact they have still not achieved completely professional standards, and that they are neither widely known to the public or attractive and inviting to patients."[105] To local organizers, however, PPFA's constant stream of suggestions and criticisms about clinic operations could prove especially hollow. Because it functioned solely as an umbrella organization and therefore carried out no clinic work of its own, the federation's input had little substantive basis.

To make matters worse, while the federation avidly promoted its affiliated clinics and took an active interest in clinic affairs, the organization was actually trying to get out of clinic work. Consequently, for all its promotion of the family planning clinic and its desire to standardize clinic operations, the national office was increasingly pressuring local committees to focus on other matters: namely, getting contraceptive services integrated into hospitals and public health agencies (as part of what it called "The Big Push") or operating what PPFA called the "demonstration clinic," whose function was to show existing agencies the need for birth control services and how to offer them.[106] In contrast, those at the local level saw the establishment and operation of a clinic as their primary goal, a conflict of interests that thoroughly annoyed the national office. "Far too many leagues and committees," chastised one report, "still think of education as limited to the radius of an extra-mural clinic."[107] Such words could have hardly endeared the federation to local organizers.

Such conflicts aside, there were moments when local committees and the national organization worked together and even broadened the services clinics provided. One such example was the opening of an infertility facility through the Chicago affiliate. First established in May 1944, the clinic operated at the affiliate's downtown location. Both the local and national Planned Parenthood offices swelled with pride over this new facility, which, according to one account, was the first of its kind in the nation.[108] That the clinic achieved quick popularity, serving 120 couples in 1949 alone, reveals the demand for this kind of help.[109] Smaller affiliates, such as those in Champaign, Illinois, began to offer referrals for those who wished assistance on infertility matters as well. In addition, marriage and sex counseling services also on occasion made their way into local clinics. Probably the most intensive, and certainly the most famous, was the one offered through Sanger's Clinical Research Bureau in New York City, which Gordon described.[110] But affiliates in Illinois did the same, and by the end of the 1950s, Chicago as well as Champaign had instituted their own marriage education workshops.[111]

Nevertheless, infertility and marriage counseling programs remained either spotty or, more commonly, supplemental to the clinics' main goal of providing contraceptives. In other words, for all the places that offered such services, there were often just as many that did not. In Illinois, for example, although Chicago and Champaign had marriage and infertility services, Springfield and Danville did not.[112] Nationwide, the numbers reveal a similar pattern.[113] Furthermore, that such work consisted largely of referrals to outside agencies still meant that daily clinic activity was primarily to provide women with birth control. Basic clinic service, as was defined by PPFA's 1956 standards for certification, still included only two things: "Advice on conception control" and a "complete pelvic exam," both of which generally coincided with the diaphragm fitting.[114]

Finally, even the change in language from "birth control" to "family planning" was incomplete. Evidence of this can be seen in the letter referenced at the start of this section, in which the Champaign office insisted on using the term "birth control" rather than "family planning" on its educational pamphlets. An incident that took place in the late 1930s also hinted at the problems the organization would continue to encounter. When in 1939 members of the Minnesota Birth Control League entitled their state fair exhibit "Planned Parenthood" so as to assuage any potential conflicts, they quickly learned that the term "birth control" carried popular recognition and support. As one local member explained, although they offered many pamphlets, it was the *Birth Control Review* (the movement's newsletter) that garnered the most interest, though ironically it contained the least practical advice. "What the public wanted was 'birth control,'" she concluded, and therefore took anything that bore those words.[115] Instructions from a 1944 clinic manual about the use of telephone directories illustrates this point further. When advertising contraceptive services in the local directory, the manual advised that the clinic appear under the heading "birth control."[116] In other words, where people would look for it. That such advice came from the national office reveals how it too sometimes appreciated the popularity of the term Sanger coined, despite its more recent preference for the depoliticized term "family planning."

What all this suggests, therefore, is: Although PPFA was trying to change its image and its reputation, trying even to get out of what Sanger herself was increasingly calling a contraceptive clinic "rut," the institution born in the 1920s and 1930s persisted into the 1940s and 1950s essentially unchanged.[117]

Unwanted Babies Are Born

If little changed in daily clinic routines, then why bother examining the rhetoric of family planning? The answer lies in the dichotomy such language promoted: the creation of planned families and wanted children created in turn a darker side—unplanned families with all their unwanted children. And so, just as family and society would benefit from the planned family, everybody would suffer from that which was not planned. And just as the ability to plan one's family had become a sign of a strong marriage, good parenting, and happy family ties, the reverse also took root: those who failed to plan were nothing more than irresponsible parents who burdened society with yet another unhappy, unproductive, and dysfunctional citizen. In addition, although Planned Parenthood regularly argued that the poor could raise happy, healthy families, money remained at the heart of the matter. In the end, then, those from impoverished backgrounds—those who raised large families and had apparently too many "unwanted children"—regularly shouldered much of the blame for the problems in postwar America.

According to image and rhetoric, unplanned families were generally poor, and having a baby every year became synonymous with lack of education and poverty: in short, those unable to plan.[118] Pictures speak a thousand words. Stark images, which often appeared side-by-side in educational pamphlets and exhibits, contrasted the planned family with the unplanned one, revealing a striking dichotomy. On the planned side stood the happy mother and father in front of their nice home, surrounded by their handful of well-spaced, well-shod, and smilingly well-adjusted children. On the unplanned side there appeared the bedraggled parents (or parent) with their equally bedraggled, raggedly shod, unkempt, ill-spaced, and unsmiling children, all of whom stood inside or in front of broken-down shacks, decorated on occasion with newsprint wallpaper.[119] Matching African American versions regularly appeared as well. However, although Planned Parenthood's efforts to present the same message to diverse audiences indicates the organization's sensitivity to racial issues, that images of unplanned black families always moved to planned black ones, just as white went to white, underscores the racial as well as the economic divide that continued to separate many Americans.[120] Put another way, segregated pamphlets reflected segregated America, and when ordering posters, clinics were advised to "specify white or Negro families" in their request.[121]

Just as planned families were supposedly full of love and affection, unplanned ones were not. "Studies of delinquents," argued one pamphlet, "have shown that for many the need for love and security was unmet. They feel rejected by those very persons—*their parents*—whom they most wanted to be close to."[122] Such sentiments appeared in other places as well. As the title of the biography of Edna Bertha McKinnon, once head of the Chicago affiliate, later suggestively read, *Too Many People, Too Little Love.*[123] Unplanned families therefore—those who lacked not only material comfort but also love and affection—were the reasons why life in America had become so turbulent.

Unwanted children were particularly criticized. Indeed, Planned Parenthood's desire to help parents raise happy children meant more than ensuring a pleasant childhood, one that sons and daughters could fondly recall when reaching adulthood. Rather, it meant strengthening society by producing individuals who avoided such things as juvenile delinquency. For boys, this seedy path generally included petty criminal activity such as "car thefts, burglaries, and arson." For girls, "sexual delinquency." Hanging out at juke joints, which no doubt only encouraged such behavior among both groups, was something for which they were all chastised, as the following educational image depicted. A "policewoman check[s] up on" one such place and observes disapprovingly the scene she finds: boys smoking cigarettes and girls dancing to the music playing on the jukebox.[124] Even the word "delinquent" had become synonymous with unwanted. The "law calls them 'delinquents,'" explained an article in *Look* magazine, "but psychiatrists call many of them 'unwanted,' children rejected by their parents."[125]

These unwanted children could find themselves wandering down other dangerous paths as well, such as alcoholism and mental illness. "Two Doctors and the audience meet Benny," explained a 1945 proposal for a Planned Parenthood movie. Benny, everyone then learns, was an "unwanted child who had become an alcoholic." That Benny had a penchant for the bottle was by no means coincidental; his unhappy upbringing led him to drink. That he was also a "psychiatric case" further proved what lack of planning could do: poor unwanted Benny was a loser in every way, with little to be proud of personally and even less to offer society.[126] In fact, other educational materials went so far as to argue that types like Benny should never "have been born" at all.[127]

The parents of these unwanted children fared little better, and just as the planned family began with mom and dad, so too did the unplanned ones. As another PPFA pamphlet reminded its readers, delinquent children were raised by what it called "delinquent parents."[128] In addition, according to marriage counselor Walter R. Stokes, such moms and dads were lacking in virtually every way. They were emotionally immature and ill suited for marriage entirely. In the case of broken marriages at least one member of the couple (if not both) exhibited "markedly infantile characteristics."[129]

Parents of these unwanted, unloved babies also supposedly contributed to relief rolls, which burdened society not only with another dependent citizen but also a completely useless one. One Planned Parenthood fundraising flier illustrates this vividly. "A New Baby is Born!," its title gleefully announced and then went on to speculate as to the baby's destiny: "A Future President; A Second Thomas A. Edison; Another Florence Nightingale; The Home Run King of 1970; author of the Great American Novel; or—A Public Charge?" A similar yet more threatening version put out by the Chicago office began more ominously: "Every 10 Seconds a Baby is Born in America."[130] In addition, the following headline—"Unwanted Babies Taxing County Hospital Space"—deliberately cut across the discussion of clinic activities in a 1954 Chicago affiliate newsletter, driving home further the link between unwanted babies and welfare relief.[131] Hardly isolated examples, such cautions appeared regularly and suggest how children born to the poor were a detriment to society, not just because they were a financial burden to taxpayers but for other reasons as well. Indeed, by pitting income against intelligence and talent, as the "A New Baby is Born!" flier did, such messages conveyed even less flattering assumptions about what those of less comfortable means had to offer society. Those who were public charges would never become presidents, inventors, nurses, baseball players, or writers.

Discussions about infertility programs further show the ways in which class and intelligence underpinned the family planning ideal. Dr. Mary S. Calderone and Margaret Sanger, for example, engaged in vigorous debate over whether the poor ought be allowed access to such services. While Calderone argued on behalf of those of modest means, Sanger argued against, noting how the women she interviewed were "uncouth and untidy" and held "anything but ideal" attitudes about parenthood.[132] Calderone and Sanger were not alone in their divisiveness. For example, Dr. John Rock (who would later help develop and promote the pill) regularly provided infertility treatment to the poor in his clinics.[133] Many others, however, likely sided with Sanger. As one clinic manual explained in its brief mention of infertility services, the "center should encourage child bearing among those who are suitable parents."[134] Likewise, the popular press regularly reminded educated women to bear many children. Such was the case with a 1946 issue of *Ladies' Home Journal.* Complaining about high fertility rates among the poor and low ones for "college-educated parents," the women's magazine then chided educated women for squandering "their genetic inheritance."[135]

Nevertheless, although many of the claims about family planning were embedded in money, Planned Parenthood also regularly tried to argue that the planned family need not be rich. Happy, loving marriages did not require lots of money and even those of comfortable means could find themselves in divorce courts, as the theatrical melodrama "Sunday Afternoon" depicted. Even in "homes where there is enough money to take care of a well-planned family," Helen explains to Terry and Jim, "people are so apt to turn to divorce."[136] Nor did good parenting, thus well-adjusted children, necessarily hinge upon income. "These same roots of delinquency can begin their twisted growth in any home, rich or poor," announced another flier.[137] Yet that Planned Parenthood, both at the local and national level, regularly pitched its message to organizations that worked with impoverished communities attests to its belief that such behaviors were problems especially among the poor.[138] Or, as I argued in the first chapter, the more it's pitched that way, the more it becomes that way.

Of course, not all of the images were quite so grim. The rhetoric of wanted versus unwanted children occasionally took on humorously unrealistic proportions. The angelic qualities of planned babies are comical, as one account of a planned baby party sponsored by the Chicago Planned Parenthood suggests. "Contrary to expectations, not a baby cried during the afternoon," the local affiliate's June 1950 newsletter gushed. "They were Planned Parenthood babies, you see, and perfectly content and happy."[139] Similar claims appeared in another issue. Quiet little angels, the "infant guests of honor" were neither seen nor heard, a March 1948 Chicago newsletter announced, and boasted how it "takes planned babies to do that."[140] Given that such events were only for planned babies, one might wonder if mothers had to leave any of their unplanned babies behind. Similarly, the string of "Ma and Pa Kettle" movies, a series of Hollywood comedies that poked fun at the exploits of the very large and obviously unplanned Kettle family, suggests a humorous take on the family planning theme, even if some viewers may have been put off by the premise.[141]

Likewise, not everyone was impressed with the rhetoric of family planning. Catholics, for example, were quick to pick up on the negative implications embedded in Planned Parenthood's message. "How limited in vision, for instance, is their favorite slogan: 'every child a *wanted* child,'" criticized Frances Jameson in a 1942 issue of *Reader's Digest.* "Many a child not planned or even particularly desired has later become his parents' greatest happiness and in many instances an ornament to society."[142] Certainly, much of the Catholic Church's opposition to birth control hinged upon fears of sexual immorality and antagonism toward female autonomy, as Linda Gordon argued.[143] But Catholic accusations of Planned Parenthood's middle-class elitism need to be taken seriously. Just as some historians of labor and religion have in recent years argued that labor activists often drew as much from religious moralism as they did from class concerns, the same ought be said (though in reverse) about Catholic opposition to family planning rhetoric and initiatives.[144] The poor, in other words, had just as much a right to large families as anybody else.

In the end, then, the ideal of the planned family was a double-edged sword. By promoting a mission that helped mothers and fathers plan their marriage and their family, Planned Parenthood hoped to help Americans achieve a new household ideal, an ideal that was as good for the individuals in the home as it was for the wider community. Moreover, although such messages only partially materialized in clinic practice, that Planned Parenthood promoted its clinics as the place where the poor especially could learn about family planning suggests the organization's belief that everyone, regardless of background, should have such opportunities. Nevertheless, by rhetorically chastising those of modest incomes who continued to raise large families, the planned family ideal simultaneously held them accountable for all that was wrong in America. And as the following chapter reveals, by the 1960s the notion of the unplanned family would take on a new and racialized reality, thereby helping to facilitate the movement's second wave of clinic growth, dismantle its rigid definition of birth control, and contribute to the dramatic transformation of the rationale of charity that lay behind clinic work.

Chapter Four

New Habits Are Formed

When turning to what might be described as the revolution of birth control in the 1960s and early 1970s, retrospect affords me a feeling that what took place during these years had somehow already taken place once before. Indeed, many of the events in these years bear eerie resemblance to those of the 1930s. Much like the 1930s, for example, there was an explosion of growth in the contraceptive manufacturing industry. Much like the 1930s, there were new laws and initiatives that reflected a growing endorsement of birth control on behalf of the state. Much like the 1930s, there was a dramatic expansion of the birth control clinic movement, both by those interested in associating with Planned Parenthood and those beyond its doors.

For all the similarities to be noticed, however, there are at least two important distinctions (beyond of course the revolution of the pill) that shatter this warm familiarity. First, while in the 1930s it was alliances with doctors and eugenicists that gave the charity clinic movement the legitimacy it needed, by the 1960s it was alliances with the pharmaceutical manufacturing industry that would be an important strategy, ensuring its financial stability and scientific legitimacy. Second, while in the 1930s the movement worked to establish its authority by narrowly restricting the definition of birth control and the birth control clinic, by the 1960s and early 1970s it blew these definitions wide open again: it threw out its opposition to openness about various birth control techniques, it threw out its opposition to service to the unwed, it even threw out its opposition to abortion. And what is especially striking about the whole process is this: while Planned Parenthood was in part adopting the marketplace's penchant for loudness, directness, and the consumer choice message, it was continuing to employ its mission of charity to bolster its claims to authority. The only difference now was that the organization was using charity to argue precisely for what it once used charity to argue against.

Indeed, during the 1930s, the birth control movement argued that successful charity birth control work meant asserting the authority of doctors, the sanctity of marriage, the power of the diaphragm, and an end to abortion; it also meant maintaining an aura of quiet respectability. By the 1960s, Planned Parenthood used charity to make radically new claims. Successful charity birth control work now required the promotion of a wide variety of contraceptive techniques (including those from commercial sources), the abandonment of the singular emphasis on the authority of physicians, the open discussion of the specifics of birth control (including among minors), and even the provision of abortion. Only then, Planned Parenthood argued, could the poor truly be helped; and only then could society be saved from the tragedy, harm, and burden of unwanted children.

With the Planned Parenthood affiliate in Champaign, Illinois, serving as my starting point, this final chapter begins with an analysis of Planned Parenthood's relationship to the pharmaceutical manufacturing industry more generally. I focus initially on the impact of the pill, the power of the market, and the demand of consumers, and then proceed to a more in-depth investigation of an important cornerstone of this new relationship: the use of Planned Parenthood clinics to engage in biomedical research. My analysis then makes its way up to the Chicago area Planned Parenthood affiliate. Here we find the influx of blacks in the Chicago family planning movement and the undercurrent of domestic-style colonialism underpinning the organization's aggressive new birth control initiatives. Here we also see how Planned Parenthood's definition of birth control was expanding in dramatic new ways—though charity remained at the heart of its legitimating core activities. The chapter then turns to the subsequent emergence of two important flash points: first, from blacks who questioned the proliferation of clinics within their communities; and second, from within Planned Parenthood itself as battles began to rage internally about the use of clinics to engage in scientific research, a situation that came to a dramatic head at a Planned Parenthood affiliate in San Antonio, Texas. The chapter then closes with two short sections that wrap up a few loose ends about the implications of service to the unwed, the provision of abortion, and the presence of research in the local clinic, ultimately hinting at future battles with which Planned Parenthood would have to develop new mechanisms to cope.

Birth of a New Method but Especially a New Benefactor

In 1980, the Planned Parenthood office in Champaign County, Illinois, decided to commemorate its fortieth anniversary by holding a luncheon celebration. Member Dorothy Baker concluded that a presentation on the history of the affiliate would be a good way to mark the occasion. The talk she put together was illuminating. Baker had a remarkable ability to capture the scope and complexity of the various reasons behind the birth control revolution and second clinic wave. As she explained to her audience, "The year 1960 marked the beginning of a revolution in family planning [whose] reverberations were felt in dramatic changes in the scope and direction" of the Champaign affiliate. "The appearance of the contraceptive pill; the first rumblings of alarm about a global population explosion; radical changes in society's views on traditional moral issues; the beginnings of federal funding of birth control services; the advent of the so-called 'youth culture'—all contributed," she perceptively concluded, "to the growth of Planned Parenthood beyond the wildest dreams of its founders."[1] More than a few historians (myself included) would be inclined to agree.[2]

But it was the two stories she recounted that revealed even more. The first had to do with the introduction of the pill. It seems that when discussion of making this method available inside the Champaign clinic first arose in 1960, just when the pill itself had been introduced on the market, the affiliate's medical advisory board was much opposed, citing such things as "high cost, the need for medical supervision, and the necessity for daily use." A year later, however, it relented, though not without tacking on a few new restrictions of its own: not only did the patient have to bring "a prescription from her private physician," but also "there would be no publicity" announcing the availability of the pill inside the Champaign clinic. Consequently, when the first "pill patient" was accepted in May 1961, Ruth Dobbins (president/volunteer) purchased only a "small notebook to record" just how many requests for the pill there would be. She expected only a "few." "How wrong she was," Baker told the audience and provided the following numbers (drawn probably from Dobbins's notebook):

Nov. 1961	34 patients
Nov. 1962	183 patients
Nov. 1963	225 patients
Nov. 1964	309 patients

It was a dramatic jump indeed.[3]

In this first story we can see a great deal. We can see the power the local medical advisory board (which often meant the local medical society) could wield in the functioning of local Planned Parenthood affiliates. Although it was a power that clinic workers and patients constantly negotiated, the advisory board could, if it wanted, effectively hamstring clinic operations. In fact, although the Champaign affiliate was able to get the county medical society's support when it first began operations in 1940—a support that was necessary if it was to organize the required advisory board—it still chafed over the years against the restrictions the county medical society saw fit to impose. For example, even though the national Planned Parenthood office had in 1948 relaxed its recommendation that clinics serve only the indigent poor, Champaign's medical advisory board held fast to this rule, illuminating not only the persistent fear among physicians that clinics might serve as competition in the medical marketplace but also another moment of malleability within Planned Parenthood's organizational model.[4] For here was a difference in policy the national organization allowed. A scenario at an affiliate in Indiana reveals yet another burden the mandated medical advisory board could pose. When its entire board quit en masse as a result of coercion by the local Catholic hospital, the affiliate was thereby noncompliant with federation rules, resulting in a period of probation for the much-beleaguered office.[5] Thus the required medical advisory board required a lot of work to organize and maintain, and the rules that came with it were often tricky and idiosyncratic.

Yet Baker's story also reveals the power of women to consume and the power of the market to sell, regardless what some in the medical community had to say. Despite the Champaign medical advisory board's insistence that there be no publicity about the pill's availability in the local clinic, women came in by droves and asked for it by name, even if "that baby aspirin" was the phrase some migrant workers used.[6] In short, the pill was big news, and although technically the specifics about contraceptive products were only to be discussed in medical print, detailed articles about oral contraceptives appeared regularly in the popular press—in *Newsweek, Mademoiselle, Esquire, Ebony, Reader's Digest, Good Housekeeping,* and *Business Week,* to name just a few magazines—prompting women (and sometimes men) to act, and to act quickly, on the news they received.[7]

Letters reprinted in Elizabeth Siegel Watkins's social history of the pill illustrate this point well. "When I read this article," wrote one woman in reference to an early piece on the development of the pill in a 1957 issue of *Science Digest,* "I couldn[']t help but cry, for I thought there is my ray of hope." Or as another said, "Like thousands of others my wife and I bought a recent issue of *Coronet* because of the blurb on the cover concerning birth control pills."[8] Certainly, media coverage of the pill was not always glowing, particularly once questions about its safety arose in the mid-1960s, but it was consistently good enough to prompt consumers to believe that this was the answer they were looking for.

For pill manufacturers, the massive media attention was no doubt the answer they were looking for as well. With the help of widespread coverage in the popular press, combined with manufacturers' continued use of ethical channels to disseminate information—reaching physicians directly through thousands of detail representatives, direct-mail advertisements, and advertisements in medical journals—the pill had become quickly and wildly popular. As Watkins noted, within five years of its introduction on the market, "six and a half million married women" had gotten a prescription, with probably "hundreds of thousands of unmarried women" getting one as well.[9] Significantly, the pill's popularity was also felt inside local Planned Parenthood clinics. Within two years the pill was well on its way to becoming the organization's most prescribed birth control method, leaving the almighty diaphragm, which had for four decades dominated clinic work, to become for many a distant memory of an old-fashioned era.[10]

The advent of such methods as the pill also ushered in a new business arrangement between Planned Parenthood and pharmaceutical houses, one that centered on the purchase of clinic supplies. In the past, because of the illegality, taboo, and cost of contraceptives, clinic organizers often devised creative ways to get the goods they needed. In the 1920s, for example, Sanger smuggled hers in from Germany in containers from her husband's Three-in-One Oil Company.[11] During the 1930s and 1940s, activists in Cleveland used another route. As Jimmy Elaine Wilkinson Meyer explained, fearful that the wholesale goods they had purchased from their New York supplier would get confiscated during shipment, Cleveland activists accompanied "their husbands on business trips to New York City," carrying with them empty suitcases, which were then filled with diaphragms and tubes of contraceptive jelly and transported back home on passenger trains.[12] Clinic workers in Champaign, Illinois, got their supplies through a doctor's wife, who used her husband's discount card when purchasing them at the local drugstore.[13]

Thus when the national Planned Parenthood office began in the mid-1960s to hammer out wholesale purchase arrangements with pharmaceutical companies—like the Pill Purchase Plan—it was a big deal for local affiliates. Not only were supplies easier to get, but they also came at discounted rates.[14] As one Illinois Planned Parenthood worker remarked, "this was a great move on [the national office's] part."[15] Not everyone was happy with these new arrangements, though. An incident in West Lafayette, Indiana, reveals that some local druggists viewed the wholesale prices Planned Parenthood clinics received as unfair competition, adding another new twist to the story about business, medicine, and birth control.[16] While in previous decades doctors complained about the competition posed by clinics, by the 1960s it was druggists who felt the squeeze in the contraceptive marketplace.

However, for all the significance of this new birth control method, and for all the din and subsequent demand generated by its corresponding publicity, it was Baker's second story that drove home the significance of the new relationship between clinics and pharmaceutical manufacturing companies. As Baker spoke of the massive increase in patients receiving the pill, she noted how "a good part of [the increase] was due" to the Champaign affiliate's participation in a clinical research project sponsored by the pharmaceutical manufacturing giant Eli Lilly.[17] Eli Lilly, in other words, was looking to jump in on this latest birth control boom by testing its own version of the pill; and Eli Lilly, like pharmaceutical companies across the nation, was as a result on its way to becoming a central part of clinic operations.

Indeed, Champaign's "Lilly Project" was hardly unique. According to one PPFA report put out sometime in the mid-1960s, of its approximately ninety-five affiliates, thirty-seven were carrying out projects in conjunction with seven different pharmaceutical companies: Ortho Pharmaceutical, G. D. Searle, Eli Lilly, Parke-Davis, Mead Johnson, Upjohn, and Breon Laboratories. Research at an individual affiliate, moreover, was not always confined to a single project with a single company. To the contrary, only eleven said they were participating in one study while the rest reported more than that; the Detroit Planned Parenthood topped the list with fifteen different projects sponsored by six different companies. Other institutions pursued cooperative research endeavors with clinics as well. Studies done in conjunction with the Population Council, the FDA, as well as state agencies made their way into local clinics, though even these often had pharmaceutical company support.[18] These numbers were, however, only the tip of the iceberg; many affiliates failed to keep the national office apprised of their local activities, much to the frustration of the federation, which tried to regulate the work of the local clinics.[19]

Given the magnitude of this new arrangement, it is surprising just how little about it has been written. Of the three affiliate histories that took their local Planned Parenthood stories to the present, only two mentioned the new collaboration between clinics and manufacturers specifically, and these only in passing.[20] Notably, Marcia Meldrum offered a more sustained account.[21] But because she was more concerned with several projects sponsored at the national level and the scientific legitimacy they generated for the Planned Parenthood organization, she overlooked the larger phenomenon now taking place. But in light of what my book has laid out, it is clear that a dramatic new relationship was now emerging between Planned Parenthood and the pharmaceutical manufacturing industry, bringing with it some obvious new benefits plus a few surprising ones too: in sum, hampered by the limits of charity, hampered by restrictive medical societies, and hampered by internal policies and governmental laws, the organization at all its levels saw in pharmaceutical companies an amazing source of power, not only to overcome some of the charity birth control movement's toughest obstacles but also even occasionally some of its oldest rules.

None of this would have happened were it not for at least three important developments. First, after a long history of contentious relations, by the 1950s the medical community and the pharmaceutical industry had become great friends. The golden age of the pharmaceutical company was at hand, and manufacturers were able to project an image of themselves as the purveyors of science and the embodiment of benevolence, an image not too unlike the one carefully crafted by the regular medical profession in previous decades.[22] However, because manufacturers of contraceptives still remained on the ragged edges of respectability, the rise of the pill as well as renewed interest in such methods as the IUD made the manufacture of contraceptives scientific and therefore respectable. This new image constituted in turn the second necessary development; now even the major manufacturing houses were rushing to get their versions of contraceptives on the market. For Planned Parenthood, these were crucial developments because to cultivate direct ties with the

contraceptive manufacturing industry no longer carried the risk of alienating the medical profession, as it did back in the 1930s.

Yet were it not for the rise during World War II of large-scale clinical
investigation programs and the ascendance of quantitative statistical analysis, which in turn required large pools of data, pharmaceutical companies might still have remained only marginally interested in clinic work.[23]
Therein lies the significance of these developments in collaboration because
for anybody interested in engaging in contraceptive research, as the pharmaceutical industry now most certainly was, where better to find such a wealth
of clinical material than the Planned Parenthood Federation of America.
It was an opportunity not lost on those in the birth control organization.
"These centers," wrote PPFA's national medical director Mary Calderone to
a pharmaceutical house in June of 1959 in solicitation of a major research
project, "have a total of 10,000 new patients yearly," numbers that would
surely whet the appetite of anyone interested in conducting large-scale clinical research.[24]

Given their dramatic new presence within clinic operations, it is worth
describing the nature of some of these projects and who was behind them.
Some of the larger studies were initiated for the most part by the federation and worked in this way. As Meldrum explained, the primary objective
of the Clinical Investigation Program (CIP)—a project that lasted from
1959 to 1962—was to study the effectiveness and acceptability of the dia-
phragm/spermicide regimen versus the spermicide regimen alone, a project that reflected the organization's long-standing efforts to resolve women's
dissatisfaction with the method they usually got in the clinic. The man in
charge of the operation was Dr. Christopher Tietze, who then developed a
series of questionnaires to determine for each study participant the following: her sociology and demographics, her contraceptive history and moti-
vational response, and finally, her contraceptive practices for the duration
of the study. Clinic workers then administered the questionnaires. For the
patient, this meant she was to be no older than thirty-seven; she was to be
married and living with her husband, partner, or fiancé; and she was also
to be given a choice in which method of contraception she wanted to use.
Once enrolled, she was then monitored more closely through home visits,
which was also how she received additional supplies, and she was occasionally asked to return to the clinic for additional examinations. The collected
information was then sent back to Tietze, who analyzed the data and determined the results. All told, in this study 2,782 women participated from
seven different Planned Parenthood affiliates.[25]

Even more massive was the study that would begin a few years later: the
25-Month Club. With the backing of the FDA and the support of Searle,
Inc., this project lasted four years (from 1962 to 1966), and its purpose was
to learn more about the long-term effects of the pill by observing women

who had been using for two years the first oral contraceptive put on the market, Searle's Enovid.[26] It was conducted as follows. Once a clinic patient had reached her two-year anniversary and was entering into her twenty-fifth month of pill use, local affiliates were to approach the woman and solicit her participation in the project. If she consented, they would then monitor her closely. For the patient, this meant she was to return to the clinic every six months for a history and an examination; the occasional few would undergo even more specific procedures, such as blood, urine, and thyroid tests. What the woman received in return is not entirely clear. But what the affiliates got was both money to cover the costs of the study and discounts on Enovid supplies, which they were then expected to pass on to study participants. In this case, the 25-Month Club involved thirty-eight Planned Parenthood affiliates, including over eleven thousand of their clinic patients.[27]

Then there were all the research deals hammered out at the local level, often at the impetus of manufacturers themselves. Representatives from Holland-Rantos, for example, approached a Detroit clinic about testing its contraceptive jelly, Koromex-A.[28] Representatives from Ortho Pharmaceutical approached clinics in Virginia to participate in studies on its version of the pill (Ortho-Novum) and other contraceptive crèmes and foams. Representatives from Eli Lilly, of course, approached the clinic in Champaign, Illinois, about testing its oral contraceptive, a product marketed as C-Quens. And so on and so on.[29] The offers were, in other words, coming in fast and furious, so much so that the federation began in 1957 to insist that all affiliates register their projects with the national medical committee. Then in 1963 it insisted that all affiliates consult with its national medical committee before embarking on any new study.[30] But these would be rules difficult to enforce.[31]

This is not to say that there weren't reservations about this shift to using charity clinic patients as research subjects. Although the occasional study had in previous decades appeared, the prospect of research inside the clinic was often eyed with some suspicion, both at the local level as well as the national. As the national office's 1938 standards for procedure reminded its clinics, while "clinical research in improved techniques is of vital importance," patients were still to get the "most reliable information available" and "not be used for experimental purposes.[32] Local affiliates often shared such views. Dr. Shirley Collins of Ortho Pharmaceutical noted that not only were local clinics "still diaphragm-minded," but they were also "hesitant to prescribe simpler methods," which, as Collins concluded, they considered "experimental."[33] There were also those who wondered what these new activities meant for the clinic institution itself. As the executive director of the St. Louis office firmly stated in 1959, we "are not primarily a research center." Service, her words suggested, was the clinic's main function.[34] Still others voiced more concerns. For example, although she would eventually become one of the biggest proponents of research, in the mid-1950s Calderone herself offered a number of reasons why research could not (or should not) take place in the local clinic, arguing in part that "patients simply will not take a chance" but also that "we are not legally able to use them experimentally."[35]

But the incentives that came with research were simply far too enticing to pass up. In part the desire for scientific legitimacy was a major draw. As Meldrum explained about the Clinical Investigation Program, although Planned Parenthood had secured the backing of the AMA and the World Health Organization, it still remained on the fringes of scientific respectability. Thus the establishment of CIP, she noted, was not simply to test the diaphragm against other methods but also to serve another function: "the scientific legitimation of Planned Parenthood itself."[36] Such motivations could also be found at the local level, though in slightly different ways. At a clinic in San Antonio, Texas, because the study was sponsored by a prestigious physician who apparently held considerable clout among local doctors, the affiliate's medical committee eagerly participated in the projects he promoted.[37] Sentiments such as these were expressed proudly by the Chicago office in *Planned Parenthood News* of May 1959: to be "designated as one of PPFA's official clinical testing center[s] is a great honor . . . and shows how highly considered is the calibre of our centers."[38] For many affiliates, then, the chance to participate in projects sponsored by the federation was a validation of their efforts and a feather in their cap.

However, perhaps the most important incentive was a practical one: the injection of much-needed money and supplies. For local affiliates, many of whom had long struggled to make ends meet, the chance to fill meager coffers with precious funds and bare medicine cabinets with the latest in contraceptive supplies must surely have seemed like manna from heaven. The peace of mind such arrangements could afford is evident in the field report submitted about the much-beleaguered Indiana affiliate whose difficulties I described earlier in this chapter. After recounting the litany of problems it was slowly trying to resolve—the poor relations with the medical community, the en masse resignation of its entire medical advisory board because of pressure from the local Catholic hospital, and the punishment of probation imposed by the federation because of these difficulties as well as its failure to pay federation dues—one can almost hear the relief when there is at least one piece of good news to report: "A research grant from Mead-Johnson is in process and this will help the financial stability."[39]

Such support was significant. While there was money to be had from charitable organizations and now also money from the federal government, this funding was not always easy to get, and it often came with strings attached. As Maria H. Anderson explained in her history of the Houston affiliate, the money available through the Office of Economic Opportunity (in 1964) and Medicaid (in 1965) was a "double-edged sword" because, in order to get it, the affiliate was expected to expand its services, which was difficult given that it was already struggling to provide the services it did. As a result, "Planned Parenthood found itself simultaneously in the hard-won position of 'universal acceptance' at the federal level and increased involvement with government agencies, and the unwanted position of subjugation to the very agencies offering funding."[40] Federal money also brought with it other hassles, as the advice offered in 1972 by one of Planned Parenthood's regional directors to the affiliate in Decatur, Illinois, suggests. As Terrence P. Tiffany explained to Betty Forbes (Decatur's executive director):

> Current Federal project grants do not allow for such important Planned Parenthood activities as population education, abortion counseling and referral and sex education. Unless you can demonstrate that your participation in such activities are totally outside of the grant program, you could conceivably find yourself in hot water with the Federal government.[41]

Consequently, even if the money was awarded, the logistical headache and bureaucratic nightmare had only just begun.

In contrast, pharmaceutical companies held their purse strings far more loosely, and unlike other sources of funding, they could also offer real supplies. These were no small matters. As the director of an Iowa affiliate remarked, pharmaceutical company support had ensured the clinic's survival and enabled patients to receive the best available contraceptives from what he described as "an excellent staff of nurses, doctors and other needed personnel."[42] With research, in other words, came the opportunity not only to improve services for the clinic patients but also to keep the clinic going in the first place, motivations that could draw in even those who remained committed to the organization's old-fashioned mission of making contraceptives available to those too poor to afford them.

Notably, with research also came a few unexpected opportunities, not the least of which was the chance to get out from under the thumb of conservative local medical societies and even circumvent one of Planned Parenthood's oldest rules. Again, Baker's fortieth anniversary talk is instructive. As she explained the significance of Champaign's participation in the Lilly Project, she noted that it had another "far reaching effect." In Eli Lilly's desire to have unbiased samples, the company insisted that the clinic accept all women who wanted to participate in its project, regardless of marital status. For the first time, the Champaign clinic was able openly to serve unmarried women, an opportunity upon which it quickly seized; it would extend this policy by the mid-1960s to all women who attended the local clinic, as a result of other developments that I shall soon discuss.[43] Thus it was a curiously subversive challenge, not just to the rules of Planned Parenthood but also to the nation's laws.[44]

Ironically enough, therefore, the commercial world was in fact helping to legitimate sex among the unwed. It's just that in this case it was happening in ways far different from what the 1930s charity movement had imagined: when the clinic movement's quest for status, autonomy, and resources collided with the pharmaceutical industry's desire to participate in this latest birth control boom by engaging in the most scientific research methods of the day, a loophole in the rules about service to the unwed had been found. And for those who wanted such rules to be changed, it was an unexpected benefit indeed.

But the rise of research was not the only way the presence of business was felt inside the local clinic. Nor was the subversive challenge to the necessity of marriage the only way to get around this long-standing rule about not providing birth control to the unwed. As the next section reveals, there were more.

Another Clinic Boom, but with a Whole New Birth Control Way

Meanwhile, just as this new relationship with pharmaceutical companies was picking up steam, the clinic movement itself was surging ahead with new strength and new vigor. One look at the many letters Planned Parenthood was receiving from individuals looking to establish clinics in their own communities makes this plain.[45] Another look at the number of new affiliates that opened during this period makes this even more apparent. According to one report from the late 1960s, while only 6 new affiliates were established during the 1940s and 1950s, the period from 1960 to 1967 saw the rise of 60, bringing the total for the Planned Parenthood organization to approximately 153 offices across the nation, many of which operated at least 1 clinic if not more.[46] Thus, Sanger's dream of old—that there would one day be a "glorious 'chain' of clinics"—had by the 1960s become a vast reality.[47]

But it was a reality with a radically different vision. Gone for the most part was the charity movement's sweeping hostility toward over-the-counter methods; largely gone too were the charges of greed-driven profiteering and the exploitation of unwitting consumers, particularly the young and unwed. Nor, for that matter, did such methods as the pill or the IUD occupy the same hallowed ground as the diaphragm once did in the organization's rhetoric of old. Part of this shift, of course, was a product of the birth control manufacturing industry's newfound prestige, which enabled Planned Parenthood to cultivate an alliance with pharmaceutical companies without alienating the medical profession. But a larger cultural shift was at work here as well. As historian Lizabeth Cohen noted, America had become a "consumers' republic." Consequently, to pit oneself against the marketplace was no longer the useful tool it once was, because the Progressive-era hostility toward consumerism—still lingering in the 1930s—had by the 1940s and 1950s given way to a new set of values. As Cohen described them, these included "an economy, culture, and politics built around the promises of mass consumption, both in terms of material life and the more idealistic goals of greater freedom, democracy, and equality."[48] Consumption, in other words, not only enriched people's lives through commercial goods, but also promised to make possible the nation's larger social and political values. And like everybody else, Planned Parenthood was stepping right in line, eagerly embracing this new liberatory philosophy.

Nevertheless, the rhetoric and mission of charity remained central to Planned Parenthood's rationalization process. Although the organization now had close ties with birth control manufacturers and was adopting the language of the marketplace, the organization still used charity to justify its authority and its expanded new vision of birth control services. First, because its mission was to reach the uneducated poor, it was imperative that its charity services be openly discussed, easily understood, and available directly to consumers. Second, because charity eased the burden of what the organization now called the nation's unwanted children, it was also imperative to reach in particular the poor, *unwed* women in the nation's urban slums—presumably these were the women to whom unwanted children were born. Third, because it was the organization's moral duty as a charity to make available to the poor all the methods of birth control they might be denied (an argument it once applied exclusively to the diaphragm), this mission now included the provision of a variety of contraceptives, and even abortion. Thus the shift—from the organization's narrow definition of birth control in the 1930s to something far more expansive by the 1960s and 1970s—was a dramatic one; it was also one the organization expected others who engaged in the provision of birth control to follow. Here again, Chicago offers a useful place to begin.

After years of hostility, by the 1960s the Chicago affiliate had become the apple of the federation's eye; this sentiment found full expression in the field reports submitted to the national office. "Chicago is truly leading the country," enthused Jean Trisko in her 1962 report, and was apparently so "impressed" that she even "made out a pledge card" herself.[49] That same year Miriam Garwood wrote with enthusiasm in her report that the "excitement of the fast, onward moving program in Chicago has brushed off even on the office boy."[50] Also impressed were other local affiliates who regularly turned to the midwestern office in search of advice.[51] Given the federation's long history of conflict with this local affiliate, these were significant words of praise. What was the cause for all this excitement?

Part of it had to do with the growth of the local office. Not only were its demographics changing dramatically (as will become clear in the section to follow), but also by the mid-1960s it had become the largest affiliate in the entire Planned Parenthood organization. With over twenty thousand patients annually attending its more than twenty different clinic locations, the Chicago affiliate had within a few short years tripled its number of centers and quadrupled its caseload, an increase that Jane C. Browne, the affiliate's executive director, proudly announced at its local annual Planned Parenthood meeting.[52] The affiliate's physical size, moreover, was matched only by its financial resources. With an annual budget of more than six hundred thousand dollars, the Chicago office boasted the largest income in the Planned Parenthood organization, one that was even larger than that of the Sanger Bureau, which came in second.[53]

Yet the enthusiasm about the Chicago affiliate also had to do with the fact that birth control services more generally were being reconfigured in important new ways. Indeed, despite the massive growth of the number of clinics and the renewed faith of the federation in the utility of the local clinic, there was a simultaneous effort to move beyond the "clinic idea," beyond, in other words, the very bedrock upon which the institution was founded: the direct delivery of contraceptives under the supervision of a physician. In Chicago, much of this was coming from the affiliate's participation in a University of Chicago-sponsored study called the Bogue Project, whose purpose was to investigate and implement ways to make contraceptive services more widely available to impoverished communities. Or, as its official title read: "The Chicago West Side Experiment to Accelerate the Adoption of Birth Control by a Mass Communication Campaign."[54]

The Bogue Project involved a variety of initiatives. Among its most successful was the "Coffee Sip" program. Women held small gatherings in their homes for neighbors and friends to discuss birth control. They also explained the mechanics of reproduction using plastic anatomical models.[55] Another Bogue Project activity involved mass-mailed invitations—done through the local settlement house—to the poor women of the neighborhood encouraging them to attend the newly established clinics. Also mailed out was a short two-page birth control pamphlet (which mentioned various contraceptive techniques) as well as a "get-acquainted" discount coupon that promised one dollar off the purchase of clinic supplies. Still another program was the rise of the affiliate's mobile-unit service—which temporarily brought all the makings of a clinic to locations where none existed—a program for which the Bogue Project provided start-up funds.[56]

Each of these programs is remarkably telling. For example, although the goal of the "Coffee Sip" hostess was ultimately to encourage clinic attendance, that the lay housewife (rather than a physician, or at least a nurse) might serve as an authority on such matters marked a dramatic shift from the organization's message of old, which touted the expertise and the moral authority of physicians. Moreover, that mobile units were frequently manned by nurses (as was the case in Reading, Pennsylvania, and Trenton, New Jersey, in migrant worker campaigns) or a minister (who distributed supplies to his congregation in Kentucky) suggests further this shift away from the authority of the doctor.[57]

Indeed, getting lay people in particular involved had become an important strategy not just in Chicago but also throughout the country. A memo written by Elsie Jackson in 1965 to Fred Jaffe of Planned Parenthood–World Population about a position tellingly referred to as the "Indigenous Neighborhood Worker" illustrates this well. Our understanding of this person's role, Jackson wrote, is as follows:

> [The Indigenous Neighborhood Worker is] one who is indigenous to the community by virtue of his knowledge and roots therein, who has no training, background or experience in a professional capacity and who is of comparable economic and social standing as the potential patient group with which he will work. Workers of this nature could probably sweep across the whole range of American life. . . . When all other communication has failed—Person to Person is still left as a strong information and education tool. Neighborhood cooperation and group action are old American methods of getting a job done. Community people serve the purpose of getting a job done by themselves for themselves.[58]

Her words are striking. While the language of good old-fashioned American gumption and know-how rings throughout her description, the necessity of experts does not. Hence it is significant for two more reasons. The first is that it runs completely counter to the messages put forward by the charity clinic movement of the 1920s and 1930s, which continued to bear the lingering effects of the Progressive era and its preoccupation with science, expertise, and the necessity to enlighten the unenlightened. The second is that it bears an uncanny resemblance to the politically radical language of Sanger's "Family Limitation" pamphlet of the 1910s, in which she had great faith in the ability of the poor not only to use birth control but also to teach others.

That these Bogue Project initiatives were aggressively overt is suggestive as well. Not only do they run completely counter to the organization's strategies in the 1920s and 1930s—which insisted upon quietness, discretion, and a general air of secrecy about the specifics of birth control—but they were also remarkably commercial; the initiatives liked to be direct, enticing, and above all loud. The mass-mailed invites sent out by the Chicago Planned Parenthood office in its participation in the Bogue Project were little more than direct-marketing campaigns; the birth control booklet an advertisement for contraceptive methods and local Planned Parenthood clinics; and the "get-acquainted" discount coupons nothing more (and of course nothing less) than discount coupons. Thus the trick was to entice the recipient of the letter to attend one of the affiliate's new clinic locations with the promise that she would save an additional dollar when purchasing her already price-reduced charity supplies. As the invitation read, "You will find our service is FRIENDLY, RELIABLE, CONFIDENTIAL, and INEXPENSIVE." To which it added, "The cost of our service is never more than you can pay. We give FREE service to mothers on public assistance."[59] Never before, perhaps, had Planned Parenthood's charity services been advertised so noisily.

In short, the market's desire for loudness, directness, and easy availability increasingly held great appeal for local clinic organizers and those at the national level. For example, although manufacturers were still technically unable to advertise directly to consumers, a letter written in 1958 by the head of the Champaign, Illinois, affiliate to the national office makes clear her envy about the publicity they received nonetheless. "If *Newsweek* can come out with the names of drugs available without prescription to persons wishing birth control methods," wrote Mrs. Van Cleave with a hint of annoyance to Mary Calderone, "I see no reason why Planned Parenthood cannot have a short mimeographed letter to mail out to women asking for help in planning their families." She attached a version of how it might look. In addition to describing a variety of methods—including the diaphragm, the condom, contraceptive jelly and foam, as well as the rhythm method—it also mentioned specific brands for the jelly and foam, along with the advice that they could be "bought at many drug stores without a prescription."[60] The reply Van Cleave received echoed her sentiments. "Your suggestion could not have come at a more opportune time," wrote Johanna von Goeckingk, because we are "just now drafting an easily understood letter which describes various methods including products which may be purchased in a drugstore without a prescription."[61]

Bogue Project initiatives shared this new line of thinking. Promoting visibility of its informational materials, and in turn frank discussion of the information, was key. "The program of distributing information from drug stores, beauty shops, and doctors' offices is highly useful," its interim progress report explained. To which it added with a hint of pride, "Some beauty operators complain that with the booklets on display they don't get to talk about much during the day except birth control."[62] Once the project was fully underway, it expanded its original, mass-mailed, two-page pamphlet to one that was more detailed and included descriptions of all the contraceptives available with or without a doctor's prescription. It was an illustrated pamphlet as well with simple line drawings depicting various contraceptive methods, the female reproductive anatomy, and several diaphragm insertion techniques. The stamped message on the front: "Please Lend This Booklet to Your Neighbors—It May Interest Them, Too."[63] Consequently, although doctor authority was still regularly touted, such pamphlets bear remarkable resemblance to those distributed by the politically radical Sanger in the 1910s and those distributed by entrepreneurs like Rufus Riddlesbarger in the 1920s and 1930s—they all display strategies that the charity clinic movement had for decades vehemently disavowed, only to change its mind by the late 1950s.

At work here, I would argue, was the marketplace ethos of consumer choice, which had become a prominent feature, if not also a common expectation, of American life. Another of the Bogue Project booklets, which described a visit to a local clinic in the early 1960s, demonstrates this well. Much of it echoed what Martha Martin experienced in her imaginary trip to a local clinic in the 1930s. "When you go to a Neighborhood Planned Parenthood Center, you will receive a friendly welcome. Everyone there will be courteous and understanding and willing to help." But there the message diverged. After describing how "a trained nurse or social worker" will ask a "few health questions" and explain the various contraceptive techniques, the booklet had this to say: "*She will then ask you if you know which method you would like to use.*" So intent were the authors in conveying this last bit of information that they italicized it. The booklet even had a chapter titled: "Which Method Should You Choose?"[64] For prospective patients this new message was no doubt reassuring because Planned Parenthood long had the reputation of being a place where you literally had *no choice* in the method you were given. Bogue Project materials were not alone in conveying such sentiments. As PPFA's president, Dr. Alan Guttmacher, wrote in his 1969 birth control manual: "This chapter is designed not to choose a method for you, but to help you and your spouse make that selection."[65]

The ethos of the market notwithstanding, the language and mission of charity work remained a driving force. The necessity for simple language and spare line drawings, for example, lay in the fact that it was the uneducated poor that in particular needed to be reached. As Mrs. H. J. Van Cleave argued in her 1958 letter to the national office in regard to how to respond to the many letters her Champaign office received, "it seems increasingly clear that we are not giving these women the help they need so desperately. The pamphlet by Dr. Stone, 'The Prevention of Conception,' while excellent for the person of education, is useless for a large majority of those writing for information." In addition, her letter revealed the limits of doctor-prescribed methods. In areas where there were no sympathetic doctors, or no doctors at all (a problem common in rural areas), drugstore methods were especially vital. For this reason, over-the-counter methods had to be described and in ways anybody could understand them, regardless of education level.[66] It was a philosophy the Bogue Project shared. When it justified in its interim progress report the necessity of its expanded, illustrated pamphlet, it argued that "pictographic techniques" would "effectively . . . help inform semi-literate populations."[67]

Of course, how to navigate the whole issue of marriage and the possibility that such information would reach minors in this mass-marketing blitz remained a tricky issue. Doubly tricky because it was this openness that the charity movement had once railed so vocally against, precisely because of the possibility that it might promote sex among the unwed. As a result, although Planned Parenthood's policy on service to the unwed was by the late 1950s changing, it still tried to keep quiet about it. But by the 1960s the organization was becoming more daring, protecting itself in part by a front of legalese but also by a new use for the language of family planning. For example, while the birth control pamphlet called "Read and Remember" contained lists of contraceptives that patients were then to ask for by name at their local drugstores, it also included the following disclaimer at the end: "for the use of persons over 21 or married, who are seeking this information on the advice of a physician or to meet a specific health need."[68] Guttmacher's revised and updated birth control manual from 1969 did much the same. "This book has been prepared for persons twenty-one years of age or older or married," read the injunction on the book's opening pages, "who are seeking birth control information on the advice of a physician or to meet a specific health need." In addition, the language in Guttmacher's manual also implied its reader was married, because its advice usually went not to a man or woman but rather "the spouse."[69]

Further revealing still are the ways in which the Chicago Planned Parenthood handled the issue of marriage in the literature developed specifically for teens. Here the 1964 pamphlet, "What Teen-Agers Want to Know About Family Planning," is illustrative. Much as was the case in the examples above, a legal disclaimer was in place. "IMPORTANT NOTICE," the pamphlet stated on its second page, and below it was the following:

> This booklet has been prepared under medical auspices for distribution to parents of older teen-agers (15 years of age or over). *It is to be placed in the hands of teen-agers only via the parent or a physician, social worker, or minister.*
>
> It is intended to help young people understand the health, economic, and social problems associated with bearing and rearing children. In all cases, the reading of this booklet must be approved by the parent or guardian of the young person.

But on the next page—the one that people might actually read—came the following. "This booklet is written for teen-agers *and their parents . . .* because this organization is trying to accomplish two things of great importance." The first was to "help young adults to get ready for a lifetime of married happiness." The second was "to help young people guard and protect a person whom they do not even know yet, but who will someday be a most important person in their life. This person is: THEIR FIRST BABY."

The emphasis on marriage, in other words, is unmistakable, as is the desire promote childbearing; the rhetoric of family planning, moreover, is equally unmistakable if not also completely unavoidable. After the pamphlet made its

"THEIR FIRST BABY" pronouncement (complete with a bouncing baby illustration) came the following message: "Planned Parenthood is founded on two major beliefs":

1. A child should be brought into the world only when the parents are able to give it a good home and the loving care it needs.
2. Every child born should be a *wanted* child, and not just an accident of sex.

"This, we believe, is true morality," its lesson concluded, to which Jane C. Browne added her endorsement-like signature below. In the event that its message wasn't clear enough, a flow chart appearing on a later page drove home the idea that the values of family planning were relevant to teens: "FIRST finish school; SECOND get the job you want; THIRD get married and fix up your home; THEN have your first baby." Then, and only then, were the specifics about contraception discussed.

Still, the line the pamphlet walked was a fine one. On the one hand, all of its stories were ultimately about marriage and childbearing, and it referred regularly to "couples" in its advice. It also included the following exhortation in its Q&A section: "Does Planned Parenthood Favor Sexual Relations Before Marriage? DEFINITELY NOT!!" was the reply. But other messages made it confusing because when its Q&A section posed this question: "Does Planned Parenthood give service to unmarried people?" The reply was "Yes." To which it added: it was given in part to "young engaged couples who want to plan their family from the very start"; but it was also given "*Under special circumstances . . .* to an unmarried girl if she is accompanied by a responsible adult." So which was it? In addition, that the pamphlet still clearly listed all the methods that could be purchased—or, in the case of clinic services, be obtained largely for free or at reduced rates— suggests that the organization's concerns that such information might be misused were diminishing.[70]

However, for all that Planned Parenthood was doing to push at the marriage boundary, where the case for birth control could be made the most loudly, and the most effectively, was when it was connected to unwed motherhood, particularly among those on welfare relief. Here again the events of Illinois are illustrative because by the early 1960s the Illinois Public Aid Commission (IPAC) controversy was ready to explode. The issue first emerged in 1962 when, in an effort to alleviate the plight of the urban poor as well as to relieve the financial burdens of relief rolls, the IPAC commissioner, Arnold H. Maremont, instituted a new policy. Not only would the state cover the cost of contraceptives for those on relief, but it would also expand the program to include the unwed. Not surprisingly, it set off a firestorm of debate, resulting in the immediate dismissal of Maremont from office as well as the adoption of counterresolutions in the Illinois state legislature.

Planned Parenthood was not about to let this opportunity slip away, however, and it rallied to get the expanded version of the policy back into place. As legal historian C. Thomas Dienes noted, Planned Parenthood secured in part "the services of speakers who presented overwhelmingly favorable testimony about Maremont's policy" in subsequent hearings about the case. The organization also helped create an "independent citizens' committee," which "obtained the support of social, religious, and medical associations" as well as sponsored "letter-writing" and "lobbying" campaigns. Its efforts paid off; by 1965 the state adopted a new policy that allowed any public aid recipient who was over fifteen and a mother to obtain contraceptive services regardless of marital status. The first of its kind in the nation, the resolution marked a dramatic legal challenge to long-standing laws that limited contraceptives to those who were wed.[71]

That this successful challenge began with welfare recipients is significant. The state approved the expansion of birth control to unmarried welfare recipients not because they had a right to have sex, but rather because limiting the number of children poor women bore alleviated the financial burden of relief rolls. Moreover, and as will become clear in the following section, fears of rising birth rates among blacks and other ethnic populations contributed to the resolution's palatability nationwide as well. Indeed, despite the controversy it generated, it stuck, and publicly so. While the *Washington Post-Times-Herald* proclaimed that the "World Eyes Birth Control Project," other big-city newspapers and small-town gazettes regularly described what was going on in Illinois.[72] Even television took notice; the IPAC controversy served as the subject of a major CBS documentary entitled "Birth Control and the Law."[73] This was, in other words, big news, news apparently that more people than ever before were willing to accept, despite its potential immoral implications.

Finally, also worth noting in this dramatic reconfiguration of birth control services are the ways in which Planned Parenthood was still trying to get others to provide birth control services while at the same time looking to keep itself on top. The battle in Chicago, for example, to get Cook County Hospital to offer contraceptives in its newly established obstetrical wing (the Fantus Clinic) was among the affiliate's biggest campaigns. First begun in the late 1950s, the often heated negotiations lasted ten years, during which time the local office even resorted to guerrilla-style tactics by occasionally parking one of its new mobile units just outside the city's public hospital.[74] Consequently, when in 1968 Cook County Hospital finally began to offer contraceptive services, this was heralded by the affiliate as a great achievement, one it proudly announced in its newsletter.[75] Likewise, the city's opening in 1965 of a string of six birth control clinics of its own, which operated under the purview of the Board of Health, constituted yet another landmark shift in Chicago's birth control policy, about which the local Planned Parenthood office was thrilled.[76]

But these were still developments that Planned Parenthood monitored with great care, much as it had done in the 1930s when the competition it faced came from those irregular clinics. In other words, although pleased that such facilities were now available, the organization was determined to assert its authority; its model of birth control services was the one to follow. As Dr. Day, medical director of Planned Parenthood–World Population, remarked at a 1965 Chicago medical advisory board meeting, "There are a great many new recruits doing family planning work for the first time, and making the public more and more aware of the urgency of the program of birth control." Using striking language, he added, "Planned Parenthood has the most know-how to do the job of 'brain washing' that needs to be done." Chicago's Browne supported this view, chiming in, with a hint of territoriality, "that if we didn't get on the ball, someone would take the job away from us."[77] Likewise, the language found in a report submitted in 1970 by an Iowa affiliate reveals a similar imperative. If "good" clinics were to remain in operation, Robert L. Webber insisted, Planned Parenthood clinics needed to serve as "watch dogs'" to facilities established by others.[78]

Given its aspirations, what were Planned Parenthood's concerns about what others were or were not providing? One was that Chicago's Board of Health clinics were reputedly offering only the pill, and only for reasons of health. As Dr. George Langmyhr (of Planned Parenthood–World Population) remarked in 1966 to Browne, "This is only one straw in the wind as to why we should not relinquish our service clinics," a sentiment that suggests the national office's renewed faith in the utility of the local clinic and its centrality to Planned Parenthood's authority.[79] That the Chicago Board of Health clinics might demand too many medical tests was raised as well. As Mary-Jane Snyder of Chicago commented, although these city-sponsored clinics were "a giant step forward," she expressed concerns about the rumor she heard that they would "demand blood tests and urinalyses each month." She also expressed concern that they would "screen the patients very carefully," a point that may have been in reference to marital status.[80] In fact, Chicago's Board of Health clinics did limit its services to the wed, as one undercover Chicago reporter learned in her 1965 investigation for the *Chicago Sunday Star*. "No Pill for the Single Girl," its headline boldly read, as she recounted her visit to the city-run clinic.[81] But when she went to one operated by Planned Parenthood (though this time posing as an engaged woman), her efforts were met with success: "Our Single Girl Gets Birth Control Info," the paper's headline announced the following week.[82] Notable here is the position the city's Board of Health clinics took with regard to Planned Parenthood's aggressive new strategies. As Dr. Sam Andelman, Chicago's commissioner of health, explained, "the city's careful attitude was to merely offer the pills, foams and injections and let groups such as Planned Parenthood actually advertise and promote their use."[83] Let Planned Parenthood be the one making all the noise.

Interestingly enough, when others were making an even greater ruckus, Planned Parenthood was less than pleased. Its reaction to the birth control activist William Baird—the man behind *Eisenstadt v. Baird*, the 1972 Supreme Court ruling that legalized contraceptives for the unwed—is illustrative. "Mr. Baird is a self-styled crusader," wrote Planned Parenthood's Lucie Prinz in December 1967 to Miss Irene Nordine of Illinois' Department of Children and Family Services, "and although he is, I think, quite sincere about wanting to get the laws revised and make contraceptives available to all, his methods of operation are often questionable." So what was Baird doing? According to Prinz's letter, a lot. In New Jersey, for example, "he sought to get the law concerning [the] display of contraceptives changed by renting a truck and inviting ladies in to see the methods." He was arrested. In Massachusetts, he was "trying to get the law prohibiting prescription of contraceptives to unmarried women changed" by generating "a lot of publicity." He was arrested again. He was "now even more concerned about abortion," Prinz explained, "and openly has defied several abortion laws in many states" by telling women where an illegal one might be had.

Yet her criticisms about his work are somewhat misplaced; Baird's activities, though bold and innovative in their own right, simultaneously echoed some of Planned Parenthood's latest efforts. For example, while Planned Parenthood was using mobile units to make contraceptives more easily available, so too was Baird, who drove around in his Plan Van, which he parked on city streets and invited women inside to learn about the various birth control methods available. In addition, while Planned Parenthood was generating lots of publicity and looking to extend contraceptive services to the unwed, so too was Baird. Of course, it didn't help matters that Baird also "delight[ed] in attacking Planned Parenthood," as Prinz explained in her letter, "accusing us of not giving birth control to the poor and of being 'establishment' and not interested in anything but spending our 'large budget' frivolously."[84] But maybe Baird had a point. Much as was the case in the 1930s, Planned Parenthood was again circling its wagons and looking to establish itself as the one true authority on birth control and how best to make it available. Consequently, for all its efforts to make respectable what were once radical strategies, it didn't suffer lightly the presence of others who interfered with its authority-making game.

Spreading the Word with Missionary Zeal

Meanwhile again, in December 1959 the following headline appeared on the cover of the Chicago affiliate's official newsletter: "63rd Street Center To Open Full Time." Brimming with excitement, the article described how the clinic's rapidly growing caseload necessitated this shift to full-time operations. Alongside the article the newsletter ran a photograph. Taken somewhere in the reception area of the newly expanded facility, it showed four women seated around a desk, three of whom listened carefully to what the fourth, an older woman clad in a white medical coat, had to say. The caption below it read, "Mrs. Rebecca Young, social worker at 63rd St. Center, gives careful explanation to patients." Though perhaps staged, as many of these photographs often were, its image is telling because, with the exception of one of the patients, all the women were African American.[85] Indeed, by the 1960s the black community occupied an important place in Chicago's family planning movement, yielding in turn a major shift in what was once the local office's busiest clinic. No longer was the downtown facility, which had in the 1920s and 1930s served mainly white middle-class women, the affiliate's major draw. Instead, it was now the 63rd Street Center, which operated deep in the heart of the vibrant black belt district.

There is, however, another side to this story; the missionary zeal of the black community was matched by the missionary zeal of another sort. For all the demand for birth control in the black community and compassion behind this expansion of services, it did seem as if certain communities were being singled out, revealing in turn how a thread of colonialism underpinned the domestic family planning movement. In other words, when racialized concerns about overpopulation abroad collided with racialized concerns about overpopulation at home, the northern industrial city had become the equivalent of the third-world slum, an analogy that served as a powerful legitimating tool in the organization's aggressive new birth control initiatives, particularly its desire to reach the unwed. Thus the story in this section has two parts: it begins with the influx of blacks in the Chicago family planning movement and then turns to the darker side of the story.

Part of the story behind the photograph described above can be traced back to the second great migration of African Americans in the 1940s and 1950s, who, in search of work and an escape from the oppression of Jim Crow, packed up their bags in the South and headed north. As a booming industrial center, Chicago was one of their destinations, precipitating in turn a dramatic transformation in the city's population. As historian Arnold Hirsch explained, while in 1920 blacks accounted for less than 4 percent of the city's population, by the mid-1960s the number had risen to 30 percent. With such growth, moreover, came a major recomposition of the city's many distinct neighborhoods. On the west side, for example, what was once a small African American enclave had become a major neighborhood. And on the South Side, the already prominent black belt district had grown even more, pushing its main business district roughly two miles to the south, from Forty-Seventh Street to Sixty-Third, the street that was now home to the bustling full-time Planned Parenthood clinic that was glowingly described on the front page of the Chicago office's 1959 newsletter.[86]

That the Chicago affiliate was reaching so many African Americans was not simply a product of its prime location; it was also a product of the black community itself. Although it is difficult to determine just how many worked at the Chicago office, the social worker Rebecca Young was not alone in her efforts; African Americans occupied positions throughout the local organization and at all levels.[87] Some worked as nurses. Betty Perez, for example, not only put her training into practice by working inside the clinic, but she also served on the affiliate's speaker's bureau, which regularly spoke about family planning at local schools.[88] Others served as volunteers, as was the case with Evelyn Thompson, a Chicago resident who hailed from one of the city's poorer neighborhoods. For her work in the affiliate's 1963 "Help Your Neighbor Help Herself" campaign, she received first prize at the volunteer luncheon.[89] Still more served on the affiliate's newly inaugurated Patients' Auxiliary.[90] Then there were African Americans who occupied more prestigious positions. While Marion Hampton worked as the Chicago affiliate's coordinator of social services, Shirley Arnold was the coordinator of research.[91] In addition, Dr. Lendor C. Nesbitt worked as one of the physicians, and Reverend Edgar Ward, pastor of Grace United Presbyterian Church, served on the board of directors.[92]

African Americans made their presence known in other ways as well. When in the summer of 1962 the Chicago affiliate began its Bogue Project-sponsored "Coffee Sip" program, Rebecca Young and Vivian Moore reportedly held them all over their Lawndale community on the city's west side.[93] When the organization began its Bogue Project-financed mobile units, African Americans worked inside as nurses and volunteers.[94] When Cook County Hospital continued to refuse to provide contraceptive services in its newly established obstetrical wing, African Americans picketed outside.[95] Furthermore, when the Illinois Public Aid Commission controversy began to heat up, the African American Illinois State Representative, William H. Robinson, testified on behalf of the extension of birth control to unwed welfare recipients and continued to work "to see that birth control services became public policy," for which he was later honored by the Planned Parenthood organization.[96]

Indeed, the whole community seemed to be involved. The city's black newspaper, the *Chicago Defender*, regularly ran glowing articles describing Planned Parenthood activities and even instituted in the mid-1960s an advice column entitled "Keep Your Family the Right Size," which then served as the "voice of the Chicago Planned Parenthood Association."[97] National black publications, such as *Ebony*, ran congratulatory articles as well, complete with photographs depicting clinic work in Chicago.[98] Moreover, organizations such as the Chicago Urban League, as well as its parent office, threw their support behind contraceptive programs for the poor.[99] Even local black politicians lent their support in tangible ways. Alderman

Benjamin Lewis not only endorsed birth control, but he also helped pub-licize local services among his constituents by displaying pamphlets in his office, encouraging local "Coffee Sips," and voting with his precinct cap-tains "to distribute door-to-door 10,000 samples of one simple birth con-trol device."[100]

There was also an eager embrace of birth control from poor black women themselves, which could be seen in clinic attendance records and heard in the public housing projects. For example, when the *Chicago Defender* asked twenty-five projects tenants their thoughts on local birth control initiatives, nineteen expressed support. Furthermore, and in response to what appears to be the IPAC controversy, one of the respondents, a mother of six, said this "is a blessing for people like us. I don't see why they have to do so much arguing about it. If some of them folks had to live like this, they would think a lot different about the idea."[101]

That blacks supported birth control was of course not new; nor were their efforts to make it available within their communities. As Jessie Rodrique demonstrated in her study of the black community in the early days of the birth control movement, despite the racism of the movement many African Americans had long embraced fertility control, viewing the practice not only as a tool for gender equality but for racial equality as well. As Rodrique wrote, blacks "saw birth control as one means of freeing themselves from the oppression and exploitation of white society through the improvement of their health and their economic and social status." She noted that intellectu-als such as W. E. B. Du Bois preached its importance as early as the 1910s, and African American organizations—including "health professionals, civic groups, and women's clubs"—spent the 1930s establishing contraceptive programs within their communities.[102]

That such work accelerated in Chicago with the rise of the modern civil rights movement also makes sense because organizations for racial equal-ity increasingly made their way into the city's many neighborhoods.[103] As the sentiments of the Chicago Urban League suggest, black activism and birth control continued to go hand-in-hand: "to fight poverty without birth control," its members officially announced in the mid-1960s, "is to fight with one hand tied behind the back."[104] Likewise, such organizations as the Southern Christian Leadership Conference (SCLC) threw its support behind birth control. SCLC eagerly embraced contraceptive programs in black communities, and, on at least one occasion, it worked directly with a Planned Parenthood affiliate in Tennessee to make contraceptive services available to poor blacks, a program about which Martin Luther King and his colleagues expressed great support.[105] In fact, in 1966 and on behalf of her husband, Coretta Scott King would be the first to accept Planned Parent-hood's newest and highest honor: the Margaret Sanger Award.[106] Thus the influx of African Americans made for a powerful new movement, revealing how the energized birth control movement in Chicago was as much born of the efforts of the black community as it was the white.

But alongside such efforts, racial strife was also building and the reaction among many whites to the massive demographic shift of the 1940s and 1950s was a hostile one. One way they expressed their animosity toward this black "invasion" was to get out of the city, and those who could afford it often fled to outlying areas, an exodus that contributed to the massive suburbanization boom of the postwar era. Those who could not leave stayed behind, determined to fight, however, to protect their homes, their jobs, and their white racial purity. And fight they did. Adopting such slogans as "white people must control their own communities," white residents of these neighborhoods in transition often backed up their rhetoric with action and regularly targeted African Americans with violence, as was the case in the ethnic uprising in Chicago's Trumbull Park Homes in 1953–54. Other neighborhoods, indeed other northern industrial cities, experienced similar racial conflicts in the postwar era, and although the close of the 1950s brought with it abatement in violence, tensions still festered below the surface.[107]

Here then emerges the significance of the 1940s and 1950s-inspired family planning motif, which placed the blame for America's problems in the lap of the unplanned family and all of its unwanted children; within the context of these massive demographic shifts, unplanned families seemed increasingly to reside in the northern industrial slums. Or, as historian Laura Briggs might put it, they were simply having "the wrong sort of family."[108] Such sentiments appear vividly in the remarks made in 1960 by Dr. Philip M. Hauser of the University of Chicago. While increases in urban population yielded some cultural benefits, he argued, they were far outweighed by the problems they produced, which included "family disorganization, delinquency, alcoholism, drug addiction, [and] unemployment," characterizations that bear striking resemblance to those used to describe unplanned families in the preceding chapter.[109] That welfare had also become increasingly racialized only made matters worse. As scholar Daniel Walkowitz explained, "the inequity of the 'affluent society' [of the 1950s] had a racial cast to it, increasingly leaving African Americans and Hispanics behind and dependent on welfare."[110]

Yet it was the "evil" of illegitimacy, to quote another observer—the ultimate violation of the family planning ideal—that regularly took center stage, revealing why birth control for the unwed took on a new urgency.[111] For example, when two youth services representatives in Chicago described potential clinic clientele to Planned Parenthood members, they made reference to unwed motherhood. The "average block has 250 families," Jeannette Hall and Barbara Bell reported about one Chicago neighborhood, the "average size family is nine, with no father in the home—no father image. 86% are on ADC [Aid to Dependent Children]." Worse still, they added, "74% are second generation illegitimate."[112] When Planned Parenthood offices talked about the liberalization of admission policies, the term "illegitimate" came up again. "We recognize that there are those who would take advantage for immoral purposes the greater availability of birth control," an Ohio affiliate wrote, "but we feel that dangers of such abuse are not as great as the dangers to individuals and the community that arise from a continued growth in illegitimacy."[113] Furthermore, when talking about the need to provide contraceptive services in Chicago's Cook County Hospital, the reference to illegitimacy came up there too. "I hope the program helps reduce the number of illegitimate children," explained Fred Hertig, the hospital warden. "One month there were 90 illegitimate births by unmarried girls 16 and under at the hospital. I'm pleased Planned Parenthood has opened an office in our neighborhood."[114] Significantly, although women of all racial and economic backgrounds experienced out-of-wedlock pregnancy, blame for illegitimacy and the problems it posed often fell squarely on the shoulders of poor, unwed, black women. Or, as historian Rickie Solinger once noted, the blame fell on their "wombs."[115]

It was in this environment, therefore, that the inner city as third-world metaphor emerged. A new program instituted by the Chicago affiliate illustrates this well. In an effort to see firsthand the impoverished communities it served, in the early 1960s the local office initiated the rolling board meeting. Rather than simply conduct their business in a meeting room, far removed from the nitty-gritty tasks of daily clinic affairs, board members and other Planned Parenthood representatives sometimes did their work aboard a rented bus, which toured the slums of the city and occasionally made stops to visit particularly noteworthy locations. Certainly such meetings served important functions. The passengers got a firsthand glimpse of clinic operations, and they also became at least somewhat acquainted with the impoverished communities they wished to assist.

Yet these meetings also suggest a strange sense of safari, a titillating expedition for the middle class to see "how the other half lived."[116] Consider, for a moment, how a 1962 report described one such excursion:

> As the group of about thirty men and women rolled through the "gray" sections of the city, items on the agenda were presented. Stops were made at a number of the branch clinics and Mobile Unit Clinic Locations, including a hasty trek through the receiving floor of the Cook County Hospital. . . . The $3.00 fee for each passenger covered the expenses of the ride, as well as the price of a box lunch and coffee. . . . One of the advantages of this type of Board meeting was that it enabled the Trustees of the organization to examine the clinic locations, view the slum areas from which their patients are recruited, and envision expansion of the program as we rolled though miles of housing developments, which will in time be demanding the attention of our Chicago Affiliate.[117]

The image is a striking one, and when combined with other bus tour accounts—which described how "friends and relatives" sometimes joined in or how microphone-delivered commentary provided colorful details about the neighborhoods through which they toured—conveys a sense of voyeuristic tourism, the middle class peering from behind the safety of glass windows on the world of those who toiled below.[118]

Still others made the connection between the "third world" overseas and "third world" at home explicitly. "People do not exist to live all their undernourished lives in the illiterate ignorance of an Asian village," quoted *Newsweek* magazine from remarks given at a 1959 Planned Parenthood meeting. Nor do they exist "to be condemned to a distressing and nerve-racking existence of bustle in and out of monstrous cities."[119] Likewise, when columnist Georgie Ann Geyer sympathetically reported on the "Coffee Sips" held in one neighborhood on Chicago's west side, the community took on the flavor often reserved for third-world nations. The "place was West Side Lawndale," she wrote, "teeming, crime-ridden, alienated, and with a birth rate . . . as high as India's and higher than Puerto Rico's."[120] So pervasive had this analogy become that it even made its way into Dienes's historical account of the Illinois Public Aid Commission controversy.[121]

Within this context, therefore, there did seem to be a concerted effort to target "third world" residents of America's inner cities and to get them in particular to reduce their numbers. The goals of the Bogue Project, for example, were articulated in this way: we are "undertaking to speed up the adoption of birth control by high fertility populations," which it later defined as impoverished "Puerto Rican, Negro, and white" communities. And although whites appeared as a targeted population, that the study began in an African American neighborhood on the city's west side could easily be perceived by critics as an emphasis on minority populations.[122] Furthermore, at least one newspaper was unapologetically direct about the targeting of ethnic minorities. When the *Washington Post* reported on the Illinois Public Aid Commission controversy, it described the new policy as an effort to curtail "the alarming Negro and Puerto Rican birth rate of Chicago."[123]

The language used to describe these new outreach programs also conveys a sense of coercion. While one rolling board meeting report explained how participants could "view the slum areas from which their patients are *recruited*,"[124] the Chicago Planned Parenthood instituted a new program as part of the Bogue Project called the Captive Audience Motivation and Education Campaign, which worked through bedside visits to promote birth control among Cook County Hospital's newest mothers. The project explained its effectiveness in this manner: "When a woman goes to the hospital for her confinement, the fact that she is immobilized for several days provides an opportunity to contact her at low cost and with a small chance of refusal."[125] The words suggest not compassionate assistance, but rather aggressive pushiness.

That middle-class African Americans themselves seemed interested in singling out poor blacks suggests how a sense of colonialism underpinned their efforts as well, the enlightened missionaries seeking to educate the unenlightened masses. As Reverend Ward, local pastor and Chicago Planned Parenthood board member explained, the "lack of birth control services is keeping the lower class Negroes from bettering themselves . . . [and] . . . the middle class Negro has got to realize that his lower class brother is the weakest link in his own chain of advancement." "Coffee Sips" sponsored by African Americans conveyed this sentiment as well. Geyer's 1962 article on birth control in the *Chicago Scene* described how in an effort "to urge lower class Negro women in Chicago to slow their birth rate by using birth control," Mrs. Young "chides, cajoles, pleads and dares the women to plan their families."[126] Another account depicted the efforts of Young and her colleagues in this way: "These missionaries of modern motherhood have been spreading their teaching throughout the Chicago area, with a concentrated attack in Negro and other less privileged neighborhoods."[127]

Nevertheless, despite these paternalistic attitudes, many poor black women themselves saw in the family planning ideal great promise and expressed much frustration with those who seemed blatantly to ignore it. They too wanted to give their children all that money could offer. As one African American mother explained as she cooked for her eight children, "I've been wondering what could be done in a situation like mine. I just can't take care of all these kids like I should. I worry all the time because they can't have some of the things they really need."[128] Another project resident had this to say to the *Chicago Defender's* family planning advice columnist: "I live in a project where a lot of the women don't care how many children they have. Their kids run wild and they use half of their relief check for booze for their boyfriends. . . . Shouldn't they be forced to use birth control or cut off the relief?" In reply, Leontyne Hunt said that she did not think this was a good idea.[129]

Then too there were the occasional few who, when addressing America's overpopulation problem, pointed the finger directly at the middle class. "Make no mistake about it," author Marya Mannes remarked at the Chicago affiliate's 1965 annual meeting, our "threatening crowds are not the result of large families on welfare" but rather the "third child of the average middle-class American couple." Mannes then shifted the blame away from the cities and squarely upon what she described as "the bumper-to-bumper, shoulder-to-shoulder, suburb-to-suburb world" of the "selfish" middle class. What her listeners thought is unclear, but that one newspaper account described her message as "touchy" suggests that not all were pleased.[130]

And so, as all these stories about Chicago suggest, the situation truly was a complicated one. For all the demand among blacks for the city's many new birth control initiatives, and for all that the black community did to help bring these new initiatives about, there also seemed to be a concerted effort to single certain communities out; and while sometimes the motivations were noble, at other times they were not. As a result, there emerged from other members of the black community a growing opposition, the intensity of which seemed to increase with each and every birth control success. By the late 1960s these tensions could no longer be ignored; as the decade drew to a close, it was becoming painfully apparent to the Chicago affiliate that its relationship with the African American community was deteriorating rapidly.

Tempers Explode

On February 29, 1968, the Chicago office's board of directors gathered together for its regular meeting to discuss affiliate affairs. On this leap-year day, however, business as usual was superseded by a more pressing matter. Despite the many ties the local office had with the black community, there was a growing hostility among many other African Americans against the organization, a hostility that now manifested itself in personal and direct ways against Planned Parenthood workers themselves. To illustrate the severity of the situation, the committee called upon Betty Perez, an African American, to "describe her recent unfortunate experiences in the Negro community." A long-time staff member, Perez had worked as a Planned Parenthood clinic nurse for eight years and as a speaker in the organization's educational division.

Perez described three incidents to the board of directors, all of which she found deeply troubling. The first took place at the Washburne Trade School, where Perez had delivered an educational speech about birth control, only to find herself interrupted by one of the black female students in the audience. "Birth control pills [are] killing people," the girl challenged. "Negro women want to be let alone."[131] Perez's efforts to address her remarks only angered the student more, and later that day the Planned Parenthood nurse found herself confronted by the girl's boyfriend, whose hairstyle and clothing, according to Perez, were commonly worn by black nationalists. After asking "Is she is the one," he "studied [her] face carefully in a threatening way," which Perez said "frightened her." In the second incident, which took place the following day, she encountered "another group of young people similarly dressed" and heard one of them say, "There's that lady from Planned Parenthood again. Instead of telling us about birth control, why doesn't she tell those hunkies something?" Again, Perez admitted, their "hostility frightened her."

The third and final incident took place at a local black entertainment venue. When the master of ceremonies proclaimed during one of the shows that we "all know that birth control is just another scheme of the white man's to keep us down," the audience applauded in agreement. For the third time Perez admitted that she was afraid and added that, despite her shared racial heritage, she feared "being attacked by these militants . . . because of [her] affiliation with Planned Parenthood." She was perceived to have become nothing more than "someone who has been brainwashed by the white man in order to spread his message among them."

Nurse Perez's experiences touch therefore upon the rising tide of criticism among many within the African American community toward these new birth control initiatives, criticism that had long been brewing but that Planned Parenthood could no longer ignore. In fact, her testimony was part of the Chicago board's larger agenda to figure out how best to improve the affiliate's deteriorating relations with the black community. For this reason, she was not the only person invited to speak at the meeting. So too was Douglas Stewart, an African American and the director of community relations for the national Planned Parenthood office.

Yet Perez's experiences also suggest the emergence of a deeply troubling dilemma for blacks themselves. Birth control had long been a tricky issue for African Americans, and throughout the 1960s the community found itself ever more splintered over the subject, with conflicting opinions cutting across political, religious, gender, and class lines. So fractured, in fact, were the differing views that to draw neat lines of division between the older more conservative civil rights groups and the newer more militant ones is virtually impossible. For those African Americans who worked for Planned Parenthood, the dilemma was particularly difficult. While these individuals had gotten involved in the family planning movement in an effort to counter racism in America, as the 1960s drew to a close their work was increasingly seen by other members of the community as yet another manifestation of racism, though this time one that bored its way into the community from within.[132]

Much like African American support for birth control, resistance was hardly new. As Rodrique noted in her study of the early birth control movement, while such leaders as Du Bois embraced the cause, Marcus Garvey opposed it, driven by fears of the survival of the black race in addition to his staunch Catholic views. Other African Americans expressed early on their opposition toward sterilization programs.[133] Still more were reluctant to attend local contraceptive facilities, as was the case with Sanger's Harlem-based clinic (also known as the Clinical Research Bureau), for fear they might be used as the subject of scientific research, an ironic concern given what this chapter describes.[134]

As the decades passed, such resistance persisted, fueled in part by concerns about particular methods but also by continued reservations about clinics themselves. For example, despite the seeming popularity of contraceptive facilities among blacks in Chicago, getting women to come in was still no easy task. When in the mid-1960s African Americans in Cleveland opened a clinic in a poor black neighborhood, they were surprised when the "only scarce commodity" in their well-equipped facility was patients. Black women, the organizers soon learned, stayed away for a variety of reasons. While some "didn't know about birth control," others were concerned about childcare or worried about the shabbiness of their clothing, that it might be inappropriate for a visit to a local medical clinic. Then there were those who "had been badly frightened by tales of embolism, cancer, or permanent sterilization."[135] In other words, the long history of black suspicion of white medicine remained in full force, and the widely publicized controversies about the safety of oral contraceptives only added to their reservations.[136] In fact, worries about the pill appeared regularly in this rising tide of African American criticism.[137]

Many more, however, opposed birth control outright, some for religious reasons and others because they favored economic solutions to the inequities blacks faced. As one woman from Chicago's public housing projects explained, "Leave it to man to try to control the Lord's work. That's why man's in so much trouble in the world today. I'm not thinking about it." Another resident, a laborer's wife and the mother of seven, had this to say about the IPAC controversy: "They don't need to talk about birth control. What they need is some jobs for the men to take care of their families. That's your control."[138] Embedded in their critiques therefore are two more important issues. The first is the possibility that not all women want to use birth control (another story that needs to be written). The second is that faith-oriented critiques were hardly the purview of a white Catholic constituency; they often underpinned black opposition as well.

Indeed, particularly where the IPAC controversy was concerned, African Americans of a variety of religious denominations drew regularly upon moral concerns about sexual propriety, which they then blended with larger political critiques of social injustice and even race genocide. For example, while one southern Baptist minister, who also happened to be president-elect of his local NAACP, complained that the IPAC decision was "only adding to the breakdown of moral standards," another African American delivered an even harsher critique.[139] To "direct this type of program toward a race already unjustifiably stigmatized as being basically immoral would only promote promiscuity, fornication, and immorality," challenged Paul Twine of the Lake Meadow Council of Catholic Men in his testimony before the

Illinois Public Aid Commission. What was needed instead were "programs more specifically directed at eliminating the cause than the result."[140] Even more direct in its critique was the Catholic Interracial Council. "Illinois' free birth-control program for women on relief" was driven by "strong anti-Negro motivations," reported one newspaper account, and was a program that only served to "eliminate Negroes."[141]

In light of these criticisms, it's hardly surprising that Perez was not alone in her experiences. When in the following year another Chicago Planned Parenthood representative—David Mann, whose racial background is, admittedly, not clear—went to find out how the residents of another African American neighborhood felt about birth control, he was met with great hostility. Although the leader of the community group, Reverend Curtis Burrell, was apparently sympathetic enough to Planned Parenthood's work to allow him to speak before the group, many of its members could not be swayed from the opinion that birth control was simply another way for "'whitey' to depopulate the neighborhood." As Mann explained, tensions ran high, with the general attitude of the meeting being "the hell with Planned Parenthood." So harrowing was his experience that he concluded his report with the recommendation that "no further attempts [be made] by Planned Parenthood into black communities at the present time," and that any future "work planned for these communities be done through already established channels, such as Urban Progress Centers, Model Cities, health departments, etc."[142]

As Mann's conclusions suggest, many blacks had become deeply frustrated with Planned Parenthood's aggressive new initiatives; they were also quick to pick up on the subtexts of the family planning rhetoric. The emphasis on birth control, for example, seemed to suggest that only family size and structure was the source of black problems. As Stewart, the black representative from the national Planned Parenthood office, tried to explain to Chicago's board of directors in its February 1968 meeting, black communities regularly face "high rates of unemployment, unequal, poor quality of education, squalid housing conditions, . . . bad streets, no playgrounds, no comprehensive health services—then, shiny and bright, birth control! This really makes it look bad." Likewise, the connection between lack of family planning and juvenile delinquency was also not lost on the African American community, who saw the not-so-subtle connection the rhetoric implicitly drew between blacks and criminality. As Stewart remarked, although birth control might in fact reduce juvenile delinquency, "We don't have to shout it from the rafters."[143]

It did not help matters that the Chicago office's predominantly black clinic, the 63rd Street Center, was by the end of the 1960s in a state of utter disarray, which even began to generate criticism from within the local office itself. Indeed, life inside the Sixty-Third Street clinic bore little resemblance to the glorious depiction of the facility that graced the cover of the affiliate's newsletter ten years earlier. As Dr. Nesbitt, one of the affiliate's African American physicians, explained, "Everything seemed disorderly." While nurses "charged about," patients endured long waits, only to find that when their turn came, they were allotted only several minutes with the staff clinician. The clinic itself was also run down, with nothing more than "cheap plastic [and falling apart] folding doors" separating it from the street, which he saw as a dire security risk. Nesbitt's frustration may have in part been a product of his doctor's training, in that he might have been offended by the clinic's failure to adhere to standards of medical professionalism. But he was also deeply concerned with the well being of the people inside. As Nesbitt remarked, it is no wonder that blacks are so "sensitive" about the issue and "abhor the old 'cannon-fodder' clinics with all their force."[144]

Thus the situation was a complicated one, but what made it even more difficult for the black community was the paradox upon which it was built: the missionary-like efforts to promote birth control among African Americans was born as much of the efforts to counter racism in America as it was of racism itself. In other words, because blacks in Chicago and elsewhere in the nation took up the cause of birth control and made it one of racial uplift, birth control increasingly had a racial cast, particularly when it was blended with the rhetoric of overpopulation and unwanted children. Consequently, when the African American students asked Perez why she seemed more interested in getting blacks rather than whites to use birth control, they had a point: Perez was indeed looking to reach African Americans. Conversely, when Perez found herself accosted by members of her own community, it marked a bitter blow to all that she and her fellow African Americans had worked so hard to accomplish. No longer were they humanitarians who brought new hope to their black community. Instead, they were nothing more than the unwitting dupes of a racist white society. For people like Perez, therefore, this must have been a bitter pill to swallow; confrontations could yield not only fears about one's physical safety but also, in all likelihood, internal dilemmas within the hearts and minds of black family planning workers. For even if they still believed what they were doing was right, they had to come to terms with the fact that others within their community perceived their work in a much different light.

Another Pot Boils Over

In the spring and summer of 1971, another troubling story unfolded. Sometime in 1968, the Planned Parenthood affiliate in San Antonio, Texas, referred a number of its patients to a nonprofit research organization known as the Southwest Foundation. The foundation then embarked on a study of oral contraceptives, one involving 398 women, many of whom were drawn from the neighboring Latino community. As a double-blind research project, its purpose was to determine the existence of pill side effects; to assess, in other words, whether they were real or figments of women's imaginations. Subsequently, and unbeknownst to them, the more than 70 members of the control group received only placebos, not oral contraceptives, and although they were also given vaginal preparations to use as backup, at least six of the women in the control group found themselves pregnant.[145]

When news of this broke, several months before the study was to appear in the September 1971 issue of *Human Fertility*, the president of Planned Parenthood went down to San Antonio to determine what exactly had taken place. What Guttmacher found was a dire situation indeed, one that revealed all the ethical dilemmas such experiments could provoke. Yet Planned Parenthood's interest in resolving this local problem belied far deeper concerns. Although the situation in Texas was by all accounts an extreme one, it was but one example of the now massive trend within Planned Parenthood: the use of local clinics to engage in biomedical research, and the use of charity clinic patients as subjects of scientific investigation. Thus, a domestic-style colonialism manifested itself in this situation as well. Like the third-world women abroad—who, for example, were the subjects of early tests on the pill and other methods of birth control in Puerto Rico—the third-world women here at home also found themselves at the center of contraceptive research.[146]

Consequently, for all the benefits these new arrangements yielded, the upsurge of research inside the local clinic wrought equally significant problems. Many were simply the rehashing of old frustrations between the national and local offices, in which pharmaceuticals now found themselves deeply enmeshed. Other problems were more pressing. For example, because Planned Parenthood worried about how the general public would react to news about this massive new trend in using charity clinic patients as research subjects, it decided to downplay its research experiments on clinic patients. Research also provoked conflicts between doctor-run medical committees and lay members and volunteers. Most important, however, was the affect on clinic patients. Although they were not passive victims, that they were drawn by and large from poor and minority communities heightens the ethical responsibilities of those engaged in charity work.

Therein lies the paradox of this particular situation. While pharmaceutical companies certainly shoulder no small amount of the responsibility for potential unethical treatment of the poor, the ethical conflict was born not just of Planned Parenthood's new ties with business, but also of the ties the charity clinic movement had forged with scientific medicine back in the 1920s and 1930s—when the argument then was that only through the compassionate benevolence of doctor-run charity clinics could poor women be

spared the inevitable exploitation of the profit-driven commercial birth control marketplace. In short, the desire to protect the poor from commercial
greed was part of the rationale behind the charity movement's alliance with
scientific medicine.

But over the years scientific medicine changed, and by the post–World
War II era it was engaging in medical research in unprecedented new ways.
As medical historian David Rothman explained, the massive upsurge of
research yielded opportunities for tremendous scientific breakthroughs.
At the same time, however, it brought with it troubling new developments
in the culture of research, the aims of science increasingly superseding the
rights and needs of patients.[147] Given that Planned Parenthood was now
deeply enmeshed in experimental research, it was a culture that could not
help but make its way inside the local Planned Parenthood clinic, rendering
vulnerable those whom the charity organization was supposed compassionately and protectively to assist. For this reason, a closer look at what happened at the Texas office reveals the disastrous conflicts such arrangements
could provoke. However, a closer look into the climate of research within
Planned Parenthood more generally reveals how something like this was
bound to happen.

Much as was the case with affiliates across the nation and their ties to the
biomedical industry, San Antonio's relationship with the Southwest Foundation began in the late 1950s.[148] The arrangement between the two organizations worked in this way: When a new study was to be conducted under
the auspices of the Southwest Foundation, the affiliate would be notified
so that it might enlist the participation of its clientele. Patients who agreed
to participate in clinical trials were then sent downstairs from the Planned
Parenthood office to another office where the Southwest Foundation "maintained its clinical service." Though a number of studies were carried out, the
one that caused a controversial stir was the Syntex Research Project. First
begun in 1968, this study had the financial support of Syntex Laboratories
(the manufacturer of the birth control pill under investigation) and the US
State Department (through the Agency for International Development); it
also had the approval of the FDA. The man in charge of the project was Dr.
Joseph William Goldzieher, who by one account was a "big name" in the
Texas research community.[149] Hoping to break new ground, Goldzieher
decided to test the pill in new ways, which he did using the double-blind
procedures described at the start of this section. Out of more than seventy
women in the control group, at least six of them found themselves pregnant; although they all thought they were getting the pill, they were not.[150]

Problematic as the outcome was, ethical dilemmas abounded from the
very start of the relationship between the Southwest Foundation and the San
Antonio Planned Parenthood office. First, there was the matter of financial
incentives for the Texas affiliate. According to Guttmacher's report, which

he submitted in June 1971 upon returning from his trip to investigate the situation, in return for patient referrals the local Planned Parenthood received considerable financial support. This ranged from $7,500 to $9,000 a year, an amount that was "not unimportant," to quote the affiliate's treasurer, especially since at one point its total budget was only $30,000.[151]

For the patients, such financial incentives were probably even more important. For example, in return for their participation in the Syntex Research Project, they received the following: a complete medical exam; on-call doctors to "answer questions and evaluate complaints"; free rides for each clinic visit; free contraceptives and the guarantee of a year's additional supply once the project was over; and in the event of blood or urine collections, an undisclosed though apparently generous financial reward. As Guttmacher remarked, the patient was "paid well."[152] Therefore, much as it was for the participants in the Tuskegee Syphilis Study, the chance to get not only free medical supplies but also free medical attention must have mattered greatly to the participants, many of whom were impoverished Latinas.[153]

In terms of patient consent, the ethical quagmire only grew. Before joining the Syntex study, patients were informed of the "investigative nature" of the contraceptive and its "potential side-effects," whereupon they signed consent forms. But when Guttmacher pressed Goldzieher on the matter, what exactly the social workers told patients about the placebo was decidedly fuzzy. According to Guttmacher's report, Goldzieher had given the matter "much thought." At first he thought of using the word "placebo" but decided against it, since he believed it would have "no meaning" to the patients. Then he "toyed with the phrase 'dummy drug,'" but decided against that too because he thought its connection to intelligence inappropriate. Finally, he landed upon the following phrase: "unproved effectiveness," which was then what interviewers used with prospective subjects. Though perhaps technically correct, the message of the phrase hardly conveyed what the chief investigators actually knew: that the method didn't work at all. In fact, had patients heard that the method didn't work they might have reconsidered entering into what was, for all practical purposes, a game of Russian roulette with their reproductive systems. Notably, Goldzieher himself recognized the slipperiness of the phrase, yet he (along with the Syntex Advisory Committee and the FDA) reputedly believed that such a "white lie," combined with the provision of back-up methods, "was merited in view of the scientific gain anticipated from the study," as Guttmacher noted.[154]

To make matters worse, not everyone at the affiliate was happy about these research arrangements. When Guttmacher talked with the local office's executive director, Sara Prero, she reportedly broke down in tears, so stressed she was about this and other developments at the affiliate.[155] Prero also complained bitterly about the use of clinics to assist in clinical investigation programs and was especially critical of Goldzieher's influence over the affiliate's medical advisory board. "Off the record," she reportedly told Guttmacher, she did "not like research in general, and 'never particularly like[d] this one.'" Prero added that the "affiliate's medical committee is too persuasive in selling research to the Board" and believed that the committee is too "impressed with Dr. Goldzieher."[156] Several months after Guttmacher's visit, Prero quit the local affiliate.[157]

By all accounts what happened in San Antonio was an extreme situation, for which the local affiliate (and the organizations with which it chose to work) was largely responsible. But the national Planned Parenthood office also bears some of the blame. The following letter, written more than a decade earlier, demonstrates how. When in March 1958 Nurse Jean L. McNeill, clinic supervisor of a local affiliate in Detroit, Michigan, wrote to Dr. Calderone informing her of the research offer they had recently received from Holland-Rantos, she also had a question. Though she knew that a "number of studies" were being carried out in local clinics elsewhere in the nation, she wanted to make sure her organization was going about things properly and wanted especially to "know more about the Federation's policies" regarding such matters. She enclosed a copy of their offer and said that she would "appreciate any suggestions you may have."[158]

Calderone's reply is revealing. Much of it centered on the publishing and endorsement of the findings of the study; the researcher had the right to publish the findings, and the findings in no way indicated Planned Parenthood's backing of a product. Of course, Calderone also mentioned that the national medical committee would serve as a consultant to those affiliates wanting to engage in research, but she then stressed that it was the local medical advisory board who should investigate matters more thoroughly.[159] In other words, as Calderone's reply suggests, the national office had little concrete advice to offer and said even less about ethical issues—less even than it had said in previous decades. Indeed, while the 1938 standards of clinic certification emphasized the importance of research, it warned clinics not to use patients for "experimental purposes."[160] By 1948, while the emphasis on the need for research remained, the warning against experimentation had been dropped completely. Nor did it appear in the 1956 standards, precisely when research in local clinics was picking up steam.[161]

Complicating matters further, the upsurge of research had come about so quickly and from so many different directions that the federation was caught hopelessly unawares. In fact, even as it worked to rein local offices in—by insisting first in 1956, again in 1963, and then repeatedly thereafter that all its affiliates consult first with its national medical committee before embarking on any new studies—guidelines about the actual process of research itself remained largely undefined.[162] Yet even had the federation developed a concrete set of rules, it is not clear what they would have looked like because this new culture of scientific research was now firmly in place, influencing the affiliates that operated under the federation's direction. A closer look, therefore, at the two nationally sponsored projects described earlier—the Clinical Investigation Program and the 25-Month Club—reveals the models of research practice that were being issued from above.

As soon as CIP and the 25-Month Club began, questions from participating local offices immediately began to pour in to the national office. An affiliate in Georgia, for example, wanted to know how best to approach patients for participation in CIP. In her reply, Calderone said to tell them they ought feel "privileged to try a new product which has been shown to be effective and safe."[163] A similar tone can be heard in the materials sent out to 25-Month Club participants. "Congratulations on your membership in the '25-Month club,'" announced one flier excitedly. "You are one of a select group of over ten thousand women who have joined this program which is sponsored by Planned Parenthood."[164]

Then there were conversations about publicity, which quickly bled into discussions about terminology. The advice the federation gave is illustrative. "It was suggested by the Executive Committee of the Federation," Calderone wrote in a 1959 memo to affiliates participating in CIP, "that the wrong kind of publicity might well damage the program rather than help it." A "newspaper announcement could lay the center open to criticism due to misinterpretation of what clinical testing really means." She explained that a "luncheon meeting" for "carefully selected prospective donors" would be the "most productive" alternative.[165] A similar evasiveness can be found elsewhere in CIP terminology. For example, the name of the program was initially "Official Testing Centers," only to change to Clinical Investigation Program after it began. "CIP, for short," Calderone wrote. "It was felt that the word testing might carry too much of a connotation of experimentation to lay people."[166] Furthermore, it is clear that at least one local office got the message. We named our project "study group," wrote Sherwin Kaufman of a New York affiliate in March 1963, so as to be "less frightening to the patient." Calderone replied, "I agree," and added that it was "good terminology."[167]

But it was the topic of patient consent that provoked the most persistent questions within the organization. So often had this matter come up that the federation felt compelled to respond in a mass announcement. "We have received a number of inquiries," wrote Guttmacher and Calderone in the spring of 1963, "as to whether or not patients [in the 25-Month Club] should be informed of its study nature." They offered the following advice: "Although we agree that in most instances the patient should be so informed, there will undoubtedly be exceptions, as for instance the woman who might tend to react neurotically, thus possibly distorting the results of the study. In all such cases the judgment of the individual physician should prevail."[168]

For clinic workers, therefore, especially those who had direct contact with the patients, such investigation programs could be burdensome and, even more important, ethically troublesome. That research often mandated a substantial increase in paperwork for each patient—twelve pages for each participant alone in the 25-Month Club—meant more work for clinic workers. The failure to fill out such forms appropriately sparked considerable tension between Planned Parenthood and the pharmaceutical company Searle, which by the mid-1960s wished to abandon the study because of "dissatis[faction] with the quality of the information" clinics were providing.[169]

More work was only part of the problem, though. When faced with the task of combining the aims of the study with the needs of the patient, clinic workers could find themselves in a quandary about which was more important. For example, although the national office promoted patient choice upon her initial participation in CIP, things changed once she was enrolled. "Patients who wish to change products," the federation explained to local offices, "should be discouraged from doing so."[170] A similar thing happened with the 25-Month Club. When Searle introduced a lower-dose oral contraceptive—one that women might find more desirable because of its reduced side effects—the national office expressed concern that it would lose subjects and thereby compromise the project.[171] Worse still was what the Chicago office then told its prospective 25-Month Club participants. After explaining, in the affiliate's patient newsletter, that the program was sponsored by the FDA, it added that the "government requires each woman to answer [the study's] questions if she wishes to continue taking the pill."[172]

Of course, it would be unfair to suggest that the Planned Parenthood organization in its entirety was bent on deceiving its patients or that it was completely unsympathetic to the necessity of consent. That the organization had conversations about informed consent—even coming up by the mid-1960s with a "Patient Information Sheet" (that described the pill) and a "Patient Consent Form" (for prospective study participants on the pill to sign)—reveals at least some concern about the matter.[173] In addition, although Calderone and others seemed often to side with the need for limited disclosure, that their advice simultaneously pointed out the importance of consent suggests some recognition of patients' needs. Other decisions reveal even greater concern about informing patients. For example, when Tietze organized CIP he decided against the more statistically sound "randomization" technique precisely because he felt it wrong to interfere with the ethos of patient choice.[174] Then there were the actions taken by some of the affiliates themselves. St. Louis, for example, abandoned its participation in CIP precisely because the local office believed such work conflicted with the organization's mission of service.[175] Some individuals within the organization sensed the direction the organization was heading and were not happy about it.

Moreover, there is no way of knowing exactly what happened at each and every one of the studies carried out in local clinics. While some patients may have been told very little about the actual nature of the study, others may have been told a great deal. Indeed, the amount of information patients received depended on a variety of factors, not just who was in charge of designing the project, but also what any one of the people who worked in the clinic might have chosen to do regardless of the rules. Indeed, what this book as well as at least one other contemporary account of clinic work has tried to convey is this: controlling everything that happened inside the local clinic was quite simply an impossible task.[176] Equally difficult to control were clinic patients themselves. As was the case with CIP, many simply took matters into their own hands and dropped out.[177]

Nevertheless, despite the inevitable variety among local clinics, the problems posed by what David Rothman described as the "gilded age" of research could not help but make their way inside the clinics. And although research brought with it opportunities that surpassed the wildest dreams of even the smallest affiliates, it simultaneously yielded contradictions in the organization's mission of service to those from impoverished communities. By the early 1970s, then, which brought heightened debates about the ethics of human-subject experimentation, Planned Parenthood realized its new research trend required even more careful scrutiny than ever before—for the protection of its patients *and* for its own protection.

Dealing with Research

As the preceding stories suggest, by the end of the 1960s Planned Parenthood found itself waging battles on a variety of fronts. Some were the product of controversies surrounding the pill, an issue picked up by consumer rights advocates and the feminist-inspired women's health movement. As Elizabeth Watkins described, despite the pill's enormous popularity, questions about its safety regularly popped up, only to erupt in the early 1970s with congressional hearings led by Senator Gaylord Nelson to investigate the matter. As a result, Planned Parenthood found itself fending off an onslaught of criticism for its widespread prescription of the pill in its local clinics.[178] Other matters—such as the feminist outcry against state-sponsored involuntary sterilization programs on poor women of color and, of course, the growing race genocide critique among members of the African American community—only added to the scrutiny Planned Parenthood now faced.[179]

However, for our purposes perhaps the most significant issue was the pressure that was now coming from the rapidly growing movement for informed consent in human-subject research. Its roots were in Dr. Henry Beecher's exposé in the June 1966 issue of the *New England Journal of Medicine,* which uncovered widespread abuse in human experimentation; the movement caught fire in June 1972 when news about the Tuskegee Syphilis Study hit the press. Public outrage was dramatic and quickly led to Senate hearings, lawsuits, and the establishment of institutional review boards to protect the rights of potential subjects.[180] All the while, Planned Parenthood watched with growing uneasiness.

Indeed, throughout the 1960s the federation had been trying to exercise more control over its affiliates, in particular by getting them to register their many research projects with the national medical committee. In 1966, the following memo was sent out by the PPFA's national medical committee: "With the large number of Affiliates currently participating in programs of clinical research, it becomes increasingly important for us to have an accurate central records of these projects." Looking to drive home the significance of this directive, the memo went on to remind them that Planned Parenthood's standards of affiliation "require" that they do so.[181] Hoping to boost the number of affiliates who reported their research activities, the federation began sending out these reminders every six months. It also asked the organization's regional offices, which monitored affiliate work more directly, to serve as its watchdog by reporting to the federation those clinics that failed to register their clinical investigation programs.[182]

But it was only after the revelations of the San Antonio incident in 1971 that the organization took real steps to tighten its research requirements, and even these steps came after much debate. For example, although troubled by the situation, Guttmacher concluded in his investigative report that the local affiliate (and therefore the national office) was not responsible for what happened: "Planned Parenthood of San Antonio has no involvement. If it trusts the Foundation, which it had and has every reason to do, it simply refers to them those patients who volunteer to go to a medically trustworthy alternative organization. Once referred, they cease to be patients of Planned Parenthood."[183] Not everyone shared such sentiments, however. As PPFA staff member Francine Stein vehemently wrote, "As a woman and a loyal staff member, I am angered and frustrated by the whitewash of important issues involved." She criticized the national office for choosing, in its meeting with affiliates to discuss the San Antonio situation, to address only "procedural and organizational matters" rather than what she called "substantive human concerns."[184]

In the coming weeks, Planned Parenthood's national medical committee would in fact meet and review its research requirements, and would ultimately propose a series of stricter rules. In part, it called for more careful review of individual research protocols. If approved, only then could an affiliate engage in the proposed project, a provision that applied both to those projects conducted on site as well as those done elsewhere with referred patients, as was the case with San Antonio. The proposed guidelines also insisted that approval would not be granted until "informed consent had been fully drawn and implemented." However, just how effective these rules would be is open for debate. Fearful about infringing upon local autonomy and reluctant to act as a "policing or disciplinary body," the federation's medical committee chose not to centralize its approval process. As a result, permission for research need not be obtained through the national medical board; it could also be secured through research subcommittees that existed at the local level. Moreover, that Planned Parenthood continued to put the decision-making process largely in the hands of doctors demonstrates its belief that physicians made the best judgments. But even if these medical committees were rigorous in their evaluation process, there was no way of knowing or, for that matter, of making sure. Indeed, just how the organization hoped to enforce these new rules, and what possible punishments might ensue for those found violating them, remained unclear.[185]

And change, of course, rarely occurs quickly, which sparked internal worries about what outsiders might think. A memo dated December 1972, some six months after news of the Tuskegee Syphilis Study hit the press, illustrates this vividly. "Jeannie Rosoff has informally expressed some concern to me," wrote Planned Parenthood–World Population's Chief Executive Officer John C. Robbins to Guttmacher and several other Planned Parenthood representatives, "over the political risk we are running by the unsupervised conduct of research in various affiliates. She is particularly worried about the chances of work coming out in congressional hearings of the conduct of research on depo-provera, 'morning after' injections, and other sophisticated new drugs by affiliates which may fail to give patients due warning about the possible side effects." Robbins then "wonder[ed]" if it was possible to meet to talk about Rosoff's concerns and also to "decide whether we as a Federation should be taking some action to decrease our exposure."[186]

Though what came of his request is not clear, Robbins's words are suggestive. To begin with, they demonstrate how the organization's attempt at self-regulation was in many ways unsuccessful: unsupervised research continued and informed consent remained haphazard. In addition, they also reveal the desire to cover Planned Parenthood's tracks. Indeed, that some members of the organization wanted to make sure that word of its past and present research activities did not leak out to the public again highlights awareness that such work posed grave ethical conflicts. Consequently, for all the organization's attempt at internal self-reform, this too would be a task difficult to carry out. What was needed, therefore, were more stringent guidelines imposed from outside the organization, guidelines that appeared on the horizon with new federally mandated rules designed to provide protections for the subjects of scientific research. Only time would tell what effect these new regulations would have on Planned Parenthood's research practices.

In the meantime, however, it is apparent that Planned Parenthood realized it had gotten into far more than it had bargained for, despite all the benefits that clinical research in the local clinic afforded. In addition to the problems described above, others emerged. For example, one memo issued in September 1970 from the national office to affiliate executive directors reveals that the presence of biomedical research in local clinics was making negotiations "difficult" for the organization in its efforts to secure "malpractice and liability insurance." For this reason, each local office was being asked to fill out and submit an additional four-page questionnaire regarding its research projects.[187] In addition, the organization was also already fending off questions from other inquisitive outsiders who were beginning to wonder what exactly was going on inside Planned Parenthood clinics, as the following situation illustrates.

Upon returning from vacation in the fall of 1969, PPFA's Naomi Gray found an "urgent message" waiting for her from a "Dr. Louis Lomax," probably the noted African American journalist and writer who, among other things, in 1959 interviewed Malcolm X with Mike Wallace for the documentary on the Nation of Islam entitled *The Hate That Hate Produced*. There were two reasons why Lomax wanted to speak to Gray specifically: first, she was in charge of Planned Parenthood affiliates; second, she was African American. The situation, as Gray then explained to PPFA's Douglas Stewart—the black representative who in the previous year had met with the Chicago office's board of directors—was as follows: Lomax was "apparently doing a considerable amount of investigation" into the situation of "two nineteen year old Black students at Hofstra college," whom Lomax said "were placed on . . . [a] pill experimental program at Planned Parenthood of Mineola." While Lomax was concerned about the medical situation of one of the students and the welfare more generally of other "deprived Black and Puerto Rican students," he was also troubled about what this suggested about Planned Parenthood's activities more generally. As Gray explained, "He suspects that if Planned Parenthood is carrying out this kind of activity at Hofstra, Planned Parenthood centers must be doing this in other parts of the country." And this "is part of the research study he is doing."

Judging by the contents of the memo, it is obvious that Lomax's query prompted a flurry of activity within the Planned Parenthood organization. For example, with the help of another woman (Clare Brightman), Gray was in the process of "secur[ing] more information from the Affiliate" in Mineola. Gray also spoke with Planned Parenthood's Dr. George Langmyhr, who agreed to "review the research protocol." Gray then accepted an invitation for a luncheon meeting with Lomax and several other black faculty members in the hope of resolving the situation, a meeting she suggested Stewart also attend. But before this gathering was to take place, Gray thought it might be good if she, Stewart, Brightman, and Langmyhr have "a conference" to discuss "this situation."[188] What became of the luncheon meeting with Lomax is not clear, but his questions obviously rattled a number of people within the Planned Parenthood organization. And within a few short years, the organization more generally would be shaken to its core, first with the internal revelations of the Syntex Study in San Antonio, Texas, and then with the growing federal scrutiny now emerging as a result of the revelations of the Tuskegee Syphilis Study. Thus, for all the benefits that research inside the local clinic afforded, by the early 1970s Planned Parenthood found itself facing a whole new set of issues that would have to be resolved, both to protect its patients and itself.

Dealing with the Effects of Massive Growth and the Reactions to Expanded Services

Meanwhile, back in Chicago even more trouble was brewing. Just when tensions with the black community were beginning to boil over, the local affiliate entered a period of dramatic decline. Consequently, for all the excitement about the affiliate's size in 1965, this was also its peak year, only to be followed by a massive and rapid shift downward. While in 1965 more than twenty thousand women had procured the affiliate's services, by 1970 the number had dropped to just under thirteen thousand. Similarly, although it was still the Chicago office's busiest location, the 63rd Street Center saw its total caseload plummet as well, dropping from just over eight thousand in 1965 to just over five thousand in 1970.[189] Gone too by 1969 was its status as the largest office in the family planning organization; New York City now boasted the greatest number of women served.[190] Finally, the departure of its two main officers was yet another sign of the end of an era. The first to leave was its executive director, Jane C. Browne, whose letter of resignation ironically read, "I hope PPACA will always be in the lead." The second was Dr. Richard Frank, who had served as the affiliate's medical director throughout this period of growth.[191]

The reasons behind its rapid decline are difficult to determine. Perhaps the feelings within the black community contributed. Though still supportive of birth control but fed up with Planned Parenthood, African Americans may have greeted the presence of clinics within their neighborhoods less favorably. The decline in the quality of clinic services, as was the case with the 63rd Street Center, may also have contributed to the affiliate's fall from grace; patients perhaps turned to other places for their birth control needs. Finally, integrated as the Chicago office was, that Planned Parenthood more generally was still not representative of many local communities, nor more responsive to the needs of its minority patients, might also be cause for blame, as Stewart suggested before the Chicago board of directors.[192] More than likely, however, the chief cause of Chicago's decline was the intensity of its growth, which quickly outstripped the organization's administrative capabilities and financial resources. As Carl E. Speckman, a Planned Parenthood regional director, explained, "I believe firmly that many of the Chicago Affiliate's problems have been related to the rapid growth and broadening of its program." Speckman advised the office to seek "objective outside help" in reorganizing its affairs.[193] In an effort to get back on track, the affiliate stripped down its services and embarked on a massive campaign to reorganize its entire program.

The Chicago affiliate was not alone in the tumultuousness of its affairs, however. Despite the excitement of the era, not all was well in the Planned Parenthood organization. So massive was its growth that not only did new problems emerge, but old ones were also exacerbated. Much as before, local affiliates squabbled with the national office over dues. Much as before, local affiliates squabbled with the national office over bureaucracy and standards of affiliation.[194] And much as before, local affiliates squabbled with the national office about the quality of clinic programs. In light of the situation at the 63rd Street Center, the federation had good reason to be alarmed, and it regularly reminded local affiliates that, although expansion was good, it was not to come at the cost of quality of family planning services.[195]

Despite these problems, the work of Planned Parenthood, in particular the events of Chicago and elsewhere in Illinois, remain significant, especially where marital requirements were concerned. Although the organization's policy on this issue was already by the late 1950s in a state of flux, with the Illinois state legislature's 1965 expansion of birth control to unwed welfare recipients, the federation seized the opportunity to broaden its admission requirements even more, in turn encouraging local affiliates to act within state law but "be as liberal as possible in offering services to minors."[196] Of course, not everyone within Planned Parenthood agreed with these changes in marital requirements, and there remained well into the 1970s affiliates across the nation that refused to serve unmarried women, much to the annoyance of the national office.[197] Such pockets of resistance notwithstanding, the shift toward contraceptives for the unwed was undeniably in motion.

Likewise, although the Illinois 1965 IPAC decision began with the welfare recipient, four years later it was followed by legislation that made birth control available to all unwed women in Illinois, regardless of economic circumstances. With this 1969 ruling, Illinois became the first state in the nation to legalize birth control services for unwed minors, a victory about which the Chicago Planned Parenthood was "jubilant," to borrow a term from one internal memo. Having played an important role in this legislative coup, the Chicago office in turn offered to provide legal advice to other affiliates who might wish to do the same in their state.[198] Three years later, however, such lobbying efforts were no longer necessary because *Eisenstadt v. Baird* (1972) made contraceptives for the unmarried a right for all citizens. As a result, one of the cornerstones of the charity clinic movement's original claims to authority had effectively been dismantled. So too one of the nation's laws.

But what of one of the movement's other cornerstones: its opposition to abortion? Much like service to the unwed, abortion services were also beginning to make their way inside local clinics before the federal statutes had changed. But here again it was a muddy and uneven process, setting into motion a whole new set of issues to be battled over and not easily resolved. According to Leslie Reagan, by 1970 Hawaii, Alaska, and New York had decriminalized abortion, and in response women across the nation flocked especially to New York to get what was not legally available in their home states.[199] Meanwhile, and in the days leading up to 1970, Planned Parenthood's national office continued to tread carefully on the issue. As Reagan noted, while PPFA president Guttmacher had long been an advocate for abortion reform, until 1968 he shied away from calling for a repeal of antiabortion laws, seeing this as too radical a position.[200] Even more telling is what the national office said to local affiliates on the matter. As historian Simone Caron explained about the federation's late 1960s policy: "any endorsement" for abortion reform, PPFA reminded them, was to "come from staff members as individuals, not as representatives" of local Planned Parenthood offices.[201]

But by 1970 all of this changed, and the national office adopted a completely different position. In fact, it sprung immediately into action with the publication of a detailed guide intended directly for women called "Legal Abortion: A Guide for Women in the United States." Here women could find explanations about what legal abortion was, why its availability was necessary, how quickly one should get an abortion, how much it cost, and what to do after the procedure. Significantly, it also explained how to arrange for one and then offered a ten-page list of all the Planned Parenthood affiliates that existed across the nation that women could call for "abortion consultation and referral."[202]

Though not surprising, the range of responses from local Planned Parenthood offices to this latest development is striking. Some, of course, had no problem with the shift in policy, leastwise not enough to prevent them from liberalizing their own services. For example, in 1970 Planned Parenthood affiliates in New York seized upon the state's liberal ruling and began providing abortions in their clinics, first in Syracuse and then the Bronx.[203] The Rhode Island office, moreover, set out to establish its own abortion facility immediately following the 1973 passage of *Roe v. Wade.*[204] Others, however, reacted far differently. A survey conducted in 1970 by the national Planned Parenthood office regarding abortion activities at the affiliate level had this to say:

Affiliate attitudes toward abortions seem to differ greatly. Although many states have reformed or liberalized laws, and others, such as Pennsylvania, have laws which permit wide interpretation, many affiliates still act as though abortion is an entirely illicit activity. They scrupulously avoid obtaining names of patients and maintain a cover of secrecy which suggests that they do not conceive of abortion as truly legal.

Hoping to portray the situation more optimistically, the report concluded that "the national picture is confused and uncertain, yet it is not cause for despair. Even though most affiliates need a great deal of help and support in developing pregnancy counseling and abortion referral programs, they have begun to accept these activities as something which they, as Planned Parenthood affiliates, should do."[205]

But such optimism obscures the very real battles that were now being waged at the local level. As Maria Anderson noted in her history of the Houston affiliate, although the local office would eventually come around, "some Board members said they were against abortion and didn't want Planned Parenthood to perform them. Physicians on the Medical Committee were equally cautious and perhaps as divided."[206] No doubt other offices across the nation felt much the same. Consequently, and in the years that followed, there likely persisted a tremendous variety in Planned Parenthood's abortion services—some affiliates offered them (be it on site or through referral) and other affiliates did not—a variety born not just of local laws but also of individual attitudes and the resources affiliates may (or may not) have had at their disposal. Thus, as these two developments suggest—the expansion of contraceptives to the unwed and the provision of abortion—the diversity of the clinic institution of old persisted in the years that followed.

In bringing this chapter to a close, it is worth noting three points in the organization's shift to offer abortion services. The first concerns the ways in which the language of charity could now be used to justify its provision, which stood in stark contrast to the language it formerly used. Of course, the reasons behind Planned Parenthood's desire to challenge the laws against abortion were complex. But, as Reagan argued when describing the secret conference the organization held in 1955 to discuss the issue: part of it was done to "expand the practice of legal therapeutic abortion," part of it was done to "improve public health," but part of it was also to "*lessen the inequality among different classes of women in access to legal abortion and birth control.*" In other words, because of the crackdown on the procedure in the 1940s and 1950s, it was poor women and poor women of color who suffered the most, largely because they lacked the resources that "white and wealthy women" often had.[207] Thus, to provide abortion, and to provide it safely and cheaply to these groups in particular, was increasingly seen by at least some within the organization as an act of humanitarianism and not, as the charity movement once argued, the greedy desire to make money. Further illustrative of this position are the remarks made by Guttmacher at a PPFA–PPWP board of directors meeting held in February 1973, shortly after the *Roe v. Wade* decision. Insisting that Planned Parenthood especially needed to begin offering on-site abortion services (rather than simply rely upon referral or wait for state agencies to fill the need), Guttmacher implored the board to consider the following:

> What opportunity does the poor person have? Does she have equal opportunity for abortion as the affluent? I am not interested in the fact that private practitioners are changing their criteria for doing abortions because the law has changed. My only interest in this is what opportunity does the [poor] woman with the undesired, unplanned and rejected pregnancy have . . . to get the same services that her affluent sister now has attainable. This, I think, is the basis for action. And unless this organization takes a strong stand in this area, I can't believe that we are going to really have a successful program in the United States.

His words were met with applause.[208]

And so, as Guttmacher's remarks suggest, a strikingly new scenario was now in place: just as the provision of the diaphragm was born of the organization's initial desire to democratize what it saw as the rich folk's birth control, the same could now be said about its justification for the provision of abortion. The poor, in other words, had just as much a right to it as anybody else, and as a charity organization it was Planned Parenthood's duty to ensure that even the poorest had access to this often expensive procedure.

The second point worth making in the shift to provide abortion services is that for all that Planned Parenthood did to expand its definition of "birth control" from the narrow construction of the 1930s to a broader concept by the 1960s—that it could be used by the unwed; that it could be openly displayed and discussed; and that it could come from individuals other than physicians, even including commercial vendors—the notion that it was only preventative in function remained firmly in place. Guttmacher's 1969 birth control manual is illustrative. In a chapter entitled "What Birth Control Is—And Isn't," he went through all the various questions people might ask, including:

Is Birth Control Harmful?
Will It Prevent a Woman From Having a Baby When She Wants One?
Will It Interfere with Sex Pleasure?
Is It Illegal?
Is It Expensive?
Is It Immoral?
Is It Like Abortion? [To which the reply was:] No.

As Guttmacher explained, not only was birth control not an "operation," but it also prevented the "union of sperm and egg."[209] Granted, the manual was published four years before *Roe v. Wade*, but the belief that birth control is preventative only in function (thus not abortion) persists today. As Planned Parenthood's online resource (accessed in June 2008) states: "Birth control is a way for people to prevent pregnancy and to plan the timing of pregnancy. Birth control is also commonly called contraception."[210] It is a belief, I would argue, that is widely shared.

The third point worth making concerns what Planned Parenthood's newfound support for abortion also yielded: a new and energized opposition. While in the 1960s threats of violence were voiced and occasionally carried out by some members of the black community—as was the case in Cleveland, Ohio, where black militants burned down a local Planned Parenthood clinic—by the 1980s the violence escalated when it was taken up by some of the members of the newly formed pro-life movement.[211] Notably, it was clinics in particular (be it the facility itself or the people who worked within it) that were the targets of their opposition. As Linda Gordon explained, by the mid-1980s acts of violence spiked, and although they abated briefly by the decade's end, they increased again in the 1990s. The number of incidents, as Gordon described, are striking:

> From 1977 through 2001, 3 doctors, 2 clinic employees, 1 clinic escort, and 1 security guard were murdered. There were also 17 attempted murders, 41 bombings, 165 arson attempts, 82 attempted bombings or arson attacks, and 372 clinic invasions. Threats and acts of vandalism and assault number in the thousands. Anthrax threats have been coming in to clinics for years, including 480 between September 11, 2001, and the end of the year.

Certainly there were many pro-lifers who opposed such violence, choosing instead to express their views through nonviolent means. But even these methods were not without significant effect. Gordon noted that in 1985 80 percent of abortion clinics were picketed. This made patients especially vulnerable as they tried to enter or leave the facility. Staff members were also affected. As Gordon explained, "Harassment included picketing the homes of staff members, tracing patients' license plates, jamming telephone lines, sending hate mail, vandalism, and mass scheduling of fake appointments."[212] So here in this latest development, it was the clinic institution that stood at the frontline in the new battlefield over reproductive rights, and Planned Parenthood (be it at the national level or the local) would have to devise new strategies in order to protect those facilities that provided abortion services and the women they served.

As all these developments suggest, by the early 1970s Planned Parenthood found itself facing a whole new set of circumstances. And how it would negotiate them, in what was now a completely different social, political, economic, cultural, moral, legal, medical, and scientific landscape, is a story that has only begun to be written. But if history is any guide, the strategies the organization would propose would be intimately bound up with the themes I have described throughout this book: the malleable relationship between business and charity, the malleable definition of birth control, and the guerilla-style flexibility of the form and function of the local birth control clinic.

Conclusion

When I began this book I was haunted by suspicions and fearful of my conclusions; now that I have reached the conclusion, I know why. The stakes are indeed great. The three themes I laid out in the introduction—the malleable relationship between business and charity, the malleable definition of birth control, and the guerilla-style flexibility of the form and function of the local birth control clinic—remain as salient in recent decades as they did in the past, and the anxiety I felt about their implications gnaws even more deeply. Much as before, charity and business continue to intersect, and the language and practice of each continue to be deployed as tools of power. Much as before, the birth control clinic remains in a state of flux, its form and function the subject of much debate. Much as before, the very definition of birth control continues to defy fixed boundaries; its many *potential* meanings remain persistently at the heart of battles over reproductive rights. With Planned Parenthood's newly incorporated abortion services serving as a guide, what follows is a brief tracing of the ways these three themes have since the early 1970s played themselves out—though not without an appreciation of the similarities they have with the lessons of the past.

After years of telling local offices to move beyond the establishment of clinics, by the 1960s and 1970s the national Planned Parenthood office had come back around to the local clinic view. It did so in part because it saw that the need for contraceptive services remained unmet, but also because it realized that the clinic was the organization's main source of authority and power, and that its methods and message should be followed. With the incorporation of abortion into Planned Parenthood's official services, the emphasis on the clinic took on even greater urgency. In fact, it is hard to miss just how important the local clinic was to the national office. The plans set forth by Guttmacher, Robbins, and others at the 1973 PPFA–PPWP board of directors meeting (mentioned briefly at the end of the previous chapter) illustrate this well. According to Guttmacher, although abortion was now legal, there were still a number of problems to be addressed, which the "free-standing [abortion] clinic" would do much to resolve. First, there was still "tremendous resistance" within the medical profession to the procedure. Second, municipal hospitals had done little to prepare themselves and did not seem "willing to take their rightful burden" in making abortion available. Third, local affiliates seemed to be dragging their feet on the matter, preferring to send women elsewhere rather than provide the procedure themselves. Fourth, poor women especially needed access to abortion because the possibility of "financial discrimination" was great. And fifth, great efforts were being made to overturn the recent Supreme Court rulings that had made abortion legal. "The only cushion we have," Guttmacher implored, "is to rapidly implement a non-discriminatory, inexpensive [and] safe abortion policy for each and all our large communities."[1] And at the center of this plan, of course, was the local freestanding abortion clinic.

The role the national office envisioned for itself at this meeting in determining and then dictating the new policy to Planned Parenthood affiliates was substantial, and board member Robbins then laid out everything that was being planned for local offices. First, each local office had already been sent a summary of the recent Supreme Court ruling and would soon receive the full transcript. Second, "safe standards" of abortion procedures were also being devised, as were rules "for the overseeing, the inspection, [and] the approving of abortion facilities." Third, a model law for state legislatures was also being crafted, one that asserted the authority of "licensed physicians" over the abortion procedure. Fourth, each affiliate would also be encouraged to learn how to set up and run an abortion clinic of its own, using as its model the affiliates in New York City who were already performing the procedure. Fifth, local offices were also to establish "pilot" clinics in their own communities so as to serve as the model to others within their given locales. Finally, the national office would do what it could to help finance the establishment of these new freestanding abortion clinics by way of an abortion loan fund. Of course, all of this would depend on how much money the federation could raise. But Robbins was hopeful that Planned Parenthood would be able "to sell the major financing institutions in the field of fertility control on the importance of abortion programs" so that Planned Parenthood could "exert the sort of leadership that ought to be exerted in this field."[2]

Guttmacher's and Robbins's words are thus remarkably telling, and they make evident the significance of the clinic while at the same time hinting at future problems to come. For example, much as was the case with efforts to make the diaphragm available in the early decades of the twentieth century, a lot had to be done in the 1970s with the legalization of abortion: doctors needed to be won over; local hospitals and state agencies had to get involved; New York was to serve as the model; clinics needed to be established; and the charity birth control movement would have to establish and exert its authority in these matters, using its clinics as the model for others to follow. But much as before, one can already hear the rumblings of disagreement and discontent. Certainly there were local offices that no doubt appreciated this top-down guidance. As PPFA's Susan Dickler noted in a 1971 memo when the organization was still engaging primarily in abortion referral, "Since the National Abortion Service program was established, the single most insistent request from affiliates has been for a list of 'approved' clinics."[3] So desperate were some affiliates to know who the good providers were and were not that they even took matters into their own hands to find out. As Simone Caron explained about the Planned Parenthood in Rhode Island, its board members "traveled to [abortion] clinics to ensure their safety," only to be "disappointed by the disparity among them."[4]

But this top-down approach meant that the national office was not only telling local affiliates what to do but also narrowly defining what constituted appropriate abortion providers and appropriate abortion facilities. Without a doubt, the desire to protect women was part of the motivation, and the need for standards and supervision was great, as evidenced by what members of the Rhode Island Planned Parenthood found. But it was also strategic. Indeed, when it was suggested at the 1973 PPFA–PPWP board of directors meeting that it might be wise to use vaguer language in describing who could perform abortions, Guttmacher saw this proposal as completely ill advised. "The best way to turn [physicians] off," Guttmacher countered, "is to suggest that somebody else can do the job. Let's get the doctors lined up first and then perhaps we can make some accommodations."[5] And so, much as was the case in the 1930s—when the charity movement looked to win the support of the medical profession by placing both birth control and birth control clinics squarely into the hands of physicians—the same could be said of its decision to ensure that abortion and abortion clinics remained in the hands of doctors in the early 1970s. To the national Planned Parenthood, the doctor-run charity clinic and the services provided therein still served as a powerful tool in winning the right allies and legitimating the cause.

But this mission quickly became complicated. To begin with, incorporating on-site abortion services was no easy task. For example, when the Planned Parenthood in Rhode Island set out in 1973 to establish its own abortion clinic, it found itself at odds with the local health department, whose job now was to regulate this newly legalized medical procedure. Consequently, if the Rhode Island affiliate was to receive approval from the state, it had first to satisfy a number of stringent and costly new regulations. As Caron described them, "an anesthesiologist must be present, the operating room must be equipped for abdominal surgery, blood must be stored, and death certificates must be filed." If local organizers were to achieve these new standards, a new building would have to be found, which ultimately was done. But lost in this particular case was the clinic's guerrilla-style flexibility of old because with the incorporation of abortion, accommodating the rules had become far more expensive and complex.[6]

Also at risk was a pool of clinic workers and a base of financial support. As Caron noted in describing the Rhode Island affiliate's efforts, the problems they encountered in meeting state regulations were only the beginning. Other problems quickly emerged. The new residents at the local hospital didn't want to work there; the several doctors who had agreed to provide abortions backed out; and according to PPFA's Francine Stein when she visited in 1975, "the staff verbalized dread, fear, even nervous flippancy about abortion." In addition, at least one prospective intern was affected. Although the intern wanted to work at the local affiliate, she was hesitant to do anything that involved abortion. In the end, the Rhode Island office was able to open its clinic and offer quality services, but Caron put it well when she said: "Supporting abortion in the abstract was easier than providing abortions to women."[7] Of course, the national Planned Parenthood office was not oblivious to such concerns, and there were discussions about the potential "loss of local supporters if abortions [we]re provided inside" Planned Parenthood clinics.[8] After all, many supporters likely still clung fast to what had long been Planned Parenthood's mission: the establishment of contraceptive clinics so as to prevent the need for abortion—not to make it available.

By the 1980s, moreover, it was precisely the clinic's power and visibility that motivated a number of pro-lifers to seize upon the clinic idea themselves, as a way to use it for their own ends. As a result, pregnancy alternative clinics appeared all over the place. In some cases, the name of the clinic made its pro-life mission clear. The Life Clinic, for example, operated briefly in North Dakota.[9] But more often than not the names chosen (such as Pregnancy Problem Center or Crisis Pregnancy Center) were intended to confuse women who might think they were getting help in securing an abortion, when in fact they were not. As three women who attended such clinics in three different cities described their experiences, they checked in, got a pregnancy test, and then were shown graphic antiabortion slide shows.[10] Other strategies further blurred the boundaries between pro-choice and pro-life clinics. Not only were these antiabortion clinics often in close proximity to abortion-providing clinics, but they could also be found side-by-side in the Yellow Pages under "clinic" or "abortion clinics."[11] Such tactics were hardly accidental. "We need our centers to look like the abortion clinics," said Robert J. Pearson, whose organization (the Pearson Foundation) helped establish a number of antiabortion clinics, "in order to reach people."[12] It was an idea that quickly caught on. As Linda Gordon noted, by 1988 somewhere between eight hundred to two thousand such facilities were in operation across the United States.[13]

Significantly, the presence of these antiabortion facilities reminds us of the birth control clinic's malleability and that the desire to contain its function and its mission was still a source of much conflict, not just within Planned Parenthood but also beyond its doors. For example, when Faye Ginsburg, in her 1989 study of the abortion debate in North Dakota, put quotation marks around the word "clinic" when describing one of these pro-life facilities, I could not help but be reminded of what the charity movement did back in the 1930s: it too put quotation marks around the names of those irregular facilities whose practices it abhorred, precisely because it wanted to call into question their legitimacy.[14] Without a doubt, these pro-life groups are not to be commended in their efforts to deceive women as to the services provided in their clinics. But in light of this larger history, I would be hard-pressed to agree with the claim that they were *not* clinics. It was a semantic slipperiness, moreover, that these pro-lifers understood well. In fact, there is something to be said for their defense of the decision to advertise their services in the Yellow Pages under "clinic." Opponents of this practice, like the director of the PPFA office in Washington, argued that because they didn't offer medical services or that their staff lacked medical training, the advertisement was false, that it was no clinic. The organizers of these pro-life facilities immediately countered the charge of illegitimacy. "It's absolutely ridiculous," argued Curtis J. Young, whose organization operated a number of these facilities. "If you look up 'Clinic' in the Yellow Pages, there are many nonmedical agencies or businesses in there."[15] Young had a point. The idea of a clinic is a broad one, and while a clinic often operates as a medical facility, this is hardly its only manifestation.

Furthermore, equally difficult to contain is the meaning of birth control, especially the line drawn between birth control (contraception) and abortion; it persistently underpins battles over reproductive rights today. For example, when President Bush announced in 2008, shortly before he left office, the new "conscientious objection" requirement—which stipulated that any agency that wanted funds through the Department of Health and Human Services "must certify in writing that none of its employees are required to assist in any way with any medical services they find objectionable"[16]—the liberal political action group MoveOn.org had this to say in a petition drive against the requirement:

> Birth control is NOT abortion. Can you imagine living in a place where birth control is considered an "abortion" and health insurers won't cover it? Where even rape victims are denied emergency contraception? It seems unbelievable, but the Bush Administration is quietly trying to redefine "abortion" to include birth control.[17]

So, much as was the case in the 1930s, while opponents of reproductive rights look to make the line between contraception and abortion more fuzzy, supporters look to make it more distinct.

Interestingly enough, conservatives aren't necessarily wrong. The pill, for example, and other methods like it that have estrogen and progestin in their chemical composition (like emergency contraceptive pills, also known as morning-after pills or Plan B), may indeed have abortifacient capacities: that is, if one views the start of life at fertilization—which I would argue many do (just ask the lawmakers in Missouri who in August

2010 passed a bill saying as much)—and not implantation, which is the official medical line.[18] This distinction is crucial because the truth is that scientists aren't exactly sure how these methods work. As a result, medical handbooks like *Contraceptive Technology* have over the years listed a variety of possible effects, not the least of which is that "implantation is inhibited." In fact, the language found in the fifteenth (1990–92) and nineteenth (2007) editions of *Contraceptive Technology* suggests how great the stakes are in differentiating between the possible contraceptive and abortifacient capabilities of the pill and emergency contraceptive pills. For example, the fifteenth edition unequivocally states that "implantation is inhibited" or "hampered" when describing the various mechanisms of action for the two main ingredients of the pill: estrogen and progestin. Likewise, when talking about emergency contraceptive pills, this same edition states: "Presumably, high-dose estrogens work primarily by preventing implantation of the blastocyst [the fertilized egg] in the endometrium."[19]

However, with the more recent nineteenth edition, definitions get decidedly more fuzzy, defensive, and shrouded in scientific language. Now when describing the various mechanisms of action for the pill, they are placed into two different categories: those "that have been repeatedly *proven*" and those that "have never been substantiated," under which the "inhibit[ion] of implantation" now falls. The murkiness grows with its discussion of emergency contraceptive pills. It begins by saying that "some studies" have drawn the conclusion "that [it] may act by impairing endometrial receptivity to implantation of a fertilized egg." But it follows up by saying that "other more recent studies have found no such effects on the endometrium." The advice the manual then offers medical practitioners about what to tell women about the various methods available takes an even more slippery slope:

> To make an informed choice, women must know that ECPs [emergency contraceptive pills]—like all regular hormonal contraceptives such as the birth control pill, Implanon, Evra, NuvaRing, and Depo-Provera, and even like the lactational amenorrhea method—may prevent pregnancy by delaying or inhibiting ovulation, inhibiting fertilization, or inhibiting implantation of a fertilized egg in the endometrium. At the same time, however, all women should be informed that the best available evidence is consistent with the hypothesis that Plan B's ability to prevent pregnancy can be fully accounted for by mechanisms that do not involve interference with post-fertilization events.[20]

So clearly the jury is still out on the matter, despite Planned Parenthood's unequivocal disclaimer on its website: "You might have also heard that the morning after pill causes an abortion. But that's not true. The morning after pill is not the abortion pill. Emergency contraception is birth control, not abortion."[21] Of course, Planned Parenthood is right in saying that Plan B is not the abortion pill; that's RU-485. But this doesn't mean that it *might* not have abortifacient capabilities. That would depend on how the method actually worked in preventing a particular pregnancy and how one chooses to define the start of life.

Hence the pill and the morning-after pill *could* at times be abortifacients; hence birth control *might* occasionally terminate a pregnancy, rendering false, or at least muddy, the liberal line that birth control is definitely NOT an abortion. This hardly translates into a conservative victory, however. To the contrary, the many pro-life believers who continue to use such methods as the pill (which I suspect more than a few do) would have to reckon with this possibility as well. Indeed, if they believe life begins at fertilization, they will have to draw some uncomfortable conclusions about the possibilities embedded in their *own* birth control practices—whether they take the pill themselves or engage in intercourse with somebody who does—because they may not be in keeping with their pro-life views.

Finally, also reignited with Planned Parenthood's decision to offer abortion services were the old arguments about the benevolence of charity versus the evils of business. Without a doubt, the desire to engage in charitable abortion services was an important and compassionate motivation for Planned Parenthood, especially when situated within marketplace contexts. For example, when the national Planned Parenthood office proposed the mass establishment of freestanding abortion clinics in the early 1970s, part of its mission, as PPFA's Fred Jaffe explained, was "to bring the price [of abortion] down."[22] Thus, the goal was to make clear to all those who would make abortion available that it was not simply a commodity to sell. Rather, as Jaffe argued, it was a social need to be met.[23] Such a motivation also prompted those at the affiliate level. As Caron explained regarding Rhode Island's new abortion facility, although the local office had already been interested in establishing a freestanding abortion clinic, it wasn't until another group proposed opening its own—a group that the local affiliate believed was interested only in making a profit—that Rhode Island quickly sprung into action. It then justified its efforts with familiar language: a "freestanding clinic at PPRI," Caron paraphrased, "would offer lower cost and a more sympathetic atmosphere."[24] Hence only through charity could compassionate benevolence be assured.

Given that for-profit abortion clinics quickly emerged in the wake of liberalized abortion laws, Planned Parenthood's desire for vigilance is understandable. A study published in 1984 by Michael Goldstein on the rise of such facilities in Los Angeles shortly after California relaxed its abortion laws in the late 1960s is instructive. Looking at twelve physician entrepreneurs who owned or operated such clinics, Goldstein found among them a distinct set of entrepreneurial attitudes and practices. In short, they thought and behaved like businessmen: abortion was "a commodity," it was a means of "amassing great wealth," and "owning the means of mass production" was essential if you wanted to control the price and competition. Equally sugges-tive are the remarks made by one of these physician entrepreneurs:

> The whole point was to do as many as possible, back to back. Most guys couldn't line up one a day. But if you could line up say 40 a day you could pay him 20 bucks each, not the 200 he was getting for his one. Still, he'd wind up way ahead and you'd get rich. There was even money in it for the hospital. If you owned the hospital, so much the better.
>
> You got guys for 15 dollars each. You did maybe 15 to 18 an hour, especially on Saturdays—that was the biggest day. It was an assembly line. You couldn't slow down or take a break. Guys didn't like it, but tough shit. There were plenty willing to take your place. Two hundred and fifty bucks an hour wasn't bad in 1970.[25]

The fear, of course, for organizations like Planned Parenthood was that peo-ple like this would do whatever they could to make a buck, even it if meant compromising quality services and risking women's lives.

But not all physician entrepreneurs thought like this. Another spoke both of his skill in performing the procedure and his ethics. "We did high-qual-ity work—very good, very fast." But when "the others wanted to do salines [abortions during the second and third trimesters which require that a dead fetus be delivered through labor]," he drew a line. "I couldn't see that as a business like the others could." He then opened his own clinic with another doctor, explaining that only then could we "do it the way we wanted to."[26] In addition, other physician entrepreneurs found themselves ostracized not only by their physician peers but also their "ideological colleagues in the abortion movement." As one (who was a long supporter of abortion rights) lamented, "I had sacrificed everything, my income, my life for a cause"— only to be accused of being a "mercenary." Admittedly, he then "showed them about being mercenary" and amassed a tidy sum, which he was happy to rub in their faces.[27] But his point remains: because he did abortions for a living, even those who supported abortion rights had a problem with the source of his income. What they wanted instead was a clear line of division between those who provided abortions for charitable or compassionate rea-sons (which were good) and those who did so for financial reasons (which were bad).[28]

Again, though, business and charity practices are not so easily compart-mentalized. Planned Parenthood itself could not help but be drawn into the marketplace, both in ideas and practice. For example, some within the organization quickly seized upon the economic opportunities that provid-ing abortion might yield. The Rhode Island affiliate is illustrative. When staff members broke down the numbers for its abortion clinic—planning to charge $150 per abortion with the assumption that "15 percent would be unable to pay"—they went ahead with their plans anyway because it still ensured a healthy profit (more than one hundred thousand dollars), which they would then use to cover other expenses. "No one mentioned the irony," Caron wryly remarked, "of PPRI's earlier criticism" of the profit-oriented motive of the other group who also wanted to make abortion available.[29] Furthermore, economic difficulties followed closely behind. Despite Rhode Island's projections, they made far less than they hoped, a result of unanticipated expenses and a small abortion load.[30]

Others within Planned Parenthood saw right away the potential fiscal problems that offering abortion services might generate and chose another path. This was the case with the Atlanta affiliate. Originally, the local office had planned to open its own abortion clinic, but (interestingly enough) the 1973 Supreme Court ruling complicated its plans. As Mr. McCroskey, the affiliate president, explained at the 1973 board of directors meeting: although he believed the ruling was a better law because of the "complete freedom" it allowed, he feared what might ensue. Not only did it fail to "regulat[e]" what constituted "the first trimester," it also failed to regulate "the delivery of abortion services" during this undefined time. The end result, McCroskey argued, was that abortion would be "a much more competitive situation" and thereby "a much more risky situation financially." Consequently, instead of opening "a full range fertility management center," the Atlanta Planned Parenthood opted simply to "retain control of the referrals." This way, McCroskey reasoned, the affiliate could both control the "quality and the place of delivery of such services" while at the same time remaining fiscally responsible, an important consideration since New York clinics were reputedly operating at a financial loss in making the procedure available.[31]

This brings us back to those for-profit abortion facilities. Although it is not clear if the Atlanta affiliate turned to for-profit abortion clinics, at least some local Planned Parenthoods relied upon them, a source of referrals that physician entrepreneurs eagerly sought out. As one of them explained, "We wanted the Planned Parenthood business. You see, we wanted to give the community what it wanted and needed—good services for a reasonable cost." For this reason, controlling the means of production, which usually meant controlling the hospital in which the abortion services were provided, was essential in achieving this goal. As this physician entrepreneur explained, "Otherwise we could never do the numbers we needed and keep the costs down to what PP was willing to pay."[32] Thus Planned Parenthood was at least early on deeply enmeshed with for-profit entrepreneurs. Not only did it participate in the for-profit abortion trade by referring its patients to these facilities, but its demand for low-cost services indirectly contributed to the assembly lines practices at the facilities.

Of course, Planned Parenthood is hardly alone in taking this slippery slope. Pro-lifers do so as well. On the one hand, they regularly seize upon images of Planned Parenthood as a profit-making abortion mill as a way to discredit its reputation[33]—a strategy, worth remembering, the charity clinic movement used when discrediting its rivals in the 1930s. In addition, the language pro-lifers use to describe abortion clinics is deliberately intended to evoke illicit commercialism. As such, they regularly refer to them as "convenience stores," "7-11s," and "stop and chops." As Ginsburg noted, the goal is to "equat[e] abortion with undesirable commercial establishments," again not too unlike what the charity clinic movement did back in the 1930s.[34] On the other hand, pro-lifers are not immune from competitive practices themselves, nor shy about using the language of business to rationalize their strategies and goals. For example, not only did the organizers of the Life Clinic steal the name from a competing pro-life organization,[35] but the organizer of another pregnancy alternative center explained his activities in this way: "There's no crime in [making our clinics look like abortion facilities]. We're competing with them. It's like a Wendy's locating next to a McDonalds."[36]

The slipperiness of the language of business can be found elsewhere. Recent developments with Wal-Mart pharmacies illustrate how. When in 2004 the chain store refused to make Plan B (the morning-after pill) available in its pharmacies, the Planned Parenthood in Massachusetts brought a lawsuit against them for violating state law. The company lost and relented, ultimately agreeing to make the method available in its stores across the nation. Significant here is the language Wal-Mart used to justify its various positions. When asked why the company was initially opposed, its spokesperson had this to say: "it was purely a 'business decision,' . . . based on their assessment . . . demand for the product was not very high."[37] Several months later, though, when the company gave in, one of its rationales went like this: "the majority of Wal-Mart customers are women, and [they] would appreciate having it available."[38] Consequently, much as was the case with the language of charity, the language of business and consumption could be used to justify two radically different political positions. And so the story goes, which is all the more reason why so much more needs to be written about the meanings attached to business, the meanings attached to charity, and the conclusions we are to draw from each.

In bringing this book to a close, it seems appropriate to end with the words of one of the Illinois Planned Parenthood clinic workers (whom I had the good fortune to meet and interview) that tap directly into another of the main threads of this study: the shifting significance of the birth control clinic within the Planned Parenthood organization. We spoke on September 3, 1998, less than a week after my fateful visit to the archives of the AMA. She told me many stories from her roughly forty years working in the local Planned Parenthood clinic. But after describing how clinic services had in recent years improved, she stopped herself to note the irony of the situation. "It's interesting that I say that because the medical clinic [has gone] down on the rung." I pressed her to explain what she meant. "Well," she replied, "have you been in the building?" "Yeah," I said, "the second floor is quite large." She then pointed out the significance of my observation. "There's a little corner on the first floor that is the medical clinic. And they never take anybody down there." So not only was the clinic small, but it also apparently lacked the cachet of its former days, in that it was now tucked away in a corner where nobody would see it. As she noted, there is "great emphasis now on legislation," "public relations," and "education"—which she saw as "good," particularly the education part. But it was still a shift she found deeply disheartening. Her words suggested that there was no longer a feeling at Planned Parenthood that the clinic was the main source of pride, nor was there a belief that clinic operations should be the focus of the affiliate's efforts.[39]

In looking back on what she said, I'm struck by the familiarity of her lament but also curious about what had happened in recent years. Although there were times (for example, during the 1940s and 1950s) when the national office saw the establishment of clinics as an old-fashioned goal, insisting instead that local organizers focus their efforts elsewhere, those at the local level remained undeterred. The clinic was, after all, the physical manifestation of their more abstract ideals. The clinic was their pride and joy, their crown jewel in the glorious necklace of birth control clinics Margaret Sanger herself had once envisioned. It is notable, therefore, that by the 1960s and 1970s the national Planned Parenthood office had come back around to this local point of view. Indeed, to this day the local clinic clearly remains a powerful tool within the organization. In 2010 the number of Planned Parenthood clinics that exist nationwide suggest a robust movement; more than eight hundred birth control clinics operate across the nation, governed by more than eighty local affiliates.[40]

But clearly the role of the clinic remains a source of persistent contention. For this reason, I think often of the Illinois Planned Parenthood clinic worker's lament: although medical services had in recent years improved, the clinic institution itself had somehow fallen from grace within the organization. As a result, despite what the numbers might suggest, her words remind us to give her perspective careful thought and consideration. Although I have no idea how many others might have shared her views or how accurate her assessment was, I can imagine all sorts of possibilities that might explain what she observed. Perhaps in this new era of abortion services, the clinic was kept hidden as a way to minimize opposition; perhaps it was kept hidden to minimize the violence of potential opponents; perhaps too the clinic's association with abortion made it illicit, something that needed to be kept out of view. But perhaps it had nothing to do with abortion. Perhaps those other strategies the Illinois clinic worker mentioned—like public relations, legislation, and education—all held greater appeal to the younger generation of Planned Parenthood workers who, unlike the generations that preceded them, did not share in the view that the establishment of local clinics was the primary goal. But I simply do not know, which is all the more reason why I hope others will carry on the research concerning the many meanings attached to charity and business, the many definitions given to birth control, the many forms and functions of the local birth control clinic, and (what I hope the preceding pages have also made abundantly clear) the many thousands of voices embedded within the Planned Parenthood Federation of America.

Notes

Introduction

1. Tone, "Contraceptive Consumers," 485–506. These findings are now in Tone, *Devices and Desires*, in particular chapter 7.

2. John Asa Gibbons to the editors of the *Journal of the American Medical Association*, June 15, 1924, Birth Control, folder 7, box 85, Historical Health Fraud and Alternative Medicine Collection, American Medical Association Archives, American Medical Association Building, Chicago, IL (hereafter cited as HHFAMC). Courtesy of American Medical Association Archives. Gibbons practiced in Mitchell, Indiana. See *American Medical Directory* (1925), 567.

3. Though I am not certain, the book was likely *Birth Control Methods*, which was written by Bocker and published by Sanger's Clinical Research Bureau in New York City in 1924.

4. See, for example, Gordon, *Woman's Body*, 156–59. Hereinafter all future references to Gordon's *Woman's Body* will come from her recently retitled, revised, and updated edition, *The Moral Property of Women*. For another example, see Reed, *From Private Vice to Public Virtue*, 143–48, where Reed described the medical profession's hostility to Sanger and contraceptive research.

5. Sometimes the message is explicit, as evidenced by the following quote from Gordon. The "contraceptive industry of the 1930s was an extreme, if inevitable, example of commercial exploitation of popular ignorance" (*Moral Property of Women*, 313). A similar message can be found in Maria H. Anderson's local study of Planned Parenthood in Houston, Texas; words like "dangerous," "manipulative," and "brutal" appear throughout her description of the 1930s marketplace ("Private Choices vs. Public Voices," 26). At other times the message is subtler; local charity birth control clinics are described as the only source of "safe and affordable birth control" (see Lindenmeyer, "Expanding Birth Control to the Hinterland," 145–46). Or, as Marianne Leung noted in her study of the birth control clinic movement in Arkansas, "There was plenty of information available concerning different birth control methods, but few of the methods commercially promoted were effective and some were actually quite harmful" ("Better Babies" [1996], 153). Two important exceptions are Tone's more business-friendly *Devices and Desires* and Sarch, "Those Dirty Ads!" (thanks to Mickey Moran for bringing the Sarch piece to my attention). However, even Tone occasionally falls into the marketplace as evil trap, particularly when describing the commercial birth control clinics of the 1930s (see 166–69).

6. As evidenced, for example, by the ties the birth control movement forged more formally with the eugenics movement and the less formal but equally explicit racist and elitist rationales often found among clinic organizers. See Gordon, *Moral Property of Women*, 177–79, 190–203, 212–20, and 233–41. Such ties and motivations

continue to be the subject of considerable historiographic debate. For example, while McCann, *Birth Control Politics*, looked to soften the eugenic rationale, Roberts, *Killing the Black Body*, especially chapter 2, did not. Local clinic studies have regularly addressed this issue as well. For a complete list of these studies, see note 13.

7. Hall, *Inventing the Nonprofit Sector*, 1–2. For another example of the malleability of business, see Kwolek-Folland's discussion about how, when incorporating women into the history of business, one is forced to reconfigure notions of "business" and "entrepreneurship"; in *Incorporating Women*, especially the introduction.

8. For a discussion of the ways in which the middle class sought to assist only the "worthy poor," see Rosenberg, "Social Class and Medical Care in Nineteenth-Century America." For a discussion of "deserving mothers," see Ladd-Taylor, *Mother-Work*. Here she described the distinction made by Progressive-era welfare reformers between the "deserving" mothers who earned their assistance and the "lazy" ones who did not. For examples of the ways in which colonialist attitudes complicated Westerners' desire to "uplift the uncivilized," see Mohanty, "Under Western Eyes"; Briggs, *Reproducing Empire*; and Jacobs, *White Mother to a Dark Race*.

9. Joseph, *Against the Romance of Community*, viii.

10. Ertman and Williams, *Rethinking Commodification*, 4–5.

11. Tone, "Contraceptive Consumers," 501. Brief mentions, almost in passing, can be found in Gordon, *Moral Property of Women*, 225; and Anderson, "Private Choices vs. Public Voices," 26. A similar situation can be found with the commercialization of marijuana and head shops in the 1970s. However, what resulted in this case was a crackdown rather than a loosening of the law—unlike the situation with contraceptives in the 1930s. See Davis, "The Business of Getting High."

12. For an examination of the intersection between business and voluntarism, see Rosemary Steven's historical analysis of the twentieth-century American hospital, *In Sickness and In Wealth*.

13. For the early local birth control clinic more generally, see Cathy Moran Hajo's study of more than six hundred clinics across the nation, *Birth Control on Main Street*. For local birth control histories (of a specific affiliate or birth control more generally within a specific region), see the following. For Arkansas, see Leung, "Better Babies" (1996) and (1994). For Cincinnati, Ohio, see Lindenmeyer, "Expanding Birth Control to the Hinterland." For Cleveland, Ohio, see Meyer, *Any Friend of the Movement*. For Massachusetts, see Rosen, *Reproductive Health, Reproductive Rights*, chapter 4. For Minnesota, see Losure, "Motherhood Protection." For Nashville, Tennessee, see Turner, "Class, Controversy, and Contraceptives." For New York, see Rosen, "The Shifting Battleground for Birth Control." For North Carolina within a national context, see Schoen, *Choice and Coercion*. For Puerto Rico, see Briggs, *Reproducing Empire*, especially chapters 3 and 4; and Schoen, *Choice and Coercion*, 202–16. For Rhode Island, see Nicholl and Weisbord, "The Early Years of the Rhode Island Birth Control League"; and Caron, *Who Chooses?* For Houston, Texas, see Anderson, "Private Choices vs. Public Voices." For Waco, Texas, see Hulett, "Every Child a Wanted Child." For discussion of early clinic building within the black community, see Rodrique, "The Black Community and the Birth Control Movement." For an international perspective of the birth control movement, see Connelly, *Fatal Misconceptions*. In this list, the only studies of specific birth control league affiliates that took their stories to the present are the two that documented birth control groups in

Texas (by Anderson and Hulett) and Caron, *Who Chooses?*, which offered an overview of the history of birth control in America from 1830 to the present, using the Rhode Island Planned Parenthood as a case study. None, however, examined the birth control clinic institution specifically over time.

14. Gordon, *Moral Property of Women*, 138–39.

15. Ibid., 128.

16. For the history of patent medicine peddlers, see James Harvey Young's classic, *Toadstool Millionaires*.

17. For a quick introduction to the major themes of and historiographic debate about the Progressive era, see Rodgers, "In Search of Progressivism." Missing in his discussion, however, is the role of women in Progressive-era reform and their "maternalist" impulse. For this feature of Progressive-era reform, see, for instance, Hoy, "Municipal Housekeeping"; Koven and Michel, "Womanly Duties"; Ladd-Taylor, *Mother-Work*; and Curry, *Modern Mothers in the Heartland*.

18. On the institution of the clinic as it emerged in the twentieth century, there is already a rich body of scholarship. For several discussions of these early clinics more generally, see Starr, *The Social Transformation of American Medicine*, 191–97; and Rosen, *The Structure of American Medical Practice*, 32–36, 50–51, and 97–98. Many others have focused on specific types of clinics. For example, on well-baby clinics, see Curry, *Modern Mothers in the Heartland*, 18, 36, 47, 57, and 126; on social hygiene/venereal disease clinics, see Brandt, *No Magic Bullet*, 43–45, and 142–47; and Batza, "Before AIDS." On abortion clinics as they operated in the 1930s, see Reagan, *When Abortion Was a Crime*, chapter 5.

19. Morantz-Sanchez, *Sympathy and Science*. For another example of this nineteenth-century philosophy among women physicians, see Drachman, *Hospital with a Heart*.

20. For more on Sanger's shift from radical to more conservative strategies, see Gordon, *Moral Property of Women*, 3–4, and chapters 8–9.

21. For the reaction against the sexual openness of the 1920s, see D'Emilio and Freedman, *Intimate Matters*, 277–82; and Chauncey, *Gay New York*, chapters 11 through 12.

22. For Gordon's discussion of the ties the birth control movement forged with doctors and eugenicists, see *Moral Property of Women*, chapter 9. For James Reed's discussion of the medicalization of birth control, particularly by way of Dr. Robert L. Dickinson's efforts to secure medical support of birth control, see chapters 11 through 13 in *From Private Vice to Public Virtue*.

23. For this attitude among white middle-class female reformers and the battles it provoked with the young immigrant female wage earners they looked to assist, see Peiss, *Cheap Amusements*. For this moralist attitude toward the marketplace more generally, see Horowitz, *Morality of Spending*.

24. Addams, *Spirit of Youth and the City Streets*, 7.

25. Baskin, "Margaret Sanger," x.

26. Reagan, *When Abortion Was a Crime*, 36–37 and 141.

27. Although Planned Parenthood's policy toward serving the unwed was by the late 1950s quietly changing, notable is the 1967 recommendation that "each affiliate in accordance with state law . . . be as liberal as possible in offering services to minors." See Recommendations of the Executive Directors Council Meeting, held

June 26–29, 1967, Minneapolis, MN, Chicago Area, 1967, Series: Affiliates, Illinois, box 152, Planned Parenthood Federation of America Records II, Sophia Smith Collection, Smith College, Northampton, MA (hereafter cited as PPFAR II). For evidence of the changing policy toward abortion, see Langmyhr and Rogers, "Legal Abortion," which not only discussed abortion procedures but also offered a list of local Planned Parenthood offices that could provide information and referrals. In folder 4, box 20, Planned Parenthood Association Chicago Area Records, 1920–75, Chicago History Museum, Chicago, IL (hereafter cited as PPACAR).

28. For several good overviews of the shifting legal and political terrain of birth control in nineteenth- and twentieth-century America, see Dienes, *Law, Politics, and Birth Control*; and Critchlow, *Intended Consequences*.

29. Gordon, *Moral Property of Women*, 183.

30. Guthmann, *Planned Parenthood Movement in Illinois*, 4.

31. *U.S. v. One Package of Japanese Pessaries*, 13 F. Supp.334 (E.D.N.Y 1936) aff'd 86 F.2d 737 (2nd Cir. 1936).

32. *Youngs Rubber Corporation v. C. I. Lee & Co.*, 45 F.2d 103 (CCA, 2nd Cir.1930). For more on this particular case, see Gamson, "Rubber Wars."

33. *Griswold v. Connecticut*, 381 US 479 (1965).

34. *Eisenstadt v. Baird*, 405 US 438 (1972).

35. *Roe v. Wade*, 410 US 113 (1973); and *Doe v. Bolton*, 410 US 179 (1973).

36. For women during World War II and the postwar era, see Hartmann, *Home Front and Beyond*; Honey, *Creating Rosie the Riveter*; May, *Homeward Bound*; and Meyerowitz, *Not June Cleaver*. For the experiences of African Americans, see Wynn, *Afro-American and the Second World War*; and Capeci, Jr., *Race Relations*. For more on the crackdown on "deviance," see Reagan, *When Abortion Was a Crime*, chapter 6, especially 160–64.

37. On the industry's early history from the 1800s to just before the Depression, see Liebenau, *Medical Science and Medical Industry*. For the early animosity between business and medicine, particularly with respect to the patent medicine industry, see Starr, *Social Transformation of American Medicine*, 127–34; and Young, *Toadstool Millionaires*, chapters 13–14. On the significance of the industry's newfound ties with universities in the interwar period, see Swann, "Universities, Industry." On its relationship with the medical community after the passage of the Food, Drug, and Cosmetic Act in 1938, see Tomes, "Great American Medicine Show Revisited." On its image of noble benevolence (as it was crafted by Parke, Davis, and Company), see Duffin and Li, "Great Moments." Also, for a quick overview of the industry's "golden age," see the introduction by Tone and Watkins in their edited anthology, *Medicating Modern America*, 1–14; quote, 1.

38. Cohen, *Consumers' Republic*.

39. Rothman, *Strangers at the Bedside*, especially chapters 2 and 3; and Marks, *Progress of Experiment*, chapter 4.

40. Language drawn from the title of Reed, *From Private Vice to Public Virtue*. For one treatment of the growing fears of illegitimacy rates among African Americans, see Solinger, *Wake Up Little Susie*, chapters 6–7.

41. According to a 1928 report, of the 4,238 women the Illinois Birth Control League served since it began clinic operations in 1923, 2,101 attended its downtown clinic (these included predominantly white women who could afford to pay the full

price for services). The remaining 2,137 women attended its other 5 clinic locations (among these were predominantly foreign-born and black women, many of whom could pay only a limited amount, if anything). The percentage of black women was determined as follows. According to my calculations, the minimum number of black women who attended the Chicago clinics was 451 (which was the number of clients served by the predominantly black clinic); the maximum was 862 (the total Chicago caseload minus the clinic totals that served predominantly whites and immigrants). Blacks therefore constituted roughly 10 to 20 percent of the Chicago clientele. See "Brief Summary of Class and Character of Service Rendered by the Illinois Birth Control at Its Six Medical Centers," November 28, 1928, folder 1, box 8, Welfare Council of Metropolitan Chicago Records, 1914–78, Chicago History Museum, Chicago, IL (hereafter cited as WCMCR).

42. During 1966, for example, of the 5,741 new patients who attended Chicago's clinics: 72.2 percent were black (4,148); 14.5 percent white (831); 5.4 percent "Spanish" (likely Hispanic) (309); the remaining 7.9 percent (453) fell under a category defined only as "other." See Research Department: Ethnic Classification of New Patients, January 1, 1960–June 30, 1970, folder 11, box 17, PPACAR. For the numbers served on the national level, see remarks made on page 5 by Douglas Stewart in his address to the PPACA Board of Directors Meeting, February 29, 1968, Chicago Area Minutes, 1964–77, Series: Affiliates, Illinois, box 134, PPFAR II.

43. For the rise of private insurance, see Starr, *Social Transformation of American Medicine*, 290–334.

44. For the "whitening" of immigrants, see Jacobson, *Whiteness of a Different Color.*

45. "News Notes: A Fight in Chicago," 221. For another example of the use of this phrase, see Goldstein, "Birth Control Clinic Cases," 8.

46. There is a rich body of literature on the evolution of the hospital institution. See, for instance, Drachman, *Hospital with a Heart*; Gamble, *Making a Place for Ourselves*; Morantz-Sanchez, *Sympathy and Science*; Rosenberg, *Care of Strangers*; Stevens, *In Sickness and In Wealth*; and Vogel, *Invention of the Modern Hospital.*

47. Planned Parenthood Association of Champaign County leaflet, n.d. [ca. 1940s], Champaign, Planned Parenthood Association, Publicity, Pamphlets, etc., Series: Affiliates, Illinois, box 152, PPFAR II.

48. The first affiliate lasted from 1938 to the late 1950s; the second began operations in 1971. See "Forerunner of 'Planned Parenthood.' The Year 1938—And a New Kind of Clinic Was Underway," untitled newspaper clipping, December 13, 1974, page 42, folder 7, box 2, Planned Parenthood Springfield Area Records, 1938–95, MC 38, Archives/Special Collections, University of Illinois at Springfield, Springfield, IL.

49. By these national organizations, I mean: the American Birth Control League (ABCL); the National Committee on Maternal Health (NCMH); the Clinical Research Bureau (CRB), later renamed the Birth Control Clinical Research Bureau (BCCRB); and the National Committee for Federal Legislation on Birth Control (NCFLBC). For a great discussion of their many differences and conflicts between, see Hajo, *Birth Control on Main Street*, chapter 7.

50. The Tuskegee Syphilis Study was the controversial, forty-year-long study of venereal disease that lasted from 1932 through 1972 and used six hundred impoverished African American men as subjects. Those who had the disease were denied

treatment, and none were given the opportunity to give informed consent to participate in the study in the first place. For more on this, see Jones, *Bad Blood*; and Reverby, *Tuskegee's Truths*.

51. "American Medicine Accepts Birth Control," 1–2.

Chapter One

1. Tone, *Devices and Desires*, 25–26. For the persistence of abortion in the decades immediately following its prohibition in the 1860s and 1870s, see Reagan, *When Abortion Was a Crime*, chapters 1–4.

2. Sanger, "Family Limitation," 7, 9, 11, 14, 15, and 16.

3. Stuyvesant, "Brownsville Birth Control Clinic," 6. For several examples of the scholarly literature about her early advice, see Gordon, *Moral Property of Women*, chapter 8, especially 150 and 156–57; Chesler, *Woman of Valor*, chapters 5–9 (passim); Jensen, "Evolution of Margaret Sanger's *Family Limitation* Pamphlet"; McCann, *Birth Control Politics*, 24, 35–38, 42, 74, 76, 128–29, and 210–11; and Reed, *From Private Vice to Public Virtue*, chapters 6–10 (passim). Notably, Reed did mention that Sanger explained to one patient in her first clinic the cost of diaphragms available through drugstores, but he did not explore this further (106).

4. Brodie, *Contraception and Abortion*, 288.

5. Tone, *Devices and Desires*, 25–26 (Brodie's quote, 299, note 2).

6. Enstad, *Ladies of Labor*, 205.

7. Ibid., 6, 14. See also Elliott Shore's perceptive analysis of the socialist newspaper *Appeal to Reason*. As Shore explained, "the contradictions manifested by socialist goals and capitalist realities were magnified at the *Appeal*. At the *Appeal* we can glimpse the intersection of Socialist agitation and American mass culture." Shore, *Talkin' Socialism*, 4.

8. Tone, *Devices and Desires*, chapters 2–5.

9. *Chicago Medical Blue Book, 1923–1924* had approximately 1,883 listings (see 555–89). That druggists bore such names as Antoni Dziopeck, Ernest Eckhardt, U. G. McClure, and Hong Wah Tong suggests their immigrant background. See also Lynne Curry's discussion of the importance of druggists to immigrant communities in *Modern Mothers in the Heartland*, 53. Furthermore, Angus McLaren pointed out how before World War II working-class women in England preferred the advice of neighbors and the chemist (no doubt a reference to a local apothecary or druggist) for their contraceptive needs. See McLaren, *History of Contraception*, 225.

10. In the pamphlet "Why and How the Poor Should Not Have Many Children" (which was distributed by Goldman though written by Dr. William Robinson), druggists and drugstores were mentioned repeatedly. Thanks to Barry Pateman of the Goldman Papers Project at the University of California, Berkeley, for sending a copy on. Interestingly, Gordon mentioned the drugstore connection, though only in passing (see *Moral Property of Women*, 148).

11. Tone, *Devices and Desires*, 63–66.

12. Ibid., 84.

13. Gordon, *Moral Property of Women*, 156.

14. In fact, given that historians have long established that birth control was *not* medicalized until the 1920s and 1930s, it would be odd to assume it was. See Gordon, *Moral Property of Women*, chapter 9; and Reed, *From Private Vice to Public Virtue*, chapters 9 and 11–13. It's a hard habit to break though, even in Tone's great account. As she wrote, "Of course, doctors who refused to prescribe birth control were partly to blame for the proliferation of contraceptive entrepreneurs in the age of Comstockery. In the absence of medical leadership, women and men turned to the marketplace to acquire what doctors denied them" (*Devices and Desires*, 66). A similar message appeared in McCann, *Birth Control Politics*, 71.

15. For Sanger's faith in nurses, see Sanger, "Family Limitation," 4, which bore the subheading: "A Nurse's Advice to Women." For her faith in midwives, she is said to have told one patient that "a doctor or midwife may fit [the diaphragm] for you." Quote from the testimony of the policewoman who visited the clinic and later shut it down. See Reed, *From Private Vice to Public Virtue*, 106.

16. For Chase's and Farr's occupations, see Tone, *Devices and Desires*, 32 and 58, respectively.

17. The longstanding tensions between regular and irregular practitioners have been richly documented. See, for instance, Starr, *Social Transformation*, 79–144; Numbers, "Fall and Rise"; and Gevitz, *Other Healers*. So too have the tensions between the regular medical profession and the self-reliant nurse. See especially Ashley, *Hospitals, Paternalism*. Although Susan M. Reverby tempered Ashley's critique by pointing out the agency of nurses, she also found tensions between doctors and nurses. See Reverby, *Ordered to Care*, 31–33, 46, 73–75, and 130–31. And finally, equally well-documented have been the conflicts between organized medicine and the commercial marketplace, particularly patent medicine providers. See Starr, *Social Transformation*, 127–40; and Young, *Toadstool Millionaires*, chapters 13–14.

18. For Brinckerhoff's occupation, see Tone, *Devices and Desires*, 40–41; for Schmidt's, see 50–51.

19. Ibid. For Backrach, see 47; for Halleck, see 62–63. For rubber manufacturers more generally, see 61.

20. Ibid., 33–34.

21. For Sanger's motivations, see Gordon, *Moral Property of Women*, 4, and chapter 8. For the motivations of others, see Tone, *Devices and Desires*, chapters 2–3, especially 40–41 and 47–49. I would further imagine that immigrants brought with them birth control knowledge and recipes from their native lands. In fact, Norman E. Himes described a great variety of European folk remedies from the 1400s forward. While he argued that some were more magical in nature and of dubious effectiveness, he suggested that others (like the beeswax German-Hungarian women inserted into their vaginas) may have had some contraceptive value. See Himes, *Medical History*, chapter 7.

22. Details about Foote and quote in Tone, *Devices and Desires*, 57.

23. For example, Walker, *History of Black Business*; and Willett, *Permanent Waves*. As both these works demonstrated, entrepreneurship and the struggle for racial justice often went hand-in-hand within black communities.

24. For the graphicness of "Family Limitation," see 8, 11, 12, and 13, which included, respectively, one illustration for the "fountain syringe" (a douche) and the "French Pessary" (a diaphragm), plus two for the diaphragm insertion technique.

25. Tone, *Devices and Desires*, 30–32.

26. The "direct action" phrase is particularly useful because it forces us to move beyond the limited (anticapitalist) IWW definition, as described by Linda Gordon in her discussion of the early birth control radicals. "Defying such laws was a form of what the IWW called direct action, acting directly against state and capitalist power, not petitioning or negotiating but taking what was needed" (*Moral Property of Women*, 142; see 156–60 for her discussion of "direct action" techniques). But the activities of the bootleg entrepreneurs suggest the limits of this narrow definition.

27. Reprinted copies of such letters can be found in Sanger, *Motherhood in Bondage*.

28. Tone, *Devices and Desires*, 40–42. The frequent acquittal of abortionists has also been noted. See Reagan, *When Abortion Was a Crime*, 6.

29. Sanger, *My Fight for Birth Control*, chapter 8; quote, 116.

30. For this larger clinic movement, see Holz, "Nurse Gordon on Trial."

31. Sanger, *My Fight for Birth Control*, 145.

32. Untitled, *Woman Rebel*, September–October, 1914. In Baskin, *Woman Rebel*, 56.

33. For the literature on the national level, see Gordon, *Moral Property of Women*; Reed, *From Private Vice to Public Virtue*; McCann, *Birth Control Politics*; and Chesler, *Woman of Valor*. For studies at the local level, see those listed in the introduction, note 13. For the predominance of middle-class laywomen who looked to engage in local charity birth control clinic work across the nation, see Hajo, *Birth Control on Main Street*, especially chapter 3.

34. Hajo, *Birth Control on Main Street*, 2.

35. Guthmann, *Planned Parenthood Movement in Illinois*, 4.

36. Edward J. Brundage to Rachelle Yarros, February 24, 1917, folder 1, box 8, PPACAR.

37. Bundesen's initial show of support can be found in the letter from Helen G. Carpenter (president of the Parents' Clinic) to William E. Dever (the mayor of Chicago), September 27, 1923, folder 1, box 8, PPACAR.

38. Ibid. There is also evidence to suggest that the committee may have already begun clinic operations as early as February 1923, which means that it was technically operating in violation of the law. See IBCL application for membership in the Chicago Council of Social Agencies, March 2, 1925, folder 8, box 390, WCMCR.

39. His first refusal can be found in Herman N. Bundesen to Helen G. Carpenter, August 11, 1923; his second, in Herman N. Bundesen to Helen G. Carpenter, September 19, 1923. Bundesen quote from letter dated September 19, 1923. Both in folder 1, box 8, PPACAR.

40. Quotes from Helen G. Carpenter, Annual Report of the Illinois Birth Control League, April 29, 1925, folder 8, box 390, WCMCR. See also Guthmann, *Planned Parenthood Movement in Illinois*, 4.

41. As can be gathered from Chesler's account of Margaret Sanger, she faced similar obstacles and so when she resumed clinic operations in 1923, it "was run essentially as the private practice of Dr. Dorothy Bocker." Quote from Chesler, *Woman of Valor*, 274.

42. Carpenter, Annual Report of the Illinois Birth Control League, April 29, 1925.

43. Gordon, *Moral Property of Women*, 178.

44. Tone, *Devices and Desires*, 126–28; quote, 126.

45. For fees and evidence of the sale of supplies to local physicians, see the Report of the Membership Committee of the Chicago Council of Social Agencies, Regarding Application for Membership of the Illinois Birth Control League, 1929, folder 8, box 390, WCMCR.

46. Local leagues regularly reported the use of sliding fee scales in the *Birth Control Review*. For example, see Boyden, "Mothers' Health Clinic"; Salomon, "Rhode Island Clinic"; and Rennie, "Mothers Health Centers."

47. Boughton, "To Start a Clinic," 50.

48. Salomon, "Rhode Island Clinic," 280.

49. For several discussions of clinic expenses, see Rennie, "Mothers Health Centers"; and Boughton, "To Start a Clinic." Note also what one clinic manual said: the "sum needed to run the clinic will, of course, be partially covered by the fees paid by the patients." See page 4 of "How to Establish a Birth Control Clinic," 1938, folder 3, box 80, Series VII: Subject Files, Clinics, Planned Parenthood Federation of America Records I, Sophia Smith Collection, Smith College, Northampton, MA (hereafter cited as PPFAR I).

50. For example, in 1932 of the $15,635.95 the Illinois Birth Control League spent, $12,577.85 came from patient fees and the sale of supplies. See "News Notes: Illinois" (June 1933).

51. "State Organizations for Birth Control: Illinois Birth Control League."

52. For Hajo's discussion of Chicago and New York's uniqueness in this regard, see *Birth Control on Main Street*, 61.

53. Carpenter, Annual Report of the Illinois Birth Control League, April 29, 1925.

54. Indeed, among the 1,340 women who attended the Illinois Birth Control League's clinics in 1929, nearly 25 percent cited as their referral source the city's many social service agencies, numbers that clearly reveal how their participation was as vital to the success of clinic operations as was that of the medical community, which provided referrals of its own. See "State Organizations for Birth Control: Illinois Birth Control League." The list of referrals from social service agencies went as follows: the Infant and Welfare Society (167); United Charities (89); and "Social agencies and settlements" (58). Quote from same article.

55. For the support given by the Associated Charities, see "Brief Summary of Class and Character of Service Rendered by the Illinois Birth Control League at its Six Medical Centers." Also in this summary is a discussion of the patients who paid little or nothing for clinic services.

56. For discussion of the uniqueness of Chicago and New York City in their use of settlement houses, see Hajo, *Birth Control on Main Street*, 36–39.

57. Indeed, although clinics elsewhere in the nation were rarely located in settlement houses, they often made their way into public city hospitals or received funds from local philanthropic organizations. For example, the first clinic in Waco, Texas, was housed at the Child Welfare Services and worked closely with United Charities (see Hulett, "Every Child a Wanted Child," 23 and 28), and the first clinic in Cincinnati, Ohio, was located in the outpatient dispensary of the city's public hospital (see Lindenmeyer, "Expanding Birth Control to the Hinterland," 150).

58. "News Notes: Illinois" (December 1925).

59. Carpenter, Annual Report of the Illinois Birth Control League, April 29, 1925.

60. Reeves, "Birth Control Industry," 288.

61. Gordon, *Moral Property of Women*, 213.

62. Hulett, "Every Child a Wanted Child," 27.

63. For the league's continued (and unsuccessful) efforts to gain membership into the Welfare Council, largely because of Catholic opposition, see Alexander Ropchan, Summary of Applications For Membership by the Illinois Birth Control League . . . and Actions Taken on the Membership Applications by the Welfare Council, May 8, 1950, folder 10, box 390, WCMCR.

64. Yarros, "Birth Control Clinics in Chicago," 355. This article, like many others, described in great detail the backgrounds of the patients. In part, such descriptions were likely intended to provide proof that women of all different backgrounds wanted birth control and also that clinics were providing for this need. But it could hardly have been lost on those publishing such figures that the presence of Catholics indicated defiance among lay members.

65. Meyer, *Any Friend of the Movement*, 47; and Hulett, "Every Child a Wanted Child," 26–29.

66. Wenocur and Reisch, *From Charity to Enterprise*, 46–55; quote, 51.

67. Sanger, "Clinics the Solution," 6. By 1921, the language in the twelfth edition of *Family Limitation* was even losing its working-class militancy. See Jensen, "Evolution of Margaret Sanger's *Family Limitation* Pamphlet."

68. Yarros, "Birth Control Clinics in Chicago," 354.

69. Wembridge, "Seventh Child in the Four Room House," 13.

70. "Information Not Available." Signed "C."

71. "Our Correspondents' Column. Letter from E. D."

72. For example, from 1933 to 1934 the clinic in Little Rock, Arkansas, reported 46 percent of its referrals came from past and present clinic clients. See Leung, "Better Babies" (1996), 164. In her analysis of Sanger's Birth Control Clinical Research Bureau (the main New York clinic), Marie E. Kopp found that 48.3 percent were from "patients and friends." Kopp, *Birth Control in Practice*, 37. See also Hajo's discussion of this and how clinic workers saw it as a validation of their efforts (*Birth Control on Main Street*, 149–50).

73. "State Organizations for Birth Control: Illinois Birth Control League," 259.

74. Details about the clinic visit gleaned from the following manuals and analyses of clinic procedure: Dickinson, *Control of Contraception*, chapter 19; and Kopp, *Birth Control in Practice*, 145–50, and passim. Specifics about the actual diaphragm fitting come from Stone, "Vaginal Diaphragm," 123–27; quote, 123. Also helpful were the secondary source accounts of the clinic visit found in Meyer, *Any Friend of the Movement*, 95–98; and Hajo, *Birth Control on Main Street*, 63–66. The "clinic way" phrase is taken from the title of chapter 16 in Palmer and Greenberg, *Facts and Frauds in Woman's Hygiene.*

75. Gordon discussed Sanger's use of this method of diaphragm fitting in *Moral Property of Women*, 156–57.

76. For more on this stereotypical characterization of the long-suffering wife in need of birth control, see Hajo, *Birth Control on Main Street*, 126–27.

77. "I Went to a Birth Control Clinic," 77, 78.

78. Ibid., 78.

79. Both Meyer and Hajo mentioned this variety as well. See, respectively, *Any Friend of the Movement*, 61–62; and *Birth Control on Main Street*, 63. For the variety of clinic locations as operated by the Illinois Birth Control League, see "Brief Summary of Class and Character of Service Rendered by the Illinois Birth Control League at its Six Medical Centers."

80. Himes, *Medical History of Contraception*, 184.

81. Curry, *Modern Mothers in the Heartland*, 45–48.

82. Boughton, "To Start A Clinic," 49.

83. For discussion of clinic decoration, see page 4 of "How to Start a Contraceptive Center: Suggestions Offered by the American Birth Control League," n.d. [ca. 1936], folder 1, box 80, Series VII: Subject Files, Clinics, PPFAR I. For discussion of interview space and its need for privacy, see Bryant, "Clinic Interview," 52; and Dickinson, *Control of Conception*, 335.

84. For more on sexual propriety and the pelvic exam, see Reagan, "Engendering the Dread Disease"; and Kapsalis, *Public Privates*.

85. For discussions of need for privacy in the examination space, see Gaylord, "Clinical Aspects of Birth Control"; Dickinson, *Control of Conception*, 329–30, quotes, 335–36; and "How to Start a Contraceptive Center," n.d. [ca. 1936], 4. For quote about Chicago, see Kennedy, "Visit to the Medical Centers of Chicago," 26.

86. For the presence of male physicians, see Hajo, *Birth Control on Main Street*, 90–91.

87. White, "Maintaining Clinic Standards," 9.

88. "How to Start a Contraceptive Center," 3.

89. For the experiences of women doctors and their status in the medical profession, see Walsh, *Doctors Wanted*; Drachman, *Hospital With a Heart*; and Morantz-Sanchez, *Sympathy and Science*.

90. Dickinson, *Control of Conception*, 316. On the same page, Dickinson also suggested that professional discrimination against women may have contributed to women's dominance in clinic work. For another manual that identified the importance of female initiative, see Irwin and Paolone, *Practical Birth Control*, 152–54.

91. Ladd-Taylor, *Mother-Work*, 2.

92. Staff duties gleaned from "A Day at the Office"; White, "Maintaining Clinic Standards"; Boughton, "To Start a Clinic"; and "How to Start a Contraceptive Center."

93. Stone, "Essentials in Clinic Equipment," 23.

94. Helen G. Carpenter, Annual Report of the Illinois Birth Control League, April 30, 1930, frames 454–59, reel 17, Mary Ware Dennett Papers, Schlesinger Library, Radcliffe Institute, Cambridge, MA (hereafter cited as MWDP). For Dr. Ginzberg's training, see *American Medical Directory* (1929), 413. Mollenaro's background and duties in the clinic are unclear.

95. Rennie, "Some Clinic Problems," 53. See also Dickinson's discussion about the need to accommodate the presence of children, in particular his comments on the necessity of first-floor facilities, in *Control of Conception*, 323.

96. The phrase taken from the title of chapter 14 in Chesler, *Woman of Valor*, 287.

97. Rennie, "Some Clinic Problems," 52.

98. Quote from Nash, "Birth Control Clinics," 231.

99. Quotes, respectively, from Boughton, "To Start A Clinic," 50; and White, "Maintaining Clinic Standards," 9.

100. "How to Start a Contraceptive Center," 4.

101. White, "Maintaining Clinic Standards," 9.

102. Stone, "Clinical Birth Control Abroad," 321–22; quote, 321.

103. Gordon, *Moral Property of Women*, 178, 217–18.

104. Meyer, *Any Friend of the Movement*, 96; and Hajo, *Birth Control on Main Street*, 33, 65.

105. Letter to Mary Ware Dennett, February 27, 1928, frames 545–46, reel 18, MWDP.

106. "Twenty-one," in Sanger, *Motherhood in Bondage*, 310–11.

107. "Seven," in ibid., 300–301. Italics in original, though they may have been added when the letter was compiled for publication.

108. Rennie, "Some Clinic Problems," 53.

109. Hajo, *Birth Control on Main Street*, 53.

110. For example, although the clinic in Cleveland, Ohio, still had its problems, it was apparently quite successful in cultivating good relationships with the patients and a friendly atmosphere. See Meyer, *Any Friend of the Movement*, chapter 4. Nonetheless, Hajo also pointed out the variety of clinic experiences; some were good, some were not. See *Birth Control on Main Street*, 130.

111. "Brief Summary of Class and Character of Service Rendered by the Illinois Birth Control League at its Six Medical Centers." Interestingly, Irish women are strikingly absent in this and other Chicago reports. See, for example, "State Organizations for Birth Control: Illinois Birth Control League."

112. Hajo made this observation as well, in that white women in New York City were reluctant to attend the Harlem branch "because it was in the 'colored' section" of town. See *Birth Control on Main Street*, 118. See also how the clinics were described in Maria Anderson's study of Planned Parenthood–Houston: the "white clinic," the "Mexican clinic," and the "Negro clinic." Anderson, "Private Choices vs. Public Voices," 67–68.

113. Hajo, *Birth Control on Main Street*, 5, 113–24.

114. Ibid., 63–64.

115. Letter reproduced in Meyer, *Any Friend of the Movement*, 101.

116. Hajo, *Birth Control on Main Street*, 21. That much of this growth came during the 1930s suggests that the Depression marks the height of this first clinic wave.

117. Linda Gordon's introduction to the Mary Ware Dennett Papers (MWDP) offers a good account of the differences between Sanger and Dennett. However, the rivalry between them and their organizations needs further exploration. For example, the Illinois Birth Control League had deep ties with the Dennett camp, only to side formally, though somewhat reluctantly, with Sanger's American Birth Control League in the early 1930s. See Helen G. Carpenter to Mary Ware Dennett, March 18, 1930, frame 453, reel 17; and Helen G. Carpenter to Mary Ware Dennett, February 16, 1931, frame 465, reel 17, MWDP. For more on Mary Ware Dennett, see Chen, *"The Sex Side of Life"* and Rosen, *Reproductive Health*, chapter 3.

118. Mary Ware Dennett to unknown recipient in Wheaton, IL, January 16, 1930, frame 695, reel 18, MWDP.

119. Mary Ware Dennett to unknown recipient in Howell, MI, July 7, 1930, frame 729; Mary Ware Dennett to unknown recipient in Brooklyn, NY, August 12, 1930, frame 743; and Mary Ware Dennett to unknown recipient in Los Angeles, CA, February 10, 1930, frames 715–16. All letters on reel 18, MWDP.

Chapter Two

1. Benson, "Leaping on the Band Wagon," 5.

2. For the 1930s contraceptive marketplace, see Tone, *Devices and Desires*, chapters 7 and 8. For the 1930s world of abortion, see Reagan, *When Abortion Was a Crime*, chapter 5. For the irregular birth control clinic movement, see Holz, "Nurse Gordon on Trial."

3. Reagan, *When Abortion Was a Crime*, 36–37, 141.

4. Sarch, "Those Dirty Ads!"

5. Note too that this position reflects even further the ways in which the birth control organization was adopting the ways of organized medicine, since this was how organized medicine navigated the commercial world of medicine itself. For Tone's findings, see *Devices and Desires*, chapter 6. For more on what constitutes ethical manufacturers, see Liebenau, *Medical Science and Medical Industry*, 4, 109–10; and McTavish, *Pain and Profits*, 6. For more on the complexities of ethical pharmaceutical advertising, see Tomes, "Great American Medicine Show Revisited."

6. Garrett, "Birth Control's Business Baby," 269. Sanger used Garrett's article as evidence for the need for legal and regulated contraception in her statement before the unsuccessful 1934 Congressional hearings to legalize birth control. See *Birth Control: Hearings before a Subcommittee on S. 1842*, 25–28.

7. For those interested in learning more about the collection, the AMA has published an excellent guide to its contents. See Hafner et al., *Guide to the American Medical Association Historical Health Fraud*. For more on the Progressive-era campaign to regulate the patent medicine industry, see McTavish, *Pain and Profits*, chapter 5; and Young, *Toadstool Millionaires*, chapters 13 and 14.

8. Tone, "Contraceptive Consumers." See also Watkins and Danzi, "Women's Gossip and Social Change." Thanks to Mickey Moran for bringing this article to my attention.

9. Henrietta Rusin to the American Medical Association, September 1936, Lanteen, folder 4, box 465, HHFAMC. Courtesy of American Medical Association Archives. More such letters appear throughout the investigative files. See boxes 85–87, 465, and 917, HHFAMC.

10. Phrase from Himes, *Medical History of Contraception*, 352.

11. Boughton, "What 7309 'Mothers' Want," 8.

12. For the contraceptive study of the preclinic contraceptive practices of people, see Stix, "Birth Control in a Midwestern City" (January 1939): details, 84. For the prices of condoms, see advertisement reprinted in "Accident of Birth," 84. For prices of douches, see "Sears, Roebuck, and Company Catalog" (Spring–Summer 1937), 604. For the size of the diaphragm market, see Tone, *Devices and Desires*, 151.

13. Watkins and Danzi, "Women's Gossip and Social Change," 481.

14. Quote from Sanger, "National Security and Birth Control," 141. Reagan, *When Abortion Was a Crime*, chapter 5.

15. Advertisement, "'Lysol' is Safe," *Cosmopolitan*, October 1934, 143, Birth Control, folder 16, box 87, HHFAMC. Courtesy of American Medical Association Archives. See also the Lanteen circulars, "Reliable Birth Control Preparations," n.d. [ca. early 1930s]; and "Birth Control: A Health Necessity in Marriage," n.d. [ca. early 1930s]. Both in Lanteen, folder 3, box 465, HHFAMC. An ad for Ramses condoms bore a similar message. See the one reproduced in "Accident of Birth," 84.

16. Lysol ad, "We needn't *talk* about those things. . . . *Just read this little book*," *Chicago Daily Tribune*, April 17, 1929, Birth Control, folder 6, box 85, HHFAMC. Courtesy of American Medical Association Archives.

17. Woman's Bureau pamphlet, "Feminine Hygiene," n.d. [ca. 1935], Woman's Bureau, folder 5, box 917, HHFAMC. Courtesy of American Medical Association Archives.

18. Quote from Sanger, "National Security and Birth Control," 140. See also the tone in Palmer and Greenberg's discussion of feminine hygiene in *Facts and Frauds in Woman's Hygiene*, chapter 1. For one example of how this characterization has been perpetuated by the historiography, see Gordon, *Moral Property of Women*, 223–25.

19. For example, in 1937 the Sears and Roebuck catalog offered six kinds of douches, thirteen different feminine hygiene tablets, suppositories, and jellies, and a handful of manuals about sex and birth control in its books section. See "Sears, Roebuck, and Company Catalog," 604–5, 572. Likewise, the Dilex Institute of Feminine Hygiene offered La Dila—a kit that included "a universal cap diaphragm, a douching outfit, and an antiseptic douche capsule." See "Accident of Birth," 114.

20. For department store practices, see "Feminine Hygiene in the Department Store," 479. See also the "Feminine Hygiene" pamphlet put out by the Woman's Bureau. Here a nurse appears prominently on the front cover.

21. The Dilex Institute of Feminine Hygiene was one such company that had its traveling peddlers pose as nurses. See "Accident of Birth," 14. But others did as well. See the Hygienic Company of America, folder 3, box 87; and letter from Mrs. J. M. Conrad, March 12, 1937, folder 3, box 86. Both in Birth Control, HHFAMC. Worth noting is that some salespersons may have been nurses; however, more research is necessary to determine whether this was so. For the tradition of public health nursing, see Melosh, "More Than the 'Physician's Hand.'"

22. For the clinic practice of dressing lay women in whites, see Hajo, *Birth Control on Main Street*, 63, 76; as well as Leung, "Better Babies," (1996), 126.

23. Ad reproduced in "Accident of Birth," 84.

24. Ad reprinted in Tone, *Devices and Desires*, 162.

25. Names of companies gleaned from the materials in the HHFAMC collection under the heading Birth Control, folders 1–16, box 87; and "Accident of Birth," passim.

26. See, for example, "Reliable Birth Control Preparations." The desire to cultivate brand recognition, moreover, was hardly confined to Lanteen alone. As Tone described, a number of contraceptive manufacturers engaged in this practice. See *Devices and Desires*, chapter 7, especially 160.

27. The books Sears offered in 1937 included Sanger, *Happiness in Marriage*; Drs. Hannah and Abraham Stone, *A Marriage Manual*; Havelock Ellis, *Psychology of Sex*; Dr. Marie Stopes, *Married Love*; Dr. H. W. Long, *Sane Sex Life and Sane Sex Living*;

Dr. Isabel Sutton, *The Sex Technique in Marriage*; William J. Fielding, *Sex and the Love Life*; and Dr. Leo Latz, *The Rhythm of Sterility and Fertility in Woman*, and *The Modern Method of Birth Control*. See "Sears, Roebuck, and Company Catalog," 572; for feminine hygiene products, see 604–5.

28. Edith Flower Wheeler to *Journal of the American Medical Association*, May 8, 1933, Birth Control, folder 1, box 86, HHFAMC. Courtesy of American Medical Association Archives.

29. For discussion of these commercial tactics, see P. B. P. Huse to Morris Fishbein, July 5, 1929, Birth Control, folder 6, box 86, HHFAMC.

30. Murray N. Hadley to Morris E. Fishbein, March 20, 1929, Birth Control, folder 6, box 86, HHFAMC. Courtesy of American Medical Association Archives.

31. "Birth Control Revolution," 591. See also "Birth Control."

32. De Costa, "Catholic Young Woman," 555–56.

33. Vignette compiled through the following materials: Robert L. Dickinson to Morris Fishbein, February 11, 1930; R.H.S., "Advice Given by Doctor Buzza," n.d. [ca. 1930]; and an Untitled Report of Visit to Medical Bureau, n.d. [ca. 1930], Lanteen, folder 3, box 465, HHFAMC. Quotes from Dickinson to Fishbein and the Untitled Report of Visit to Medical Bureau, respectively. Dickinson to Fishbein: Courtesy of American Medical Association Archives. Untitled Report of Visit to Medical Bureau and R.H.S., "Advice Given By Doctor Buzza" © American Medical Association, n.d. [ca. 1930]. All rights reserved. Courtesy of AMA Archives.

34. Materials regarding the chain of Medical Bureau clinics can be found in Lanteen, folders 2–4, box 465, HHFAMC. Sanger quote in Sanger, *My Fight for Birth Control*, 144.

35. See listings in the 1936 and 1938 *Chicago Telephone Directory*. Directories used here are from the Social Sciences Division of the Chicago Public Library, Harold Washington Library Center, Chicago, IL. Like the commercially sponsored Medical Bureau of Birth Control Information, materials regarding the activities of the Woman's Bureau can be found in the AMA's Historical Health Fraud and Alternative Medicine Collection. See Woman's Bureau, folder 5, box 917. However, to the best of my knowledge, this collection contains nothing about the Bureau of Birth Control Information.

36. Secretary to Mrs. Sanger (Florence Rose) to Rufus Riddlesbarger, March 1, 1933, frame 694, reel 57, Margaret Sanger Papers, Filmed Collection, Library of Congress, Washington, DC (hereafter cited as MSP Filmed–LC). *Los Angeles City Directory* (1929), 1584. The listing in the Los Angeles directory reads: "Mother's Clinic Inc." The name suggests that it may have had commercial connections; its director (Nurse Freda Frost) was a nurse, which suggests that a nurse was in charge. For another possible reference to an irregular clinic, see Irwin and Paolone, *Practical Birth Control*, 158.

37. In what little has been written about these facilities, this is the message that has emerged. McCann was among the first to mention them, but she did so only in passing. See McCann, *Birth Control Politics*, 183. Tone offered a more sustained account, but her interpretation bore the same sweeping hostility toward these institutions as was voiced by the American Birth Control League and the American Medical Association (see *Devices and Desires*, 166–69). I have since tried to rectify this negative characterization. See Holz, "Nurse Gordon on Trial."

38. Many thanks to Cathy Moran Hajo, who suggested the use of this term.

39. See note 17, chapter 1.

40. For the emphasis on doctors in American clinics, see Stone, "Clinical Birth Control Abroad."

41. This was often the case in Medical Bureau clinics, particularly in its Milwaukee location, which was headed by Nurse Adele Gordon. As Gordon's work reveals, she worked on her own but in consultation with the Bureau's chief physician who made weekly visits from Chicago. See "Birth Control 'Sales' Denied" [unmarked newspaper clipping], April 4, 1935, frames 280–81, reel 108, MSP Filmed–LC. What is striking is how this practice resembles the early twentieth-century calls to justify the use of trained midwives to oversee uncomplicated deliveries. See Litoff, *American Midwives*, chapter 6.

42. For Dr. Blood's involvement, see the American Medical Association's form letter replies to those inquiring about the clinic. In Woman's Bureau, folder 5, box 917, HHFAMC. It is also possible that the clinic may have been first begun by nurses, or at least primarily staffed by them. See "Feminine Hygiene." However, whether this was the case is not clear.

43. Quote from Carpenter, Annual Report of the Illinois Birth Control League, April 29, 1925, 2.

44. For Lanteen's radio shows, see William F. Hewitt to the AMA, April 5, 1929. For form letters mailed out to private citizens, see Horner F. Sanger to Cramps, December 24, 1929; and "Dr. Mary Hall to Dear Madam," n.d. [ca. 1930]. For form letters mailed out to doctors, see "Rufus Riddlesbarger to Dear Sir," August 21, 1930. All in Lanteen, folder 3, box 465, HHFAMC. Letters, describing circulars picked up in local drugstores and elsewhere, came from Illinois, Michigan, Maryland, Ohio, New York, and New Jersey. See letters to AMA in Lanteen, folders 3–4, box 465, HHFAMC. For Lanteen flier in box of sanitary napkins, see William G. Mather, Jr. to Morris Fishbein, July 22, 1938, Lanteen, folder 4, box 465, HHFAMC.

45. For the description of leafleting, see the Woman's Bureau calling card and the handwritten note on its margin. For stacks of fliers left in downtown office buildings, see the letter of complaint from George Nichols to States Attorney Courtney, February 1, 1935. For an example of the flier itself and the image found on it, see "Feminine Hygiene," n.d. [ca. 1935]. All in Woman's Bureau, folder 5, box 917, HHFAMC.

46. Bryant, "Clinic Interview."

47. For evidence of its service to the unwed, see Untitled Report of Visit to Medical Bureau. For evidence of the discussion of female sexual fulfillment, see R.H.S., "Advice Given by Doctor Buzza."

48. One 1930 report placed the fee at $8.25 while another indicated $11. See, respectively, H. E. Hickman to American Medical Association, January 17, 1931, Lanteen, folder 3, box 465, HHFAMC; and Untitled Report of Visit to Medical Bureau.

49. Medical Bureau prescription form, frame 232A, reel 108, MSP Filmed–LC.

50. Rufus Riddlesbarger to Margaret Sanger, March 7, 1933, frame 695, reel 57, MSP Filmed–LC.

51. White, "Maintaining Clinic Standards," 9; and Gaylord, "Clinical Aspects of Birth Control," quote, 166.

52. Note, for example, the differences between the Annual Report of the Illinois Birth Control League, April 29, 1925, that was submitted to the conservative Welfare

Council of Chicago, and one that went to Mary Ware Dennett's organization, the more liberal Voluntary Parenthood League, in 1930. In the latter, the Illinois office supported an "open bill" and ridiculed the fears that if birth control "were thrown wide open" then "immorality will break loose." See Carpenter, Annual Report of the Illinois Birth Control League, April 30, 1930.

53. Chesler, *Woman of Valor*, 300–303; and Hajo, *Birth Control on Main Street*, 55–59.

54. Holz, "Nurse Gordon on Trial."

55. The names of the irregular clinics include: Bureau of Birth Control Information, Medical Bureau of Birth Control Information, and Woman's Bureau of Birth Control Information. Also in this list is the Mothers' Birth Control Clinic, which was the name Riddlesbarger first used before adopting the name Medical Bureau. All the rest designate League facilities and were taken from "Birth Control Clinics at Work" and Guthmann, *Planned Parenthood Movement in Illinois*, 4. Notable too is the fact that league clinics often changed their names as well (see Guthmann, 4).

56. Benson, "Leaping on the Band Wagon," 6. Italics mine.

57. Ibid., 5. Birth control manuals soon echoed such sentiments, even down to the use of quotation marks. See Irwin and Paolone, *Practical Birth Control*, 158–59.

58. Letter from J. M. Conrad to the American Health Association, March 12, 1937. Courtesy of American Medical Association Archives.

59. Tone, *Devices and Desires*, 169–73; and Reed, *From Private Vice to Public Virtue*, chapter 18.

60. Bromley, *Birth Control: Its Use and Misuse*, 96.

61. Accident of Birth," 110. See also ibid., 110–11.

62. For discussion of Gamble's "white lists," his faith in a wide variety of methods, and his desire to reach lay (and not simply physician) audiences, see Reed, *From Private Vice to Public Virtue*, 241–42, 244–45; quote 242. See also Briggs, *Reproducing Empire*, 102–8.

63. Quotes from "How to Start a Contraceptive Center," n.d [ca. 1936], 5, 6. For recommendation of specific birth control products by brand, see Dickinson's manual of clinic procedure, which, interestingly enough, included diaphragms, contraceptive jellies, and condoms. *Control of Conception*, 348–51.

64. "I Went to a Birth Control Clinic," 78.

65. Bromley, *Birth Control: Its Use and Misuse*, chapter 8; quote, 94.

66. Yarros quoted in ibid., 117.

67. Boughton, "To Start a Clinic," 49. See also Sanger's remarks in which she argued that the "commercial success of [feminine hygiene] products" was largely because of the demand of the "submerged class of underfed and overbred motherhood." In other words, the poor. In Sanger, "National Security and Birth Control," 140. A similar message about the susceptibility of the poor to "the charlatan, the ill-equipped," "the cheap fraud," and the abortionist can be found in Cook, "Bootleg Birth Control," 42.

68. Bromley, "Birth Control: Yes or No?," 38.

69. "Accident of Birth," 108.

70. "Ask Your Physician."

71. Ibid.

72. Cook, "Bootleg Birth Control," 42.

73. Sanger, "National Security and Birth Control," 141.

74. Garrett, "Birth Control's Business Baby," 270.

75. Stubbs, "Profits in Birth Control."

76. Investigative material found in Lanteen, folders 2–4, box 465, HHFAMC.

77. Untitled Report of Visit to Medical Bureau.

78. R.H.S., "Advice Given by Doctor Buzza." It is unclear why Buzza used the words "husband" and "wife" in her advice to R.H.S., who claimed to be unmarried. Perhaps the language was habitual or there was an assumption that the relationship would one day lead to marriage.

79. AMA to J. Rosslyn Earp, April 11, 1930, Lanteen, folder 3, box 465, HHFAMC. © American Medical Association, April 11, 1930. All rights reserved. Courtesy of AMA Archives.

80. Bryant, "Clinic Interview," 52.

81. Dickinson to Fishbein, February 11, 1930.

82. Lanteen pamphlet, "Is Birth Control Right?," 1935, Lanteen, folder 2, box 465, HHFAMC. Courtesy of American Medical Association Archives. For Riddlesbarger's pronouncements against abortion in the press, see "Voice of the People: Ruthless Nature."

83. Reagan, *When Abortion Was a Crime*, 147–59. The address of the Medical Bureau appeared on its circulars. Investigative reports from previous years indicate that the Medical Bureau may have at one point operated on the tenth floor of the same building (office number 1016); see Untitled Report of Visit to Medical Bureau.

84. For example, Dr. John C. Hill, who reputedly regularly played golf with Riddlesbarger and assisted him in the Medical Bureau, conducted his practice out of the State Lake Building at 190 North State Street. For material on Dr. Hill's relationship with Riddlesbarger, see the May 1930 series of letters as well as a letter from the Bureau of Investigation to Fishbein, September 28, 1931, Lanteen, folder 3, box 465, HHFAMC.

85. Nichols to Courtney, February 1, 1935. Nichols also forwarded a copy of this letter to the AMA and Cardinal George Mundelein. Courtesy of American Medical Association Archives.

86. Irwin and Paolone, *Practical Birth Control*, 158.

87. For the phrase "bona fide," see Benson, "Leaping on the Band Wagon," 5; and ibid., 159.

88. For clinic standards, see Required Minimum Standards for Certification of Birth Control Clinics, September 1938, folder 1, box 80, Series VII: Subject Files, Clinics, PPFAR I. For more on certification, see McCann, *Birth Control Politics*, 182–83.

89. Hajo, *Birth Control on Main Street*, 61.

90. Benson, "Leaping on the Band Wagon," 6. The exact same language appears in Irwin and Paolone, *Practical Methods of Birth Control*, 160.

91. Edwin P. Vary to *Journal of American Medical Association*, February 6, 1932, Lanteen, folder 3, box 465, HHFAMC. Courtesy of American Medical Association Archives. More such letters appear throughout this folder.

92. American Medical Association Bureau of Investigation to Mrs. Grayson Yarrington, September 30, 1932, Lanteen, folder 3, box 465, HHFAMC. © American Medical Association, September 30, 1932. All rights reserved. Courtesy of AMA Archives.

93. "Rufus Riddlesbarger to Dear Sir." Margin notes on the form letter written by R. C. Hetherington of Geneva, Illinois. Courtesy of American Medical Association Archives.

94. Appel, Review of *Facts and Frauds in Woman's Hygiene.*

95. The doctors whom the AMA described were Mildred Buzza and John C. Hill. See "Bureau of Investigation. Lanteen Laboratories, Inc.," *Journal of the American Medical Association* 94, no. 20 (1930): 1619. It is not clear how Buzza felt, but Hill was furious and vehemently denied any involvement. For more on Dr. Hill's relationship with the Medical Bureau, see the series of letters from May 1930 as well as a letter from the Bureau of Investigation to Morris Fishbein, September 28 1931, Lanteen, folder 3, box 465, HHFAMC.

96. See the ads for Lygel (a feminine hygiene product) in "Sears, Roebuck, and Company Catalog," 605; and Ramses condoms in "Accident of Birth," 84. Another company even took on the name Clinic Supply Company. As one of the nation's largest diaphragm manufacturers, it likely lived up to its name. This company was also described in "Accident of Birth," 112.

97. Tone, *Devices and Desires,* 166–69.

98. Indeed, one study appearing in a 1938 issue of the *Journal of Contraception* revealed that many physicians failed to utilize the full range of sizes when prescribing the conventional diaphragm to their patients. See Clark, "Sizes of Vaginal Diaphragms." See also "Clinic Reports. Minnesota Birth Control League." Here one Minnesota doctor suggested the size of diaphragms the local clinic was prescribing was too large.

99. Holz, "Nurse Gordon on Trial."

100. For slowness of clinic certification, see "Birth Control Marches On." For the AMA's birth control resolution, see "American Medicine Accepts Birth Control," quote, 1. Notably, Carole McCann argued that the AMA's support for the birth control clinic remained extremely cautious, both at the time of the resolution and in the decades that followed (see *Birth Control Politics,* 94–95). Nonetheless, given the profession's previous antagonism, I would argue that the AMA's resolution marked a significant breakthrough.

101. For the 1948 investigation of Riddlesbarger's Medical Bureau, see Oliver Field to Dr. Smith, May 19, 1948, Lanteen, folder 4, box 465, HHFAMC. For the AMA's continued vigilance over the Woman's Bureau, see series of letters from the 1950s in Woman's Bureau, box 5, folder 917, HHFAMC.

102. Naismith, "Racket in Contraceptives;" quotes, 12.

Chapter Three

1. Gordon, *Moral Property of Women,* 3–4 and chapter 11; quotes, 244.

2. For scholars who have repeated this interpretation, see Petchesky, *Abortion and Woman's Choice,* 92–93; Chesler, *Woman of Valor,* chapter 18; D'Emilio and Freedman, *Intimate Matters,* 248; May, *Homeward Bound,* 149–50; and Marsh and Ronner, *Empty Cradle,* 186. I often convey this interpretation in my classroom as well.

3. Quote from PPFA pamphlet, "Plan Your Children for Health and Happiness," 1943, folder 2, box 33, Series III: PPFA, 1942–62, PPFAR I. See also page 9 of PPFA pamphlet, "Planning to Have a Baby?" n.d. [ca. 1940s], folder 2, box 33, Series III: PPFA, 1942–62, PPFAR I.

4. The Chicago affiliate's new name from Guthmann, *Planned Parenthood Movement in Illinois*, 9.

5. Jennette Dowling, *Sunday Afternoon*, 1947, folder 25, box 17, PPACAR.

6. According to one Planned Parenthood report, from 1940–47 the "Federation sold 1,264,946 pieces of literature, gave away 1,318,825 pieces representing a total distribution of 2,583,771 pieces." See Milestones in Planned Parenthood, n.d. [ca. late 1940s through early 1950s], folder 6, box 78, Series VII: Subject Files, Birth Control, PPFAR I.

7. Gordon, *Moral Property of Women*, 242–55.

8. For the World War II era as a planning "renaissance," see Scott, *American City Planning*, 397. For more on the history of planning, see Sies and Silver, eds., *Planning the Twentieth-Century American City*; for an excellent historiographic overview of planning and urban histories, see their introduction, "The History of Planning History," 1–34.

9. For example, "A family, like a house, expands more successfully when the expansion is well planned." Quote in PPFA pamphlet "A New Design for Living," n.d. [ca. 1940s–50s], folder 2, box 33, Series III: PPFA, 1942–62, PPFAR I.

10. Levitt quoted in Jackson, *Crabgrass Frontier*, 237.

11. Skinner's novel discussed in Herman, *Romance of American Psychology*, 8, 268–69.

12. Koncick, "No Longer under the Mattress."

13. Whitfield, *Culture of the Cold War*.

14. See Herman, *Romance of American Psychology*.

15. For divorce as neurosis, see Lundberg and Farnham, *Modern Woman*, 38–39. For juvenile delinquency, see Kathleen W. Jones, *Taming the Troublesome Child*, a study on the rise of child guidance clinics in the 1920s that showed the early roots of juvenile delinquency as a psychological problem both in child and parents. For unwed motherhood, see Solinger, *Wake Up Little Susie*, chapter 3; and Kunzel, *Fallen Women, Problem Girls*, chapter 6. For miscarriage, see Reagan, "From Hazard to Blessing to Tragedy," 362–63. For infertility, see May, *Barren in the Promised Land*, chapter 5.

16. For concerns about juvenile delinquency in the post–World War II era, see Gilbert, *Cycle of Outrage*. For concerns about unwed motherhood in the post–World War II era, see Solinger, *Wake Up Little Susie*. Interestingly, however, divorce rates had actually stabilized during this period and worries about youth gangs and unwed motherhood had long been in existence. For the stabilization of divorce rates, see Mintz and Kellogg, *Domestic Revolutions*, 178–79. For earlier concerns about unwed motherhood, see Kunzel, *Fallen Women, Problem Girls*. For earlier concerns about juvenile delinquency, see Schneider, *In the Web of Class*. See also the Progressive-era psychology studies on juvenile delinquency, Puffer, *The Boy and His Gang*; and Thrasher, *The Gang*. Thanks to my husband Eric Buhs for pointing out these last two books to me.

17. Quotes from PPFA pamphlet "An American Drama. Act III," 1946, folder 2, box 33, Series III: PPFA, 1942–62, PPFAR I; and PPFA pamphlet "Today," 1947, folder 6, box 19, PPACAR.

18. PPFA pamphlet "The Soldier Takes a Wife," n.d. [ca. 1940s], folder 6, box 19, PPACAR.

19. Dowling, "Sunday Afternoon," 10.

20. For picture of the blueprint baby, see "The Soldier Takes a Wife." For house floor plans, see "A New Design for Living."

21. Dowling, "Sunday Afternoon," 14.

22. "A New Design for Living."

23. Quote and images found on pages 2 and 16 in "Planning to Have a Baby?"

24. PPFA pamphlet "Escape from Fear," 1956, folder 2, box 33, Series III: PPFA, 1942–62, PPFAR I.

25. "Thirteen," in Sanger, *Motherhood in Bondage*, 212–13; quotes, 213.

26. Walter R. Stokes's comments reprinted in "Medicine. How to Have Babies." A similar focus on psychological rather physical can be found in the PPFA pamphlet, "The Roots of Delinquency," n.d. [ca. 1940s], folder 2, box 33, Series III: 1942–62, PPFAR I. See especially the last three pages.

27. See chapter 3, "The Trap of Maternity," in Sanger, *Motherhood in Bondage*, 40–59.

28. Quote from Dowling, "Sunday Afternoon," 9.

29. Story printed in Illinois Birth Control League newsletter, "Better Babies through Planned Parenthood," n.d. [ca. mid 1940s], folder 4, box 2, PPACAR.

30. Letters appeared in the PPFA pamphlet "Dear Doctor," n.d. [ca. 1940s], folder 2, box 33, Series III: PPFA, 1942–62, PPFAR I. However, it is not clear whether such letters were real.

31. "The Soldier Takes a Wife."

32. Dowling, "Sunday Afternoon," 6.

33. "Escape from Fear." Italics appeared as boldface in original.

34. Dowling, "Sunday Afternoon," 16–17; and "Escape from Fear."

35. "Planning to Have a Baby?," 15.

36. For example, Strickland and Ambrose, "The Baby Boom."

37. Dowling, "Sunday Afternoon," 13.

38. Early examples were clearly born of demobilization rhetoric. See, for example, "The Soldier Takes a Wife." But even as discussion of returning veterans faded from view, this message remained. See Dowling, "Sunday Afternoon."

39. Quote from "The Soldier Takes a Wife." See also "Plan Your Children for Health and Happiness," which encouraged couples to have babies "at least two years apart."

40. Quote from Stokes in "Medicine. How to Have Babies."

41. Dowling, "Sunday Afternoon," 10.

42. Smith, "Enter Planned Parenthood," 31.

43. "Planned Parenthood Meeting."

44. McCann, *Birth Control Politics*, 193–94.

45. Quotes about unsuspecting father found in "Planning to Have a Baby?," 2. For men's participation in helping women get abortions and contraceptives, see Watkins and Danzi, "Women's Gossip and Social Change," 479–82; and Reagan, *When Abortion Was a Crime*, 31–35.

46. Although, as Andrea Tone has noted, condoms had become less popular with rising feminine hygiene sales, they remained common. See "Contraceptive Consumers," 500.

47. "Told by Clinic Nurses."

48. "Fourteen," in Sanger, *Motherhood in Bondage*, 406–7; quote, 407.

49. "Ten," in Sanger, *Motherhood in Bondage*, 255.

50. Stearns and Knapp, "Men and Romantic Love."

51. "Six," in Sanger, *Motherhood in Bondage*, 252–53; quote, 252.

52. "Eight," in Sanger, *Motherhood in Bondage*, 332–35; quote, 335.

53. "What Do You Think of Birth Control?," 7.

54. LaRossa, *Modernization of Fatherhood*, chapters 1, 4, and 7; quote, 145–46. For more on the Children's Bureau and the letters it received from women, the significance of which LaRossa did not want to diminish, see Ladd-Taylor, *Raising a Baby the Government Way*.

55. Dowling, "Sunday Afternoon," 14.

56. Sanger, "Clinics the Solution," 6.

57. Dowling, "Sunday Afternoon," 16.

58. Planned Parenthood Association of Champaign County leaflet and attached anonymous letter from Champaign affiliate to national Planned Parenthood office, n.d. [ca. 1940s]. Both in Champaign, Planned Parenthood Association, Publicity, Pamphlets, etc., Series: Affiliates, Illinois, box 152, PPFAR II.

59. According to a 1945 report, there were 584 clinics throughout the United States. See Report on Contraceptive and Fertility Clinic Services, 1945, folder 1, box 83, Series VII: Subject Files, Clinics, PPFAR I.

60. These locations taken from 1947 directory. The directory also indicated that Illinois was home to seventeen clinics, but some of these may not have been directly affiliated with PPFA. See Directory of Planned Parenthood Clinic Services, March 1947, folder 1, box 33, Series III: PPFA, 1942–62, PPFAR I. For more on Illinois affiliates and their clinics throughout the state, see Guthmann, *Planned Parenthood Movement in Illinois*.

61. For example, according to one PPFA survey, only six new affiliates emerged during the 1940s and 1950s. See Field Department to Affiliate Presidents and Executive Directors, Regarding Affiliate Historical Survey, November 8, 1968, Affiliates Historical Survey, 1967–80, Series: Affiliates, PPWP Affiliates General, box 138, PPFAR II. There was even some discussion that clinic attendance may have declined. See Field Committee Meeting, March 5, 1952, folder 1, box 15, Series III: PPFA, 1942–62, PPFAR I. Evidence of local fluctuations in Chicago can be found by comparing lists and locations of clinics for 1937 (which lists nine), 1947 (which lists seventeen), and 1959 (which lists seven). See, respectively, Annual Report of the Illinois Birth Control League, April 1937, folder 12, box, 88, Series VII: Subject Files, PPFAR I; Directory of Planned Parenthood Clinic Services, March 1947; and *Planned Parenthood News* 11, no. 3 (December 1959), folder 10, box 390, WCMCR.

62. Discussion of need for field visits in PPFA Annual Report, 1948, folder 8, box 14, Series III: 1942–62, PPFAR I.

63. K.T.—Field Department, Comments on Present Status of State Leagues, March 23, 1942, History, 1931–53, Series VII: Subject Files, Birth Control, box 78, PPFAR I.

64. Simone M. Caron documented similar tensions during this period between the Rhode Island Planned Parenthood and the national Planned Parenthood office. See *Who Chooses?*, 124, 141–47.

65. Dickinson, *Control of Conception*, 2.

66. Stix, "Birth Control in a Midwestern City" (April 1939): 157.

67. Robishaw, "Study of 4,000 Patients," page 431.

68. Kopp, *Birth Control in Practice*, 167. Notably, these were the reasons why service was deferred (i.e., the diaphragm was not prescribed). But I would argue that they suggest the reasons why the women who were prescribed the method stopped using it later on.

69. "Clinic Reports. Minnesota Birth Control League," 20. See also Matsner, "Letters to the Editor."

70. Hajo, *Birth Control on Main Street*, 65.

71. Quote from Stix, "Birth Control in a Midwestern City" (April 1939): 164. Italics mine. Table that shows postclinic methods of contraception, 166.

72. Reed, *From Private Vice to Public Virtue*, 244–45; quote, 244.

73. Tone, *Devices and Desires*, 183.

74. Ibid., 181–82.

75. Meyer, *Any Friend of the Movement*, 102.

76. Hajo, *Birth Control on Main Street*, 66.

77. Letter reprinted in Meyer, *Any Friend of the Movement*, 103.

78. Stix, "Birth Control in a Midwestern City" (October 1939): 402–4.

79. Ibid., 423.

80. Dickinson, *Control of Conception*, 5. Dickinson's inclusion of the safe period should come as no surprise because discussion of the rhythm method had become more common during the 1930s and 1940s. See Lennon, "Rhythm and Authority."

81. Dickinson, *Techniques of Conception Control*, 52.

82. Dickinson, *Control of Conception*, 6. Another PPFA manual offered similar advice. See *Case Worker and Family Planning*, 19. See also the chart entitled "Summary of Contraceptives and Their Uses," which appeared inside the front cover of Dickinson's 1950 manual, *Techniques of Conception Control*. In this same edition, Dickinson further suggested that the term "diaphragm" was too difficult for individuals with limited education and urged those who chose to prescribe this method to such individuals to use the words "cap or cup" (13).

83. Briggs, *Reproducing Empire*, 105.

84. For Sanger's 1912 vision of a pill, see May, *America and the Pill*, 21.

85. Letter reprinted in Schoen, *Choice and Coercion*, 28.

86. Quote in Briggs, *Reproducing Empire*, 105.

87. Letter reprinted in May, *America and the Pill*, 20.

88. See Mary S. Calderone, "1960 Survey of Methods Used in 73 Planned Parenthood Centers," May 16, 1961, folder 60, box 4, Mary Steichen Calderone Papers, MC 179, Schlesinger Library, Radcliffe Institute, Harvard University, Cambridge, MA (hereafter cited as MSCP). Note too Calderone's remark in this survey that "obviously this is the method of choice," though she then questioned whose choice (patients' or clinics').

89. Guttmacher's remarks, which he claimed he made in the late 1950s, taken from Guttmacher, *Birth Control and Love*, 57.

90. For the history of women's entrance into the medical profession in the nineteenth century as well as their subsequent decline in numbers by the middle of the twentieth, see Walsh, *Doctors Wanted*. For the makeup of clinic personnel, see

the following. In Chicago, the pool of clinic doctors consisted of six men and one woman. The six remaining staff members (nurses, social workers, and office help) were all women. See Mary A. Young, PPACA Membership Report, March 25, 1947, folder 9, box 390, WCMCR. In Danville, the two volunteers described at one clinic session were women, though the doctor was male. The other six people listed with the affiliate were all women. See Miriam F. Garwood to William Vogt, Regarding the Evaluation of Planned Parenthood Services—Vermillion County Planned Parenthood Assn. in Danville, Illinois, December 12, 13, 14, 15, 16, 1955, Danville, Field Trips, 1950–55, Series: Affiliates, Illinois, box 153, PPFAR II.

91. Robishaw, "Study of 4,000 Patients," 431. Calculations conducted by me: 3,264 women received the diaphragm, among them 1,504 quit (46.1 percent) and 1,760 (53.9 percent) continued.

92. Though she drew this as a possible conclusion, she also worried: "are we unconsciously resisting [other] methods and, therefore, underselling them?" See Calderone, "1960 Survey of Methods Used in 73 Planned Parenthood Centers."

93. Quoted in Valien and Fitzgerald, "Attitudes of the Negro Mother," 280.

94. See page 3 of Postgraduate Institute on Clinic Procedures, January 26, 1940, folder 1, box 81, Series: VII: Subject Files, Clinics, PPFAR I.

95. "The Fight for Better Babies." See also the Planned Parenthood clinic visit depicted in "Escape from Fear."

96. See, for example, "Plan Your Children for Health and Happiness"; and "Planning to Have a Baby?" Two exceptions are "The Soldier Takes a Wife"; and "Escape from Fear."

97. "Escape from Fear." Italics mine.

98. Dickinson, *Techniques of Conception Control.* Discussion of a variety of methods as well as illustrations appear on 13–47. Actual clinic work and the supplies they need, 50–54.

99. Postgraduate Institute on Clinic Procedures.

100. Page 2 in Minutes of the Field Committee Meeting, November 20, 1947, folder 4, box 15, Series III: PPFA, 1942–62, PPFAR I. Unfortunately, the report did not indicate who or how many actually left, though the number appears to have been substantial enough to pose "great concern" among the Field Committee members.

101. See series of reports dating from 1955 to 1956: Miriam F. Garwood to Doris L. Rutledge, Regarding Visit to Champaign-Urbana, Illinois, December 14, 1955, Champaign, Field Trips, 1950–62, box 152, Series: Affiliates, Illinois, PPFAR II; Garwood to Vogt, Regarding the Evaluation of Planned Parenthood Services—Vermillion County Planned Parenthood Assn. in Danville, Illinois, December 12, 13, 14, 15, 16, 1955; Miriam F. Garwood to Mary S. Calderone, Regarding the Situation in Danville, Vermillion County, Illinois, December 21, 1955, Danville, Affiliation, PP Association of Vermillion County, 1949–56, box 153, Series: Affiliates, Illinois, PPFAR II; and Mary S. Calderone to Mrs. William B. Derby, January 25, 1956, Danville, Affiliation, PP Association of Vermillion County, 1949–56, box 153, Series: Affiliates, Illinois, PPFAR II.

102. Garwood to Vogt, Regarding the Evaluation of Planned Parenthood Services; quotes, 4.

103. Tanner quotes in Garwood to Calderone, Regarding the Medical Situation in Danville, Vermillion County, Illinois,.

104. Quotes from page 7 in Part II: Recommendations, n.d. [ca. 1940s], History, 1931–53, Series VII: Subject Files, Birth Control, box 78, PPFAR I. Jessie Rodrique made similar findings in her study on African Americans and birth control. See "The Black Community," 149.

105. Part II: Recommendations; quotes, 7 and 8.

106. For this desire to get out of clinic work, see Outline of Work toward "Big Push," n.d. [ca. 1959], folder 1, box 5, PPACAR; and Summary of Panel Discussion: "What Do We Mean by the Big Push," November 16, 1959, "Big Push," 1959–61, Series: Affiliates, PPFA National Affiliates, box 137, PPFAR II.

107. Part II: Recommendations; quote, 7. For more on local workers' preference for clinic (rather than administrative) work, see page 9 of Answers to Questionnaire Presented by the Committee for the Study of Voluntary Health Agencies of the National Health Council to PPFA, Inc., n.d. [ca. mid-1940s], folder 5, box 78, Series VII: Subject Files, Birth Control, PPFAR I. See also the situation in Danville. Mrs. L. T. Allen was not alone in her desire to do clinic work; two other women shared her sentiments. See Garwood to Vogt, Regarding the Evaluation of Planned Parenthood Services.

108. Guthmann, *Planned Parenthood Movement in Illinois*, 9.

109. Clinic total from PPACA Highlights, 1949, folder 12, box 71, Series V: Counties and Regions, Margaret Sanger Papers, Unfilmed Collection, Sophia Smith Collection, Smith College, Northampton, MA (hereafter cited as MSP Unfilmed–SC). In a report several months after the opening, the clinic noted how it was immediately . . . swamped with patients." See "S.R.O. at New Fertility Clinic. Illinois," *News Exchange* 1 (June 1944), folder 1, box 21, PPACAR.

110. Gordon, *Moral Property of Women*, 255–78.

111. See listing of services for Champaign and Chicago in Clinic Directory–Planned Parenthood Affiliates, 1957, Directory of PP Affiliate Centers, 1957–70, Series: Affiliates, PPWP Affiliates General, box 137, PPFAR II.

112. For Springfield, they tried a marriage workshop, but very few attended. There is also no mention of infertility services. See Miriam F. Garwood to William Vogt, Work with Planned Parenthood Association of Springfield, April 23–25, 1957, Springfield, Field Trips, 1957–60, Series: Affiliates, Illinois, box 153, PPFAR II. For Danville, there is no mention of either of these services.

113. For example, a 1949 directory of services listed five pages of affiliates that offered "Conception Control Services" while "Fertility Services" had just over one page. See Directory of Planned Parenthood Clinic Services, 1949, folder 6, box 80, Series VII: Subject Files, Clinics, PPFAR I.

114. Required Minimum Standards for Certification of Clinics, June 1956, Clinics, General, 1956–68, Series: Affiliates, PPFA National, box 137, PPFAR II.

115. Borg, "Birth Control and State Fairs," 371.

116. See page 16 of Clinic Manual (third draft), November 1944, folder 10, box 80, Series: VII: Subject Files, Clinics, PPFAR I.

117. Sanger quote in Chesler, *Woman of Valor*, 298.

118. A similar tension, which assumed the poor were unable or unwilling to take into account the future impact of their current habits, could be found in anticancer campaigns in America. See Patterson, *Dread Disease*, 228–29.

119. For one description of these exhibits, see Borg, "Birth Control and State Fairs," 372.

120. For an African American version, see PPFA pamphlet "Planned Parenthood," n.d. [ca. early 1940s], folder 9, box 20, Series II: National Office, Planned Parenthood, 1925–73, PPACAR.

121. Quote from page 7 of *News Exchange* 12 (June 1945), folder 1, box 21, PPACAR.

122. "The Roots of Delinquency."

123. Dykeman, *Too Many People.*

124. "The Roots of Delinquency."

125. "The Fight for Better Babies."

126. The Story of the Picture (treatment of a proposed motion picture for PPFA), June 20, 1945, folder 5, box 86, Series VII: Subject Files, PPFAR I.

127. Quote from Lt. Col. Roy R. Grinker in "The Soldier Takes a Wife."

128. "The Roots of Delinquency."

129. Stokes quoted in "Medicine. How to Have Babies."

130. PPFA pamphlet "A New Baby Is Born!," 1948, folder 2, box 33, Series III: PPFA, 1942–62, PPFAR I; and Planned Parenthood Chicago Area pamphlet "Every 10 Seconds a Baby is Born in America," 1949, folder 12, box 71, Series V: Counties and Regions, MSP Unfilmed–SC.

131. *Planned Parenthood News* 7, no. 3 (May 1954), folder 4, box 2, PPACAR. For more on the assumption that children born into impoverished homes are mistakes, see May, *Barren in the Promised Land,* 8–9.

132. From the following exchange of letters: Margaret Sanger to Mary S. Calderone, February 25, 1956; and Calderone's reply, February 29, 1956. Both in PPFA: National, Medical Correspondence, General, 1955–58, Series: Classified Files, box 69, PPFAR II.

133. Marsh and Ronner, *Empty Cradle,* 171–98. For discussion of the economic backgrounds of his clinic clientele, see 189.

134. Quote from page 4 of Clinic Manual (third draft), November 1944.

135. "Are You Too Educated to be a Mother?" For other examples in the popular press that made similar eugenic arguments, see Thompson, "Race Suicide of the Intelligent"; and Smith, "Enter Planned Parenthood."

136. Dowling, "Sunday Afternoon," 12.

137. "The Roots of Delinquency."

138. In Chicago, for example, they talked not only to members of the medical profession, universities, hospitals, labor groups, and religious organizations, but also to "board members and staffs of social agencies, staffs and residents of Housing projects, private, state and county institutions, . . . probation officers, judges of juvenile and marriage courts." See *Planned Parenthood News* 5, no. 1 (November 1951): 4, folder 4, box 2, PPACAR.

139. Quotes from page 3 in "A Baby Party," *Planned Parenthood News* 3, no. 1 (June 1950), folder 4, box 2, PPACAR.

140. *News Exchange* 34 (March 1948), folder 2, box 21, PPACAR.

141. From 1949 through 1957, there were a total of nine "Ma and Pa Kettle" movies: *Ma and Pa Kettle,* directed by Charles Lamont (Universal International Pictures, 1949); *Ma and Pa Kettle Go to Town,* directed by Charles Lamont (Universal International Pictures, 1950); *Ma and Pa Kettle Back on the Farm,* directed by Edward Sedgwick (Universal International Pictures, 1951); *Ma and Pa Kettle at the Fair,* directed

by Charles Barton (Universal International Pictures, 1952); *Ma and Pa Kettle on Vacation*, directed by Charles Lamont (Universal International Pictures, 1953); *Ma and Pa Kettle at Home*, directed by Charles Lamont (Universal International Pictures, 1954); *Ma and Pa Kettle at Waikiki*, directed by Lee Sholem (Universal International Pictures, 1955); *The Kettles in the Ozarks*, directed by Charles Lamont (Universal International Pictures, 1956); and *The Kettles on Old MacDonald's Farm*, directed by Virgil W. Vogel (Universal International Pictures, 1957).

142. Jameson, "Catholic Mother Looks," 102.

143. Gordon, *Moral Property of Women*, 239.

144. See, for example, Jama Lazerow's historiographic review of religion and working-class history in antebellum America in "Rethinking Religion and the Working Class in Antebellum America." He noted that historians had defined the real interests of workers as better working conditions, shorter days, and better pay, while religious fervor was seen as nothing more than inconsequential trappings or hindrances to labor organizing.

Chapter Four

1. Dorothy Baker, "History of Planned Parenthood Association of Champaign County, 1940–1980;" quote, 5–6. A copy of the talk was obtained directly from the historical records maintained by the Planned Parenthood of East Central Illinois, Champaign, Illinois. This speech was then reprinted virtually word for word in a publication put out by the local affiliate in 1980. Permission for use obtained from the Planned Parenthood of East Central Illinois and is in author's possession.

2. Admittedly, to use 1960 as the benchmark for all these developments is restrictive in that it applies to the introduction of the pill on the market. But these processes were in development around this time and have all been described by historians. For the pill, see Watkins, *On the Pill*; and Marks, *Sexual Chemistry*. For concerns about overpopulation, increased federal spending, and the sexual revolution more generally, see Allyn, *Make Love Not War*; Bailey, *Sex in the Heartland*; Critchlow, *Intended Consequences*; D'Emilio and Freedman, *Intimate Matters*, chapters 13 and 14; and Gordon, *Moral Property of Women*, chapter 12.

3. Baker, "History of Planned Parenthood," 6.

4. For the Champaign Medical Society's insistence that they serve only the indigent poor, see Baker, "History of Planned Parenthood," 7. For the federation's 1948 softening of its income requirement, see William T. Kennedy and L. E. Kling to Chairmen et al., Regarding Revised Standards for Certification of Clinics," March 3, 1948, folder 11, box 80, Series VII: Subject Files, Clinics, PPFAR I. The reasons why this recommendation was eased are not clear and deserve further investigation.

5. Carl E. Speckman to Naomi T. Gray, September 13, 1965, Regarding Affiliate Renewal Report for Evansville, Indiana, Anti-Poverty from 1965, Series: Affiliates, Illinois, box 151, PPFAR II. Failure to pay federation dues was also an issue.

6. Quote in Mrs. J. McVicker Hunt to Mrs. Eve R. Dyrssen, September 16, 1964, Migrant 1964–69, Series: Affiliates, Illinois, box 151, PPFAR II.

7. List of magazines drawn from Watkins, *On the Pill*, 41–49.

8. Ibid., 50.

9. Ibid., chapter 2; quotes, 34.

10. Mary S. Calderone, "Impact of New Methods on Practice in 73 Planned Parenthood Centers," speech given at the annual meeting of the American Public Health Association, October 17, 1962, Contraceptives, 1961 Survey of 73 Centers, 1961–62, Series: Affiliates, PPFA National, box 137, PPFAR II. See also Watkins, *On the Pill*, 40–41.

11. Hajo, *Birth Control on Main Street*, 158.

12. Meyer, *Any Friend of the Movement*, 123–24.

13. Ruth Dobbins, interview by author, September 3, 1998. Tape recording and transcription in author's possession. Permission for use and IRB approval also in author's possession.

14. For documents discussing the Pill Purchase Plan, see PPACA Executive Committee Meeting, February 5, 1965, Chicago Area, Minutes, 1964–77, Series: Affiliates, Illinois, box 134, PPFAR II; Terrence P. Tiffany to Benjamin Lewis, n.d. [ca. 1971], Chicago Area, 1970–79, Series: Affiliates, Illinois, box 152, PPFAR II; and (Selected) Direct Services Provided by National Staff for Affiliates, 1971, Series: Affiliates, Affiliates General, box 137, PPFAR II.

15. Interview with Ruth Dobbins.

16. Materials can be found in the folder entitled "PPWP: Medical Department, Contraceptives, Oral, Purchase Program, 1965–1967," Series: Classified Files, box 70, PPFAR II.

17. Baker, "History of Planned Parenthood," 6.

18. Details regarding affiliate research drawn from Affiliate Research Chart, n.d. [ca. mid 1960s], PPFA National: Affiliates' Research, General, Mimeos, etc., 1962–72, Series: Affiliates, box 139, PPFAR II. The total number of affiliates is difficult to determine because of the constant fluctuation and the difficulty in obtaining solid numbers. In this case, however, they are drawn from Calderone, "Impact of New Methods." In this talk, Calderone said there were ninety-five.

19. For evidence of local offices' failure to report to the national office about research, see correspondence in folder entitled "PPWP Affiliates General: Affiliates' Research, 1970–1973," Series: Affiliates, box 139, PPFAR II.

20. Anderson, "Private Choices vs. Public Voices," 225–26, 282; and Caron, *Who Chooses?*, 150–51.

21. Meldrum, "Simple Methods."

22. See note 37 in the introduction of this volume.

23. Rothman, *Strangers at the Bedside*, chapters 2 and 3; and Marks, *Progress of Experiment*, chapter 4. Many thanks also to my statistician husband for explaining to me the mysteries of quantitative statistical analysis.

24. Mary S. Calderone to Harold, June 22, 1959, folder 69, box 5, MSCP. See also the language she used in a 1963 memo in which she remarked: "It is not too much to say that this study is of significance in the eyes of the whole medical world, and we carry a responsibility because we are the only group able to command such a large number of long-term Enovid users." Mary S. Calderone to the Chairman of the Medical Advisory Committee et al., November 14, 1963, PPFA: Subject, Enovid, Survey, Long Term Studies, from 1957, Series: Classified Files, box 68, PPFAR II.

25. Details of the study drawn from Meldrum, "Simple Methods"; PPFA Clinical Investigation Program: Operating Procedures, October 1959, folder 69, box 5, MSCP; and Sarah Tietze, PPFA Clinical Investigation Program, May 12, 1960, talk delivered before the Planned Parenthood Federation Eastern League, folder 83, box 6, MSCP.

26. The two-year duration of the study was determined by FDA rules. When the FDA first approved the pill, it limited prescriptions to two years because of its unknown long-term effects. Hence the necessity of such a study. For discussion of the pill's approval process, see Junod and Marks, "Women's Trials." For a scathing critique of the 25 Month Club at the time, see journalist Morton Mintz's discussion in his exposé on the pill in *"The Pill,"* 57–59.

27. For details about CIP, see Mary S. Calderone to All Affiliates, Regarding 24 Months Enovid Program, January 15, 1963; and PPWP News Release: Mass Oral Contraceptive Study Findings Released, June 1965. Both in PPFA: Subject, Enovid 25-Month Club, 10/5/62–10/21/66, Series: Classified Files, box 68, PPFAR II.

28. Jean L. McNeill to Mary S. Calderone, March 12, 1958, folder 77, box 6, MSCP.

29. See materials throughout the folder entitled "PPWP Affiliates General: Affiliates' Research, 1970–1973," Series: Affiliates, box 139, PPFAR II.

30. For the first call in 1957 that affiliates register their research, see Mary S. Calderone to Executive Committee, Regarding Medical Committee Recommendation, October 8, 1957, PPFA: National, Medical Correspondence, General, 1955–58, Series: Classified Files, box 69, PPFAR II. For the renewed call in 1963, see Laurie S. Strauss to Mary S. Calderone, September 17, 1963, PPWP Affiliates General: Affiliates' Research, 1970–73, Series: Affiliates, box 139, PPFAR II.

31. Indeed, by 1966 the national medical advisory board was sending out notices every six months reminding affiliates to register their projects. Medical Department (PPFA) to All Affiliates, Regarding Research Registration, September 1966, PPWP Affiliates General: Affiliates' Research, 1970–73, Series: Affiliates, box 139, PPFAR II.

32. Required Minimum Standards for Certification of Birth Control Clinics, September 1938.

33. Collins quoted in PPFA Medical Committee Meeting, September 13, 1961, folder 60, box 4, MSCP.

34. Marjorie P. Davis to Mary S. Calderone, May 22, 1959, folder 80, box 6, MSCP. Underlining in original.

35. Mary S. Calderone to Nathaniel Elias, December 29, 1955, folder 55, box 4, MSCP.

36. Meldrum, "Simple Methods," 269.

37. Memo to John Robbins, Robin Elliott, and Doris Bernheim, April 30, 1971, Regarding San Antonio Research, Affiliates General: Affiliates' Research, 1971–72, Series: Affiliates, box 139, PPFAR II.

38. *Planned Parenthood News* 11, no. 2 (May 1959), folder 10, box 390, WCMCR.

39. Speckman to Gray, Regarding Affiliate Renewal Report for Evansville, Indiana, September 13, 1965.

40. Anderson, "Private Choices vs. Public Voices," 228. See also her great discussion of the affiliate's efforts to resolve its financial difficulties during the 1960s (227–38).

41. Terrence P. Tiffany to Betty Forbes, February 25, 1972, Decatur, PP Steering Committee, 1966–79, Series: Affiliates, Illinois, box 153, PPFAR II.

42. Pages 4–5 of Robert L. Webber, "A Brief History of Planned Parenthood Iowa," October 1970, Affiliates Historical Survey, 1967–80, Series: Affiliates, PPWP Affiliates General, box 138, PPFAR II.

43. Baker, "History of Planned Parenthood," 6–7; quote, 6.

44. I would also argue that Champaign could hardly have been unique in this regard; Eli Lilly carried out research at affiliates elsewhere in the nation, probably using similar techniques. Moreover, even the rules for the Clinical Investigation Program were slippery where marriage was concerned, in that the study participant need only be living with a husband, partner, or fiancé. See PPFA Clinical Investigation Program: Operating Procedures, October 1959.

45. See the letters found in a folder entitled "Contacts from 1964," Series: Affiliates, Illinois, box 151, PPFAR II.

46. Numbers drawn from Field Department to Affiliate Presidents and Executive Directors, Regarding Affiliate Historical Survey, November 8, 1968. Another report indicated that Planned Parenthood's caseload had "more than tripled" between 1957 and 1969. See page x in "Planned Parenthood–World Population Inter-Affiliate Statistical Report, 1969 Summary," Interaffiliate Statistical Report and Summary, 1969–70, Series: Affiliates, PPWP Affiliates General, box 138, PPFAR II.

47. Sanger, *My Fight for Birth Control*, 144.

48. Cohen, *Consumers' Republic*, 7.

49. Jean Trisko to Winfield Best, Regarding CBS Report TV Program, May 18, 1962, Chicago Area, Field Trips, 1960–66, Series: Affiliates, Illinois, box 153, PPFAR II.

50. Miriam F. Garwood to Winfield Best, Field Report, June 5, 1962, Chicago Area, Field Trips, 1960–66, Series: Affiliates, Illinois, box 153, PPFAR II.

51. For a letter from St. Paul (probably Minnesota), see Mrs. Lloyd A. Larsch to Jane C. Browne, November 25, 1964. For a letter from Rochester, NY, see Linda J. Redman to Jane C. Browne, December 1, 1964. For a letter from Alameda County (probably California), see Sybil A. Dinaburg to Jane C. Browne, November 25, 1964. All three can be found in Chicago Area, PP Association, 1960–64, Series: Affiliates, Illinois, box 152, PPFAR II.

52. Numbers drawn from Biographical Sketch of Mrs. Jane C. Browne, Executive Director of Planned Parenthood Association, Chicago Area, June 1967, Chicago, PP Association, Reports, Members, 1964–76, Series: Affiliates, Illinois, box 152, PPFAR II; and the remarks made by Jane C. Browne at PPACA Annual Meeting and Benefit Dinner at the Conrad Hilton, February 3, 1966, Chicago, PP Association, Reports, General, 1964–77, Series: Affiliates, Illinois, box 153, PPFAR II.

53. In 1964, the top twenty budgets belonged to: Chicago ($610,244), the Sanger Bureau ($552,982), then Manhattan-Bronx, Baltimore, Cleveland, Pittsburgh, Detroit, San Francisco, Washington, DC, Buffalo, Oakland, Philadelphia, Denver, Los Angeles, Cincinnati, St. Louis, Rochester, Minneapolis, Dallas, and Houston (whose budget stood at $91,519). See PP–WP Fundraising Report for

1964, Chicago, PP Association, Reports, General, 1964–77, Series: Affiliates, Illinois, box 153, PPFAR II.

54. Donald J. Bogue and Jane C. Browne, "The Chicago West Side Experiment to Accelerate the Adoption of Birth Control by a Mass Communication Campaign: An Interim Progress Report," n.d. [ca. 1962], University of Chicago, Mass Communications, Reports, 1955–66, Series: Affiliates, Illinois, box 152, PPFAR II. See also Jane C. Browne and Donald Bogue, "Problems of Bearing and Rearing Children," 1961, University of Chicago, 1st Workshop, Mass Communications, 1961–63, Series: Affiliates, Illinois, box 152, PPFAR II. Here the weaknesses of the clinic approach were directly laid out.

55. Plans for Planned Parenthood Discussion Groups ("Coffee Sips"), n.d. [ca. 1960s], Public Health, Correspondence, 1963–70, Series: Affiliates, Illinois, box 151, PPFAR II.

56. Details about the Bogue Project and its methods of outreach drawn from Bogue and Browne, "The Chicago West Side Experiment to Accelerate the Adoption of Birth Control;" and Jane C. Browne, "Planned Parenthood's Campaign to Reach Families in the Slum Areas of Chicago," n.d. [ca. 1962], Cook County Hospital Situation, 1958–66, Series: Affiliates, Illinois, box 151, PPFAR II. For more materials on the Mobile Unit Program in Illinois, see folder entitled "Illinois Mobile Units, 1961–1963," Series: Affiliates, box 139, PPFAR II. For more on mobile units established in other cities, see materials in folder entitled "PPFA: Mobile Units, Miscellaneous, 1961–1965," Series: Affiliates, box 139, PPFAR II.

57. For backgrounds of those working inside the mobile units, see PP-Mobile Units, October 18, 1961, PPFA: Mobile Units, Miscellaneous, 1961–65, Series: Affiliates, box 139, PPFAR II.

58. Elsie Jackson to Fred Jaffe, Preliminary Outline "Committee for the Study and Development of Non-Professional Neighborhood Workers," September 29, 1965, Indigenous Neighborhood Workers, 1965–73, Series: Affiliates, PPWP Affiliates General, box 138, PPFAR II.

59. Letter and coupon both in Bogue and Browne, "Chicago West Side Experiment."

60. Mrs. H. J. Van Cleave to Mary S. Calderone, February 14, 1958, PPFA: National, Mothers' Letters, Procedure General from 1955, Series: Classified Files, box 69, PPFAR II.

61. Johanna von Goeckingk to Mrs. H. J. Van Cleave, February 20, 1958, PPFA: National, Mothers' Letters, Procedure General from 1955, Series: Classified Files, box 69, PPFAR II.

62. Bogue and Browne, "Chicago West Side Experiment," 26.

63. "How to Practice Birth Control Effectively." This pamphlet was included in Bogue and Browne, "Chicago West Side Experiment."

64. Donald J. Bogue and Jane C. Browne, *Successful Family Planning Easy and Inexpensive: A Birth Control and Marriage Manual* (Chicago: University of Chicago Press, 1962), Chicago, PP Association, Publicity, Pamphlets, etc., 1972–76, Series: Affiliates, Illinois, box 153, PPFAR II. Quotes and chapter title, 50–51, and 41, respectively.

65. Guttmacher, *Birth Control and Love*, 102.

66. Van Cleave to Calderone, February 14, 1958.

67. Bogue and Browne, "The Chicago West Side Experiment," 24.

68. PPFA Patient Instructions, "Read and Remember," n.d. [ca. 1960s], Cook County Hospital Situation, 1958–66, Series: Affiliates, Illinois, box 151, PPFAR II.

69. Injunction appears in Guttmacher, *Birth Control and Love*, iv. The word "spouse" appears throughout the book; see especially chapters 7 and 8.

70. Planned Parenthood pamphlet "What Teenagers Want to Know about Family Planning," 1964, University of Chicago, General Correspondence from 1964, Series: Affiliates, Illinois, box 152, PPFAR II. All italics and capitalizations in the original.

71. Details of the IPAC controversy taken from Hal Bruno, "Birth Control"; and Dienes, *Law, Politics*, chapter 9, especially 274–77; quote, 276; full text of the final 1965 resolution, 333–34.

72. Drew Pearson, "World Eyes Birth Control Project," *Washington Post-Times-Herald*, April 1963, Chicago 3/63, Series: Affiliates, Illinois, box 153, PPFAR II. More newspaper clippings can be found in same folder. For more clippings, see another folder entitled "Chicago, Newspapers, 12/62," Series: Affiliates, Illinois, box 153, PPFAR II.

73. Trisko to Best, Regarding CBS Report TV Program, May 18, 1962.

74. For early coverage of the battle with Cook County Hospital, see Ralph Simon, "Background Statement Concerning Birth Control in Chicago, Illinois," 1962, Cook County Hospital Situation, 1958–66, Series: Affiliates, Illinois, box 151, PPFAR II; and Georgie Anne Geyer, "Birth Control in Chicago: The End of the Fight Is in Sight," *Chicago Scene* (November 1962): 24–29. For discussion of the Mobile Unit outside Cook County Hospital, see "Mobile Unit Dedicated," *Planned Parenthood News* 14, no. 2 (Summer 1962), folder 4, box 2, PPACAR.

75. "County Hospital Will Open Clinic!" *Planned Parenthood News* 19, no. 2 (Second Quarter, 1967), Chicago, PP Association, Publicity, Pamphlets, etc., 1972–76, Series: Affiliates, Illinois, box 153, PPFAR II.

76. The first Board of Health clinics were located at 4350 Sixteenth Street, 6504 Cottage Grove Avenue, 10801 Racine Avenue, 4720 Sheridan Road, 1000 Lyttle Street, and 4844 State Street. For initial clinic openings in 1965, see "717 Receiving Birth Control Aid," *Chicago Tribune*, June 1965, Newspaper Clippings, 1965, Series: Affiliates, Chicago, box 152, PPFAR II. For the additional clinics that existed by 1966, see "Margaret Sanger and Chicago."

77. Comments made by Dr. Day (medical director of Planned Parenthood–World Population) at the PPACA Medical Advisory Board Committee Meeting, October 27, 1965, Chicago Area, Minutes, 1964–77, Series: Affiliates, Illinois, box 134, PPFAR II. Browne's comments in same meeting minutes.

78. Webber, "Brief History," 10.

79. George Langmyhr to Jane C. Browne, November 1, 1966, Chicago Area, PP Association, 1965–66, Series: Affiliates: Illinois, box 152, PPFAR II. It's not clear, however, if this emphasis on the pill was true. As the quote later in the paragraph suggests, the city clinics may also have offered other methods.

80. Mary-Jane Snyder to Fred Jaffe, March 8, 1965, Public Health, Correspondence, 1964–72, Series: Affiliates, Illinois, box 151, PPFAR II. Underline in original.

81. Monk, "No Pill for the Single Girl."

82. Monk, "Our Single Girl Gets Birth Control Info." See also the first in the series, which followed a married woman's visit to one of the new Board of Health

clinics. Sandra Pressman, "Our Reporter Gets THE PILL!," *Chicago Sunday Star*, n.d. [ca. April 1965], folder 7, box 23, PPACAR.

83. Andelman quoted in Irv Letofsky, "Chicago Drops to 3rd City; Birth Control No Help," *Minneapolis Tribune*, n.d. [ca. May 1966], Newspaper Clippings, 1965, Series: Affiliates, Chicago, box 152, PPFAR II.

84. Lucie Prinz to Irene Nordine, December 19, 1967, Public Health Correspondence, 1963–70, Series: Affiliates, Illinois, box 151, PPFA Papers II. For more on William R. Baird, see Allyn, *Make Love Not War*, 35–37, 263–64, 266; Dienes, *Law, Politics,* 210–15; Garrow, *Liberty and Sexuality*, chapters 5–9, passim; Wall, "A Complicated Man"; and Wall, "Foam and Fornication."

85. "63rd Street Center to Open Full Time," *Planned Parenthood News* 11, no. 3 (December 1959), folder 10, box 390, WCMCR.

86. Hirsch, *Making the Second Ghetto*, 2–3. For more on post–World War II black migration and especially its impact on Chicago, see Lemann, *Promised Land.*

87. For example, see the Chicago Planned Parenthood staff photo in which a number of African Americans appear. In "Meet Our Staff," *Planned Parenthood News* 15, no. 2 (Fall 1963), Chicago, PP Association, Publicity, Pamphlets, etc., 1972–76, Series: Affiliates, Illinois, box 153, PPFAR II.

88. Perez's work described in PPACA Board of Directors Meeting, February 29, 1968, Chicago Area Minutes, 1964–77, Series: Affiliates, Illinois, box 134, PPFAR II. Though her name might suggest otherwise, she was also of African American heritage, as the meeting minutes note.

89. "'Help Your Neighbor' Project a Success," *Planned Parenthood News* 15, no. 2 (Fall 1963), Chicago, PP Association, Publicity, Pamphlets, etc., 1972–76, Series: Affiliates, Illinois, box 153, PPFAR II.

90. See photo of Patients' Auxiliary in *Planned Parenthood News* 18, no. 2 (Spring 1966), Chicago, PP Association, Publicity, Pamphlets, etc., 1972–76, Series: Affiliates, Illinois, box 153, PPFAR II.

91. For Marion Hampton, see photo and announcement in *Planned Parenthood News* 11, no. 3 (December 1959), folder 10, box 390, WCMCR. For Shirley Arnold, see photo and announcement in *Planned Parenthood News* 16, no. 3 (Fall 1964), folder 4, box 2, PPACAR.

92. For Dr. Nesbitt, see photo and caption in *Planned Parenthood News* 16, no. 3 (Fall 1964), folder 4, box 2, PPACAR. For Reverend Ward, see caption for photo in "PPA Dedicates the New Mobile Medical Unit at Henry Booth House," *Defender* (March 31–April 6, 1962), 21, folder 5, box 2, PPACAR.

93. Geyer, "Birth Control in Chicago."

94. See photos in "PPA Dedicates the New Mobile Medical Unit," PPACAR.

95. Picket photo on front page of *Planned Parenthood News* (Winter 1964), folder 3, box 21, PPACAR.

96. For Robinson's support in 1962, see Testimony Offered Regarding Birth Control before the Illinois Public Aid Commission, November 20–21, 1962, Cook County Hospital Situation, 1958–66, Series: Affiliates, Illinois, box 151, PPFAR II. For Robinson's award from Planned Parenthood, and quote, see "Three Receive Awards," *Planned Parenthood News* 17, no. 2 (Spring 1965), folder 4, box 2, PPACAR.

97. Clippings of the column can be found in boxes 23 and 24 of PPACAR. For quote, see clipping dated September 4, 1965, folder 3, box 24, PPACAR.

98. Guttmacher, "How Safe Are Birth Control Pills?"

99. Lees, "Negro Response to Birth Control," 47.

100. Alderman Lewis's work described in Geyer, "Birth Control in Chicago," 25.

101. "Project Tenants for Birth Control."

102. Rodrique, "Black Community," quotes, 150 and 147, respectively.

103. Lemann, *Promised Land*, 101.

104. Statement from the Chicago Urban League in Lees, "Negro Response to Birth Control," 47.

105. "A Proposal: A Program to Make Family Planning Available to the Southern Negro through Education, Motivation, and Implementation of Available Services," 1963, University of Chicago, 1st Workshop, Mass Communications, 1961–63, Series: Affiliates, Illinois, box 152, PPFAR II.

106. Knowles, *Seventy-five Years of Family Planning in America*.

107. For Chicago, see Hirsch, "Massive Resistance in the Urban North"; white slogan, 548. For Detroit, see Sugrue, "Crabgrass-Roots Politics."

108. Briggs used this phrase to describe white attitudes toward Puerto Rican families (*Reproducing Empire*, 117, 165).

109. Dr. Philip M. Hauser quoted in "Birth Control Policy Urged," 117.

110. Walkowitz, *Working with Class*, 217.

111. Quote from Brownlee, "Do We Have Too Many Children?," 35.

112. PPACA Board of Directors Meeting Bus Trip to PPACA Centers, May 19, 1965, Chicago Area, Minutes, 1964–77, Series: Affiliates, Illinois, box 134, PPFAR II. Hall and Bell account on page 2.

113. Policy for Planned Parenthood in Columbus, Ohio, can be found in folder entitled "PPWP Affiliates General: Survey of Affiliates' Policy on Service to Minors, 1967," Series: Affiliates, box 140, PPFAR II. Similar language also appeared in the federation's policy. See National Medical Advisory Committee Statement of Policy on Birth Control Services to Minors, October 10, 1967, PPWP Affiliates General: Services: Minors, Teenagers, 1967–74, Series: Affiliates, box 139, PPFAR II.

114. Hertwig's remarks in Michael Royko, "Officials Disagree on Private Center," *Chicago Daily News*, May 24, 1962, Chicago, 1–9/62, Series: Affiliates, Illinois, box 153, PPFAR II.

115. Solinger, *Wake Up Little Susie*, 18.

116. Phrase borrowed from Jacob A. Riis and his Progressive-era study, *How the Other Half Lives*.

117. Miriam F. Garwood to Alan Guttmacher, Chicago Visit, November 9, 1962, Chicago Area, Field Trips, 1960–66, Series: Affiliates, Illinois, box 153, PPFAR II.

118. PPACA Board of Directors Meeting Bus Trip to PPACA Centers, May 19, 1965.

119. "Men or Maggots?"

120. Geyer, "Birth Control in Chicago," 25. Similar language can be found in Shepherd, "Birth Control and the Poor," 64.

121. Dienes, *Law, Politics*, 255.

122. Bogue and Browne, "Chicago West Side Experiment."

123. Pearson, "World Eyes Birth Control Project," PPFAR II.

124. Garwood to Guttmacher, Chicago Visit, November 9, 1962. Italics added for emphasis.

125. Browne and Bogue, "Problems of Bearing and Rearing Children."

126. Reverend Ward and Young quoted in Geyer, "Birth Control in Chicago," 26 and 25, respectively.

127. Brownlee, "Do We Have Too Many Children?," 35.

128. "Project Tenants for Birth Control."

129. Letter appeared in Hunt, "Keep Your Family the Right Size."

130. Marya Mannes quoted in Wille, "Overpopulation Blamed on 'Selfish' Middle Class." It was Wille who suggested Mannes's remarks were "touchy."

131. PPACA Board of Directors Meeting, February 29, 1968; this and subsequent quotes, 4.

132. For more on the race genocide critique as it emerged in the 1960s, see Caron, "Birth Control"; and Nelson, *Women of Color*, chapter 3.

133. Rodrique, "Black Community," 142, 144–45. For more on the early debates within the African American community, see Roberts, *Killing the Black Body*, 82–89; and Hart, "Who Should Have the Children?"

134. Roberts, *Killing the Black Body*, 87–88.

135. Lees, "Negro Response to Birth Control," 47.

136. For Black fears of white medicine, see Gamble, "Under the Shadow of Tuskegee." Thanks to Mickey Moran for bringing this to my attention. For discussion of pill controversies regarding its safety, see Watkins, *On the Pill*, chapters 4 and 5.

137. The accusations made by the African American student during Perez's birth control speech were but one example. For another, see David Mann to Mrs. Mann, Regarding Nielson Survey, Kenwood-Oakwood Community, January 27, 1969, folder 5, box 17, PPACAR.

138. Both women quoted in "Project Tenants for Birth Control."

139. Quote in "Birth Control Plan in Illinois Rapped by NAACP Leader." Another NAACP member, Reverend Henry H. Nichols, also opposed birth control for the unwed and was reportedly "unalterably opposed to any birth-control program until the youth have become moral enough not to use it for immoral purposes." See Lees, "Negro Response to Birth Control," 46.

140. Twine quote from "IPAC Birth Control Plan Touches Off Sharp Debate," *Journal Standard* (Freeport, IL), November 1962, Chicago, Newspaper Articles, 11/62, Series: Affiliates, Illinois, box 153, PPFAR II. This same article identified him as a "Negro."

141. "Birth Control Aid Called Anti-Negro."

142. Quotes in Mann to Mann, Regarding Nielson Survey, Kenwood-Oakwood Community, January 27, 1969. An earlier memo suggests they tried to get a black Planned Parenthood worker by the name of Mr. Birchette to attend the community meeting. But apparently it was David Mann who attended, though the reasons why are unclear. Also unclear is his race. See Mrs. Mann to Mr. Birchette, Regarding KOCO Presentation, January 10, 1969, folder 5, box 17, PPACAR.

143. PPACA Board of Directors Meeting, February 29, 1968; quotes, 7 and 2, respectively.

144. Lendor C. Nesbitt to Donna Shavers, "Observations and Analysis of 'Double' Clinic at Center #3," June 21, 1969, folder 10, box 3, PPACAR.

145. Details drawn from "Fake Birth Control Pills," *Washington Post*, October 1, 1971; and Guttmacher, Report on San Antonio Fact Finding Trip Regarding Southwest Foundation-Syntex Research Project, June 7–8, 1971. Both in Affiliates General:

Affiliates' Research, San Antonio, 1971–72, Series: Affiliates, box 139, PPFAR II. Number in the control group drawn from Guttmacher's remark that "one in five were on the placebo." In addition, although Guttmacher reported seven pregnancies, the *Washington Post* reported only six—perhaps because one of the women may not have been in the placebo-taking control group. Also according to Guttmacher, of the women who got pregnant, five were Latina and two were white.

146. For discussion of contraceptive research in Puerto Rico, see Briggs, *Reproducing Empire*, 135–40; Gordon, *Moral Property of Women*, 286–88, 332; Marks, *Sexual Chemistry*, chapter 4; Ramírez de Arellano and Seipp, *Colonialism, Catholicism, and Contraception*, 105–33; Reed, *From Private Vice to Public Virtue*, 359–62; Watkins, *On the Pill*, 31–32; and Vaughan, *Pill on Trial*, chapter 3.

147. Rothman, *Strangers at the Bedside.*

148. The Southwest Foundation was established in 1941. Its primary goal was to operate as a nonprofit scientific institution committed to basic biomedical research. The foundation remains in existence. For more on the organization, see http://www.sfbr.org/ (accessed December 6, 2010).

149. Joseph William Goldzieher received his medical degree in 1943 from the New York University School of Medicine and his license to practice in 1953. His specialty was not listed, but he may have been an obstetrician-gynecologist, as evidenced by his membership in the American College of Obstetricians and Gynecologists. By the 1960s, he practiced medicine in San Antonio, Texas, which is probably how he came into contact with the local Planned Parenthood. See *American Medical Directory* (1969), 3462. Quote regarding Goldzieher's status within the Texas research community in the memo to Robbins, Elliott, and Bernheim, Regarding San Antonio Research, April 30, 1971.

150. Information and quotes about the affiliate's relationship to the Southwest Foundation and the Syntex Project taken from Guttmacher, Report on San Antonio Fact Finding Trip.

151. Details and quote in Guttmacher, Report on San Antonio Fact Finding Trip.

152. Ibid.

153. What patients received in return for their participation in the Tuskegee Syphilis Study has been the subject of much discussion and debate, particularly as it related to the role of Nurse Rivers, the African American woman who helped carry the program out. See Part VI: "Rethinking the Role of Nurse Rivers," in Reverby, *Tuskegee's Truths*, 319–95. See also Smith, *Sick and Tired*, chapter 4.

154. Guttmacher, Report on San Antonio Fact Finding Trip.

155. Guttmacher, Impression of the San Antonio Affiliate, June 7–8, 1971, Affiliates General: Affiliates' Research, San Antonio, 1971–72, Series: Affiliates, box 139, PPFAR II.

156. Prero quoted in memo to Robbins, Elliott, and Bernheim, Regarding San Antonio Research, April 30, 1971.

157. John C. Robbins to Beasley, Guttmacher, Pilpel, Langmyhr, and Romney, Regarding the San Antonio Situation, September 27, 1971, Affiliates General: Affiliates' Research, San Antonio, 1971–72, Series: Affiliates, box 139, PPFAR II.

158. McNeill to Calderone, March 12, 1958.

159. Mary S. Calderone to Jean L. McNeill, March 18, 1958, folder 77, box 6, MSCP.

160. Required Minimum Standards for Certification of Birth Control Clinics, September 1938.

161. William T. Kennedy and L. E. Kling to Chairman, President, State Director and Executive Secretary, State Leagues and Local Committees, Regarding Revised Standards for Certification of Clinics, March 3, 1948, folder 11, box 80, Series VII: Subject Files, Clinics, PPFAR I; and (standards attached to memo) Required Minimum Standards for Certification of Clinics, June 1956, Clinics, General, 1956–68, Series: Affiliates, PPFA National, box 137, PPFAR II.

162. For the 1956 call for affiliates to register their research (which was apparently largely ignored by local offices), see Mary S. Calderone to Executive Committee, Regarding Medical Committee Recommendation, October 8, 1957. For the stricter call by 1963, see Strauss to Calderone, September 17, 1963. In fact, by 1966 the national medical advisory board was sending out notices every six months reminding affiliates that they were required to register their projects with the national medical committee. Medical Department (PPFA) to All Affiliates, Regarding Research Registration, September 1966.

163. Mary S. Calderone to Elizabeth Nichols, April 3, 1958, folder 60, box 4, MSCP.

164. Revised "25-Month Club" Congratulatory Letter, May 14, 1965, PPFA: Subject, Enovid "25-Month Club," 10/5/62–10/21/66, Series: Classified Files, box 68, PPFAR II.

165. Mary S. Calderone to Official Testing Centers, June 1959, folder 69, box 5, MSCP.

166. Mary S. Calderone to Representatives of the Clinical Investigation Centers, July 31, 1959, folder 69, box 5, MSCP.

167. Sherwin A. Kaufman to Mary S. Calderone, March 7, 1963; and Calderone's reply, March 14, 1963, folder 51, box 4, MSCP.

168. Memo by Alan Guttmacher and Mary S. Calderone, April 15, 1963, folder 51, box 4, MSCP.

169. Meeting with Representatives of the Searle Company, Regarding the "25 Month Club," August 1, 1966, Status Report of Long Term Enovid Users, Comments & Summary Tables, G. D. Searle & Company, Series: Classified Files, box 68, PPFAR II. Length of questionnaire drawn from attached report. Similar remarks of dissatisfaction can be found in Richard L. Day to Alan Guttmacher, August 3, 1966, Regarding "25-Month Club" Study in PPFA: Subject, Enovid "25-Month Club," 10/5/62–10/21/66, Series: Classified Files, box 68, PPFAR II.

170. PPFA Clinical Investigation Program: Operating Procedures, October 1959.

171. Mary S. Calderone to Mrs. Franklin O'Brien, November 8, 1963, folder 51, box 4, MSCP.

172. "Are You on the Pill?" *Patient News* (Winter 1963), Chicago, PP Association, Publicity, Pamphlets, etc., 1972–76, Series: Affiliates, Illinois, box 153, PPFAR II.

173. PPFA, "Oral Contraceptive Research Programs Patient Information Sheet" and "Oral Contraceptive Research Programs Patient Consent Form," October 1966. These were attached to a memo mentioned previously from Strauss to Calderone, September 17, 1963.

174. Meldrum, "Simple Methods," 286.

175. Ibid., 280.

176. Joffe, *Regulation of Sexuality*.

177. Meldrum, "Simple Methods," 287–88.

178. Watkins, *On the Pill*, chapters 4–5; for Planned Parenthood and the Nelson hearings more specifically, see 113–15. For more on Planned Parenthood's reaction to the hearings, see PPWP Medical Department (George Langmyhr and Walter C. Rogers) to Regional Directors et al., Regarding Congressional Hearings on Oral Contraceptives, January 8, 1970, folder 16, box 4, PPACAR; George Langmyhr to Lynn Landman, Regarding Planned Parenthood's Position to the Nelson Committee, January 21, 1970, PPWP: Oral Contraceptive, History, Nelson Hearings, Background Material, 1957–70, Series, Classified Files, box 68, PPFAR II; and George Langmyhr to Alan Guttmacher, March 4, 1970, PPWP: Oral Contraceptive, History, Nelson Hearings, Background Material, 1957–70, Series, Classified Files, box 68, PPFAR II. For a letter written on behalf of three women, "an associate of Ralph Nader," and the American Patients Association requesting pill package inserts for use in a lawsuit against the FDA, see Joan M. Katz to George Langmyhr, October 6, 1970, PPWP: Medical Department, Contraceptives, Oral, 6/9/69–1/31/79, Classified Files, box 68, PPFAR II.

179. For several discussions of sterilization abuses, see Roberts, *Killing the Black Body*, 89–98; Nelson, *Women of Color*, chapter 2; and Schoen, *Choice and Coercion*, especially the introduction, chapter 2, and epilogue.

180. For Henry Beecher's exposé, see Rothman, *Strangers at the Bedside*, chapter 4. For the 1972 revelations of Tuskegee, see Jones, *Bad Blood*, chapters 1 and 13. For the emergence of new research guidelines from the late 1960s through the 1970s, see Rothman, *Strangers at the Bedside*, chapter 9.

181. Medical Department (PPFA) to All Affiliates, Regarding Research Registration, September 1966.

182. Naomi T. Gray to Regional Directors, September 26, 1966, PPWP Affiliates General: Affiliates' Research, 1970–73, Series: Affiliates, box 139, PPFAR II.

183. Guttmacher, Report on San Antonio Fact Finding Trip.

184. Francine S. Stein to Jerim Klapper, Regarding Biomedical Research in San Antonio, May 17, 1971, Affiliates General: Affiliates' Research, San Antonio, 1917–72, Series: Affiliates, box 139, PPFAR II. A similar line of criticism was raised at PPFA's National Medical Committee Meeting on June 30, 1971, to discuss the situation. As Dr. Robert Berg asked, are we "simply worried about the legal implications as they relate to the Planned Parenthood of San Antonio and Southwest Research Foundation relationship?" See page 2 of the National Medical Committee Meeting Minutes, June 30, 1971, Affiliates General: Affiliates' Research, San Antonio, 1971–72, Series: Affiliates, box 139, PPFAR II.

185. National Medical Committee Meeting Minutes, June 30, 1971.

186. John Robbins to Pam Veerhusen, Ralph Woolf, and Alan Guttmacher, December 6, 1972, PPWP Affiliates General: Affiliates' Research, 1970–73, Series: Affiliates, box 139, PPFAR II. Robbins' position drawn from the letterhead upon which the following memorandum was written: Robbins to Beasley, Guttmacher, Pilpel, Langmyhr, and Romney, Regarding the San Antonio Situation, September 27, 1971.

187. George Langmyhr to Affiliate Executive Directors, Regarding Questionnaire Regarding Affiliate Biomedical Research, September 22, 1970, folder 8, box 17, PPACAR.

188. Details about this situation and direct quotes taken from Naomi Gray to Douglas Stewart, September 30, 1969, PPWP Affiliates General: Affiliates' Research, 1970–73, Series: Affiliates, box 139, PPFAR II. As to the specific identity of Lomax, in mentioning his name to Stewart, Gray said, "You know, of course, who he is."

189. Clinic Statistics All Centers, January through December 1965, 1966, 1967, 1968, 1969, 1970, March 12, 1971, folder 6, box 4, PPACAR.

190. According to one 1969 report, while the total number of patients served in Chicago was 16,342, the total was 21,935 in New York City. See "Planned Parenthood–World Population Inter-Affiliate Statistical Report and Summary, 1969 Summary," xiv, xvi.

191. For Browne's departure as well as the quote from her letter of resignation, see Jane C. Browne to Board of Directors of Planned Parenthood Association, Chicago Area, February 18, 1969, Chicago, PP Association, Reports, Members, 1964–76, Series: Affiliates, Illinois, box 152, PPFAR II. For Dr. Frank's departure, see PPACA Board of Directors Meeting, January 23, 1968, Chicago, PP Association, Reports, Members, 1964–76, Series: Affiliates, Illinois, box 152, PPFAR II.

192. PPACA Board of Directors Meeting, February 29, 1968.

193. Carl E. Speckman to Cameron Brown, January 29, 1969, Chicago, PP Association, 1969, Series: Affiliates, Illinois, box 152, PPFAR II.

194. For example, see the conflicts between the Champaign affiliate and the Federation, which can be found in folders entitled "Champaign County, Affiliation, PP Correspondence, 1958–1978" and "Champaign County, Affiliation, Audits, Budgets, Bylaws, 1946–1978," Series: Affiliates, Illinois, box 152, PPFAR II. For fights over dues, see the 1962 battle between the Chicago office and PPFA in the following exchanges: John W. Straub to Kenneth A. Ives, February 8, 1962, and Mrs. Stowe C. Phelps to John W. Straub, April 24, 1962, Chicago, PP Association, Correspondence, 1962–78, Series: Affiliates, Illinois, box 152, PPFAR II. For a dues battle between the Houston office and PPFA in 1964, see Anderson, "Private Choices vs. Public Voices," 230. In fact, by the end of the 1960s local affiliates more generally were deeply frustrated with the federation. See Jane C. Browne to Paul H. Todd, Jr., April 26, 1968, Chicago, PP Association, 1968, Series: Affiliates, Illinois, box 152, PPFAR II.

195. See, for example, Medical Department to Chairmen of Medical Advisory Committees, Medical Directors, et al., Regarding Physical Requirements for Family Planning Centers, April 1, 1968, PPFA: National, Medical, Memos to Affiliates, 1965–69, Series: Classified Files, box 69, PPFAR II.

196. By 1966, the federation's policy on serving unwed was as follows: "Medical consultation and services may be provided to minors who are married or engaged, or have been pregnant or are accompanied by a parent or guardian or are referred by a recognized social or health agency, a doctor, or clergyman or in any other circumstances where in the judgment of the physician such consultation and services should be provided." See PPWP Policy on Service to Minors, October 1966, PPWP Affiliates General: Services, Teenagers, Minors, Medical Department, Memos, State Laws, Reports, General, 1968–80, Series: Affiliates, box 140, PPFAR II. For quote encouraging local offices to adopt more liberal policies, see Recommendations of

the Executive Directors Council Meeting, held June 26–29, 1967, in Minneapolis, MN, Chicago Area, 1967, Series: Affiliates, Illinois, box 152, PPFAR II.

197. Lew Mondy to Doris Bernheim, Regarding Standards of Affiliation as Regards Service to Minors, September 18, 1972, PPWP Affiliates General Services: Minors, Teenagers, 1967–74, Series: Affiliates, box 139, PPFAR II.

198. Dorothy L. Millstone to Planned Parenthood Affiliates, October 9, 1969, Legal, 1937–70, Series: Affiliates, Illinois, box 151, PPFAR II.

199. Reagan, *When Abortion Was a Crime*, 241.

200. Ibid., 233–34.

201. Caron, *Who Chooses?*, 204.

202. Langmyhr and Rogers, "Legal Abortion."

203. Anderson, "Private Choices vs. Public Voices," 271.

204. Caron, *Who Chooses?*, 204–6.

205. Jeffrey C. Slade to Francine S. Stein, Regarding Survey of Affiliates: Abortion Related Activities, November 13, 1970, PPWP Affiliates General: Survey of Affiliate Abortion-Related Activities, 1970, box 140, Series: Affiliates, PPFAR II.

206. Anderson, "Private Choices vs. Public Voices," 240–41.

207. For the crackdown and the inequality it yielded in terms of who had access to abortion, see Reagan, *When Abortion Was a Crime*, 15, 193–215; for Planned Parenthood's secret conference, see 218–22; quotes, 220 and 193, respectively. Italics mine.

208. Minutes from the PPFA–PPWP Board of Directors Meeting, 44–45, February 17, 1973, folder 4, box 200, PPFAR II.

209. Guttmacher, *Birth Control and Love*, chapter 12; questions drawn from 137–39. Quotes about abortion, 137.

210. "Birth Control." Http://www.plannedparenthood.org/health-topics/birth-control-4211.htm (accessed June 19, 2008). More recently, the last sentence in the online definition has been dropped. But its message remains much the same. Date last accessed, July 5, 2010.

211. For the Cleveland incident, see Caron, "Birth Control," 548.

212. Quotes from Gordon, *Moral Property of Women*, 309.

Conclusion

1. Minutes from the PPFA–PPWP Board of Directors Meeting, February 17, 1973, 42–45.

2. Ibid., 45–55; quotes, 48, 47, 49, 52, 46, and 55.

3. Susan Dickler to John C. Robbins, Alfred F. Moran, and Jerim Klapper, Regarding Referrals for Abortion by Planned Parenthood Affiliates, September 30, 1971, PPWP Affiliates General: Services: Abortion-Pregnancy Counseling, 1970–75, Series: Affiliates, box 139, PPFAR II.

4. Caron, *Who Chooses?*, 204.

5. Minutes from the PPFA–PPWP Board of Directors Meeting, February 17, 1973, 99–101.

6. Caron, *Who Chooses?*, 205.

7. Ibid., 205–6.

8. Joy Dryfoos to PP Abortion Committee, February 22, 1973, folder 17, box 1, OIS–42, PPFAR II.

9. Ginsburg, *Contested Lives*, 103.

10. Uehling, "Clinics of Deception."

11. "Anti-Abortion Clinics Focus of Hearing in House Today."

12. Ibid.

13. Gordon, *Moral Property of Women*, 309.

14. Ginsburg, *Contested Lives*, 103.

15. "Anti-Abortion Clinics Focus of Hearing in House Today."

16. Quote describing the provision from Gandy, "NOW Calls on Obama Administration."

17. MoveOn.Org on-line petition, http://pol.moveon.org/contraception/ (accessed January 19, 2009).

18. For the official medical line held by the Food and Drug Administration, National Institutes of Health, and American College of Obstetricians and Gynecologists, see Hatcher et al., *Contraceptive Technology* (2007), 95. For the recently passed Missouri bill (Senate Bill 793), see Townsend, "Philosophy, Theology." The bill stipulates that the "life of each human being begins at conception" and adds: "Abortion will terminate the life of a separate, unique, living human being" (A5). For another example of the belief that pregnancy begins at fertilization, see Will, "Barbara Boxer in Context."

19. Hatcher et al., *Contraceptive Technology* (1992); quotes, 228, 426.

20. Hatcher et al., *Contraceptive Technology* (2007); quotes, 197–98, 94–95, respectively.

21. From the Planned Parenthood website http://www.plannedparenthood. org/health-topics/emergency-contraception-morning-after-pill-4363.htm (accessed August 9, 2010).

22. Minutes from the PPFA–PPWP Board of Directors Meeting, February 17, 1973; quote, 92.

23. Ibid.; quote, 91.

24. Caron, *Who Chooses?*, 205.

25. Goldstein, "Creating and Controlling a Medical Market," 520, 522, 523.

26. Ibid., 521.

27. Ibid.

28. Even such great movies as Mike Leigh's *Vera Drake* tiptoe around the issue. Although Vera Drake, the abortionist in post–World War II England, is sympathetically portrayed, she never once takes money for the services she provides, unlike the other (less sympathetic) characters in the movie, who do. Judging by the remarks I regularly get from students when they watch the movie for extra credit in my history of sexuality class, this makes all the difference to them. Had she taken money from the women she helped, they would have liked her far less. *Vera Drake*, directed by Mike Leigh (Fine Line Features, 2004).

29. Caron, *Who Chooses?*, 205.

30. Ibid., 205–6.

31. Minutes from the PPFA–PPWP Board of Directors Meeting, February 17, 1973; quotes, 84, 85, 92.

32. Goldstein, "Creating and Controlling a Medical Market," 523.

33. For example, McCabe, Letter to the Editor; and "Abortion for Profit."

34. Ginsburg, *Contested Lives*, 56.

35. Ibid., 103.

36. "Anti-Abortion Clinics Focus of Hearing in House Today."

37. Schienberg, "Wal-Mart Dealt Morning-After Pill Setback."

38. Thottam, "Why Wal-Mart Agreed to Plan B."

39. "Abby B." [pseud.], interview by author, September 3, 1998. Name withheld at request of interviewee.

40. Total numbers taken from the following Planned Parenthood website: http://www.plannedparenthood.org/about-us/who-we-are-4648.htm (accessed December 6, 2010).

Bibliography

Manuscript Collections

Historical Health Fraud and Alternative Medicine Collection (HHFAMC). American Medical Association Archives. American Medical Association Building. Chicago, IL.

Margaret Sanger Papers (MSP Unfilmed–SC). Unfilmed Collection. Sophia Smith Collection. Smith College. Northampton, MA.

Mary Steichen Calderone Papers (MSCP). MC 179. Schlesinger Library. Radcliffe Institute. Harvard University. Cambridge, MA.

Planned Parenthood Association Chicago Area Records, 1920–75 (PPACAR). Chicago History Museum. Chicago, IL.

Planned Parenthood Federation of America Records I (PPFAR I). Sophia Smith Collection. Smith College. Northampton, MA.

Planned Parenthood Federation of America Records II (PPFAR II). Sophia Smith Collection. Smith College. Northampton, MA.

Planned Parenthood Springfield Area Records, 1938–95. MC 38. Archives/Special Collections. University of Illinois at Springfield. Springfield, IL.

Welfare Council of Metropolitan Chicago Records, 1914–78 (WCMCR). Chicago History Museum. Chicago, IL.

Manuscript Collections on Microfilm

Margaret Sanger Papers (MSP Filmed–LC). Filmed Collection. Library of Congress. Washington, DC.

Mary Ware Dennett Papers (MWDP). Schlesinger Library. Radcliffe Institute. Cambridge, MA.

Oral Histories

"B., Abby" [pseud.]. Interview by author. September 3, 1998. Tape recording, transcription, and permission for use in author's possession.

Dobbins, Ruth. Interview by author. September 3, 1998. Tape recording, transcription, and permission for use in author's possession.

Government Documents

Doe v. Bolton, 410 US 179 (1973).
Eisenstadt v. Baird, 405 US 438 (1972).
Griswold v. Connecticut, 381 US 479 (1965).
Roe v. Wade, 410 US 113 (1973).
US Congress. Senate. Committee on the Judiciary. *Birth Control: Hearings before a Sub-committee on S. 1842,* 73rd Cong., 2nd sess., March 1, 20, and 27, 1934.
U.S. v. One Package of Japanese Pessaries, 86 F.2d 737 (2nd Cir. 1936).
Youngs Rubber Corporation v. C. I. Lee & Co., 45 F.2d 103 (CCA, 2nd Cir. 1930).

Conference Papers

Batza, Catherine. "Before AIDS: The Relationship between the Chicago Gay and Medical Communities, 1974–1982." Paper presented at the Missouri Valley History Conference, Omaha, NE, March 4–6, 2004.
Davis, Joshua. "'The Business of Getting High': Paraphernalia Merchandising in 1970s United States." Paper presented at the annual meeting of the Organization of American Historians, New York City, NY, March 28–31, 2008.
Koncick, Teresa A. "No Longer under the Mattress: Family Financial Planning in Post–World War II America." Paper presented at the annual meeting of the Society of American City and Regional Planning History, Oakland, CA, October 15–18, 2009.
Lennon, Patricia M. "Rhythm and Authority: Moral and Medical Debates on the Ogino-Knaus Method of Periodical Continence, 1930–1945." Paper presented at the Pew Fellows Conference, New Haven, CT, May 1999.
Wall, Jessica. "A Complicated Man, A Complicated Legacy: An Examination of William Baird, the Man Behind *Eisenstadt v. Baird,* 1972." Paper presented at the Thirteenth Annual McNair Research Scholars Symposium, Berkeley, CA, August 12, 2005.
———. "Foam and Fornication: National Identity, Bill Baird, and Birth Control Politics in the United States, 1965–1972." Paper presented at the annual meeting for the National Women's Studies Association, Cincinnati, OH, June 2008.

Published Primary and Secondary Sources

"Abortion for Profit." http://www.abort73.com/abortion/abortion_for_profit/ (accessed September 16, 2007).
"The Accident of Birth." *Fortune,* February 1938, 84–86, 108, 110, 112, and 114.
Addams, Jane. *The Spirit of Youth and the City Streets.* 1909. Reprint, Urbana: University of Illinois Press, 1972.
Allyn, David. *Make Love Not War: The Sexual Revolution: An Unfettered History.* Boston: Little, Brown, 2000.

American Medical Directory: A Register of Legally Qualified Physicians of the United States, *1925.* 9th ed. Chicago: American Medical Association, 1925 (11th ed., 1929; 25th ed., part 3, 1969).

"American Medicine Accepts Birth Control." *Birth Control Review* (June 1937): 1–2.

Anderson, Maria H. "Private Choices vs. Public Voices: The History of Planned Parenthood in Houston." PhD diss., Rice University, 1998.

"Anti-Abortion Clinics Focus of Hearing in House Today." *New York Times,* December 17, 1986, B12.

Appel, Cheri. Review of *Facts and Frauds in Woman's Hygiene,* by Rachel Lynn Palmer and Sarah K. Greenberg. *Journal of Contraception* 1, no. 10 (1936): 171.

"Are You Too Educated to be a Mother?" *Ladies' Home Journal,* June 1946, 6.

Ashley, Jo Ann. *Hospitals, Paternalism, and the Role of the Nurse.* New York: Teachers College Press, 1976.

"Ask Your Physician." *Woman's Home Companion,* September 1938, 2.

Bailey, Beth. *Sex in the Heartland.* Cambridge: Harvard University Press, 2002.

Baskin, Alex. "Margaret Sanger, the *Woman Rebel,* and the Rise of the Birth Control Movement in the United States." Introduction to Baskin, *Woman Rebel,* i–xxii.

———, ed. *Woman Rebel.* New York: State University of New York at Stony Brook, 1976. Reprint, New York: Archives of Social History, 1976.

Benson, Marguerite. "Leaping on the Band Wagon: A Caution to Bona Fide Birth Control Organizations." *Birth Control Review* (September 1935): 5–6.

"Birth Control." *Commonweal,* March 4, 1931, 479.

"Birth Control Aid Called Anti-Negro." *New York Times,* April 16, 1963.

"Birth Control Clinics at Work." *Birth Control Review* (February 1930): 48–49.

"Birth Control Marches On." *Birth Control Review* (February–March 1937): 3–4.

"Birth Control Plan in Illinois Rapped by NAACP Leader." *Charleston (SC) News and Courier,* January 6, 1963.

"Birth Control Policy Urged." *Science News Letter,* August 20, 1960, 117.

"The Birth Control Revolution." *Commonweal,* April 1, 1931, 589–91.

Bogue, Donald J., and Jane C. Browne. *Successful Family Planning Easy and Inexpensive: A Birth Control and Marriage Manual.* Chicago: University of Chicago Press, 1962.

Borg, Virginia. "Birth Control and State Fairs." *Survey,* December 1939, 371–72.

Boughton, Alice C. "To Start a Clinic." *Birth Control Review* (April 1934): 49–50.

———. "What 7309 'Mothers' Want," *Birth Control Review* (January 1933): 8–11.

Boyden, Mabel Gregg. "The Mothers' Health Clinic of Alameda County." *Birth Control Review* (October 1931): 286–88.

Brandt, Allan M. *No Magic Bullet: A Social History of Venereal Disease in the United States since 1880.* New York: Oxford University Press, 1985.

Briggs, Laura. *Reproducing Empire: Race, Sex, Science, and US Imperialism in Puerto Rico.* Berkeley: University of California Press, 2002.

Brodie, Janet Farrell. *Contraception and Abortion in Nineteenth-Century America.* Ithaca: Cornell University Press, 1994.

Bromley, Dorothy Dunbar. *Birth Control: Its Use and Misuse.* New York: Harper & Brothers, 1934.

———. "Birth Control: Yes or No?" *Woman's Journal,* June 1931, 20–21, 38.

Brownlee, Lestre. "Do We Have Too Many Children?" *Sepia,* April 1961, 34–35.

Bruno, Hal. "Birth Control, Welfare Funds, and the Politics of Illinois." *Reporter*, June 20, 1963, 32–35.

Bryant, Carolyn. "The Clinic Interview." *Birth Control Review* (April 1934): 52.

"Bureau of Investigation. Lanteen Laboratories, Inc.," *Journal of the American Medical Association* 94, no. 20 (1930): 1619.

Capeci, Dominic, Jr. *Race Relations in Wartime Detroit: The Sojourner Truth Housing Controversy of 1942.* Philadelphia: Temple University Press, 1984.

Caron, Simone M. *Who Chooses?: American Reproductive History since 1830.* Gainesville: University Press of Florida, 2008.

———. "Birth Control and the Black Community in the 1960s: Genocide or Power Politics?" *Journal of Social History* 31, no. 3 (1998): 545–69.

The Case Worker and Family Planning. New York: Planned Parenthood Federation of America, Inc., 1943.

Chauncey, George. *Gay New York: Gender, Urban Culture, and the Making of the Gay Male World, 1890–1940.* New York: Basic Books, 1994.

Chen, Constance M. *"The Sex Side of Life": Mary Ware Dennett's Pioneering Battle for Birth Control and Sex Education.* New York: New Press, 1996.

Chesler, Ellen. *Woman of Valor: Margaret Sanger and the Birth Control Movement in America.* New York: Simon & Schuster, 1992.

Chicago Medical Blue Book, 1923–1924. 38th ed. Chicago: McDonough & Company, 1923.

Clark, Le Mon. "The Sizes of Vaginal Diaphragms Prescribed in American Clinics." *Journal of Contraception* 3, no. 2 (1938): 33–36.

"Clinic Reports. Minnesota Birth Control League." *Journal of Contraception* 2, no. 1 (1937): 19–20.

Cohen, Lizabeth. *A Consumers' Republic: The Politics of Mass Consumption in Postwar America.* New York: Alfred A. Knopf, 2003.

Comstock Act. 1873. Reprinted in *Women's America: Refocusing the Past,* 7th ed., edited by Linda K. Kerber, Jane Sherron De Hart, and Cornelia Dayton Hughes, 314–15. New York: Oxford University Press, 2011.

Connelly, Matthew. *Fatal Misconceptions: The Struggle to Control World Population.* Cambridge: Harvard University Press, 2008.

Cook, Robert C. "Bootleg Birth Control." *Colliers,* July 15, 1939, 12–13, 41–42.

Critchlow, Donald T. *Intended Consequences: Birth Control, Abortion, and the Federal Government in Modern America.* New York: Oxford University Press, 1999.

Curry, Lynne. *Modern Mothers in the Heartland: Gender, Health, and Progress in Illinois, 1900–1930.* Columbus: The Ohio State University Press, 1999.

"A Day at the Office." *Birth Control Review* (November 1929): 316–17.

De Costa, Ellen. "A Catholic Young Woman Looks at Birth Control." *Catholic World,* February 1934, 553–59.

D'Emilio, John, and Estelle B. Freedman. *Intimate Matters: A History of Sexuality in America.* 2nd ed. Chicago: University of Chicago Press, 1997.

Dickinson, Robert L. *Control of Conception.* 2nd ed. Baltimore: Williams & Wilkins, 1938.

———. *Techniques of Conception Control,* 3rd ed. Baltimore: Williams & Wilkins, 1950.

Dienes, C. Thomas. *Law, Politics, and Birth Control.* Urbana: University of Illinois Press, 1972.

Drachman, Virginia G. *Hospital with a Heart: Women Doctors and the Paradox of Separatism at the New England Hospital, 1862–1969.* Ithaca: Cornell University Press, 1984.

Duffin, Jacalyn, and Alison Li. "Great Moments: Parke, Davis and Company and the Creation of Medical Art." *Isis* 86, no. 1 (1995): 1–29.

Dykeman, Wilma. *Too Many People, Too Little Love: Edna Rankin McKinnon: Pioneer for Birth Control.* New York: Holt, Rinehart & Winston, 1974.

Enstad, Nan. *Ladies of Labor, Girls of Adventure: Working Women, Popular Culture, and Labor Politics at the Turn-of-the-Twentieth Century.* New York: Columbia University Press, 1999.

Ertman, Martha M., and Joan C. Williams, eds. *Rethinking Commodification: Cases and Readings in Law and Culture.* New York: New York University Press, 2005.

"Feminine Hygiene in the Department Store." *Drug and Cosmetic Industry* 40, no. 4 (1937): 479, 482.

"The Fight for Better Babies." *Look,* April 1, 1947.

Gamble, Vanessa Northington. *Making a Place for Ourselves: The Black Hospital Movement, 1920–1945.* New York: Oxford University Press, 1995.

———. "Under the Shadow of Tuskegee: African Americans and Health Care." *American Journal of Public Health* 87, no. 11 (1997): 1773–78.

Gamson, Joshua. "Rubber Wars: Struggles over the Condom in the United States." *Journal of the History of Sexuality* 1, no. 2 (1990): 265–82.

Gandy, Kim. "NOW Calls on Obama Administration, Congress to Undo Harmful HHS Rule." National Organization for Women. http://www.now.org/press/12-08/12-19.html (accessed January 12, 2009).

Garrett, Elizabeth H. "Birth Control's Business Baby." *New Republic,* January 17, 1934, 269–72.

Garrow, David J. *Liberty and Sexuality: The Right to Privacy and the Making of Roe v. Wade.* New York: Macmillan, 1994.

Gaylord, Gladys. "Clinical Aspects of Birth Control." *Birth Control Review* (July 1933): 166–67.

Gevitz, Norman, ed., *Other Healers: Unorthodox Medicine in America.* Baltimore: Johns Hopkins University Press, 1988.

Geyer, Georgie Anne. "Birth Control in Chicago: The End of the Fight Is in Sight." *Chicago Scene,* November 1962, 24–29.

Gilbert, James. *A Cycle of Outrage: America's Reaction to the Juvenile Delinquent in the 1950s.* New York: Oxford University Press, 1986.

Ginsburg, Faye D. *Contested Lives: The Abortion Debate in an American Community.* Berkeley: University of California Press, 1989.

Goldstein, J. J. "The Birth Control Clinic Cases." *Birth Control Review* (February 1917): 8.

Goldstein, Michael S. "Creating and Controlling a Medical Market: Abortion in Los Angeles after Liberalization." *Social Problems* 31, no. 5 (1984): 514–29.

Gordon, Linda. *The Moral Property of Women: A History of Birth Control Politics in America.* Urbana: University of Illinois Press, 2002.

———. *Woman's Body, Woman's Right: Birth Control in America.* New York: Grossman, 1976. Rev. ed., New York: Penguin, 1990.

Guthmann, Bernice J. *The Planned Parenthood Movement in Illinois.* Chicago: Planned Parenthood Association, Chicago Area, 1965.

Guttmacher, Alan F. *Birth Control and Love: The Complete Guide to Contraception and Fertility.* Rev. ed., Toronto: Collier-Macmillan Canada, 1969.

———. "How Safe Are Birth Control Pills?" *Ebony,* April 1962, 123–28.

Hafner, Arthur W., James G. Carson, and John F. Zwicky. *Guide to the American Medical Association Historical Health Fraud and Alternative Medicine Collection.* Chicago: American Medical Association, 1992.

Hajo, Cathy Moran. *Birth Control on Main Street: Organizing Clinics in the United States, 1916–1939.* Urbana: University of Illinois Press, 2010.

Hall, Peter Dobkin. *Inventing the Nonprofit Sector: And Other Essay on Philanthropy, Volunteerism, and Nonprofit Organizations.* Baltimore: Johns Hopkins University Press, 1992.

Hart, Jamie. "Who Should Have the Children?: Discussions of Birth Control among African-American Intellectuals, 1920–1939." *Journal of Negro History* 79, no. 1 (1994): 71–84.

Hartmann, Susan M. *The Home Front and Beyond: American Women in the 1940s.* Boston: Twayne, 1982.

Hatcher, Robert A., Felicia H. Stewart, James Trussell, Deborah Kowal, Felicia Guest, Gay K. Stewart, and Willard Cates. *Contraceptive Technology, 1990–1992.* 15th ed. New York: Irvington, 1992.

Hatcher, Robert A., James Trussell, Anita L. Nelson, Willard Cates, Jr., Felicia H. Stewart, and Deborah Kowal. *Contraceptive Technology.* 19th ed. New York City: Ardent Media, 2007.

Herman, Ellen. *The Romance of American Psychology: Political Culture in the Age of Experts.* Berkeley: University of California Press, 1995.

Himes, Norman E. *Medical History of Contraception.* 1936. Reprint, New York: Schocken Books, 1970.

Hirsch, Arnold R. *Making the Second Ghetto: Race and Housing in Chicago, 1940–1960.* Cambridge: Cambridge University Press, 1983.

———. "Massive Resistance in the Urban North: Trumbull Park, Chicago, 1953–1966." *Journal of American History* 82, no. 2 (1995): 522–50.

Holz, Rose. "Nurse Gordon on Trial: Those Early Days of the Birth Control Clinic Movement Reconsidered." *Journal of Social History* 39 (Fall 2005): 112–40.

Honey, Maureen. *Creating Rosie the Riveter: Class, Gender, and Propaganda during World War II.* Amherst: University of Massachusetts Press, 1984.

Horowitz, Daniel. *The Morality of Spending: Attitudes toward the Consumer Society in America, 1875–1940.* Baltimore: Johns Hopkins University Press, 1985.

Hoy, Suellen M. "'Municipal Housekeeping': The Role of Women in Improving Urban Sanitation Practices, 1880–1917." In *Pollution and Reform in American Cities, 1870–1930,* edited by Martin V. Melosi, 173–98. Austin: University of Texas Press, 1980.

Hulett, Denise A. "Every Child a Wanted Child: The History of Planned Parenthood in Waco." Master's thesis. Baylor University, 2000.

Hunt, Leontyne. "Keep Your Family the Right Size." *Chicago Defender,* August 28, 1965.

"I Went to a Birth Control Clinic." *Physical Culture,* January 1938, 12–13, 76–78.

"Information Not Available." *Birth Control Review* (January 1929): 17.

Irwin, Rita, and Clementina Paolone. *Practical Birth Control: A Guide to Medically Approved Methods for the Married.* New York: Robert M. McBride, 1937.

Jackson, Kenneth T. *Crabgrass Frontier: The Suburbanization of the United States.* New York: Oxford University Press, 1985.

Jacobs, Margaret D. *White Mother to a Dark Race: Settler Colonialism, Maternalism, and the Removal of Indigenous Children in the American West and Australia, 1880–1940.* Lincoln: University of Nebraska Press, 2009.

Jacobson, Matthew Frye. *Whiteness of a Different Color: European Immigrants and the Alchemy of Race.* Cambridge: Harvard University Press, 1998.

Jameson, Frances. "A Catholic Mother Looks at Planned Parenthood." *Reader's Digest,* December 1943, 102–4.

Jensen, Joan M. "The Evolution of Margaret Sanger's *Family Limitation* Pamphlet, 1914–1921." *Signs* 6, no. 3 (1981): 548–67.

Joffe, Carole. *The Regulation of Sexuality: Experiences of Family Planning Workers.* Philadelphia: Temple University Press, 1986.

Jones, James H. *Bad Blood: The Tuskegee Syphilis Experiment.* 1981. Expanded ed., New York: The Free Press, 1993.

Jones, Kathleen W. *Taming the Troublesome Child: American Families, Child Guidance, and the Limits of Psychiatric Authority.* Cambridge: Harvard University Press, 1999.

Joseph, Miranda. *Against the Romance of Community.* Minneapolis: University of Minnesota Press, 2002.

Junod, Suzanne White, and Lara Marks. "Women's Trials: The Approval of the First Oral Contraceptive Pill in the United States and Great Britain." *Bulletin of the History of Medicine* 57, no. 2 (2002): 117–60.

Kapsalis, Terri. *Public Privates: Performing Gynecology from Both Ends of the Speculum.* Durham: Duke University Press, 1997.

Kennedy, Anne. "A Visit to the Medical Centers of Chicago." *Birth Control Review* (January 1927): 26.

Knowles, Jon. *Seventy-five Years of Family Planning in America: A Chronology of Major Events.* 1986. Rev. ed., New York: Planned Parenthood Federation of America, Inc., 1991.

Kopp, Marie E. *Birth Control in Practice: Analysis of Ten Thousand Case Histories of the Birth Control Clinic Research Bureau.* 1933. Reprint, New York: Arno Press and The New York Times, 1972.

Koven, Seth, and Sonya Michel. "Womanly Duties: Maternalist Politics and the Origins of Welfare States in France, Germany, Great Britain, and the United States, 1880–1920." *American Historical Review* 95, no. 4 (1990): 1076–1108.

Kunzel, Regina G. *Fallen Women, Problem Girls: Unmarried Mothers and the Professionalization of Social Work, 1890–1945.* New Haven: Yale University Press, 1993.

Kwolek-Folland, Angel. *Incorporating Women: A History of Women and Business in the United States.* New York: Twayne, 1998.

Ladd-Taylor, Molly. *Mother-Work: Women, Welfare, and the State, 1890–1930.* Urbana: University of Illinois Press, 1994.

———. *Raising a Baby the Government Way: Mothers' Letters to the Children's Bureau.* New Brunswick: Rutgers University Press, 1986.

LaRossa, Ralph. *The Modernization of Fatherhood: A Social and Political History*. Chicago: University of Chicago Press, 1997.

Lazerow, Jama. "Rethinking Religion and the Working Class in Antebellum America." *Mid-America* 75, no. 1 (1993): 85–104.

Lees, Hannah. "The Negro Response to Birth Control." *Reporter*, May 19, 1966, 46–48.

Lemann, Nicholas. *The Promised Land: The Great Black Migration and How It Changed America*. New York: Alfred A. Knopf, 1992.

Leung, Marianne. "'Better Babies': The Arkansas Birth Control Movement during the 1930s." PhD diss., University of Memphis, 1996.

———. "'Better Babies': Birth Control in Arkansas during the 1930s." In *Hidden Histories of Women in the New South*, edited by Virginia Bernhard, Betty Brandon, Elizabeth Fox-Genovese, Theda Purdue, and Elizabeth H. Turner, 52–68. Columbia: University of Missouri Press, 1994.

Liebenau, Jonathan. *Medical Science and Medical Industry: The Formation of the American Pharmaceutical Industry*. London: Macmillan, 1987.

Lindenmeyer, Kriste. "Expanding Birth Control to the Hinterland: Cincinnati's First Contraceptive Clinic as a Case Study, 1929–1931." *Mid-America* 77, no. 2 (1995): 145–73.

Litoff, Judy Barrett. *American Midwives: 1860 to the Present*. Westport, CT: Greenwood Press, 1978.

Losure, Mary. "'Motherhood Protection' and the Minnesota Birth Control League." *Minnesota History* 54, no. 8 (1995): 359–70.

Lundberg, Ferdinand, and Marynia F. Farnham. *Modern Woman: The Lost Sex*. New York: Harper & Brothers, 1947.

"Margaret Sanger and Chicago." *Chicago Sun-Times*, September 13, 1966.

Marks, Harry M. *The Progress of Experiment: Science and Therapeutic Reform in the United States, 1900–1990*. Cambridge: Cambridge University Press, 1997.

Marks, Lara V. *Sexual Chemistry: A History of the Contraceptive Pill*. New Haven: Yale University Press, 2001.

Marsh, Margaret, and Wanda Ronner. *The Empty Cradle: Infertility in America from Colonial Times to the Present*. Baltimore: Johns Hopkins University Press, 1996.

Matsner, Eric M. "Letters to the Editor. Fitting the Diaphragm." *Journal of Contraception* 3 (June–July 1938): 130–31.

May, Elaine Tyler. *America and the Pill: A History of Promise, Peril, and Liberation*. New York: Basic Books, 2010.

———. *Barren in the Promised Land: Childless Americans and the Pursuit of Happiness*. New York: Basic Books, 1995.

———. *Homeward Bound: American Families in the Cold War Era*. New York: Basic Books, 1988.

McCabe, Pam. Letter to the Editor. *Lincoln Journal Star*, November 24, 2003, B5.

McCann, Carole R. *Birth Control Politics in the United States, 1916–1945*. Ithaca: Cornell University Press, 1994.

McLaren, Angus. *A History of Contraception: From Antiquity to the Present Day*. Cambridge: Basil Blackwell, 1990.

McTavish, Jan R. *Pain and Profits: The History of the Headache and Its Remedies in America*. New Brunswick: Rutgers University Press, 2004.

"Medicine. How to Have Babies." *Newsweek*, February 4, 1946, 94.

Meldrum, Marcia L. "'Simple Methods' and 'Determined Contraceptors': The Statistical Evaluation of Fertility Control, 1957–1968." *Bulletin of the History of Medicine* 70, no. 2 (1986): 266–95.

Melosh, Barbara. "More Than the 'Physician's Hand': Skill and Authority in Twentieth-Century Nursing." In *Women and Health in America: Historical Readings*, edited by Judith Walzer Leavitt, 482–96. Madison: University of Wisconsin Press, 1984.

"Men or Maggots?" *Newsweek*, November 30, 1959, 90–91.

Meyer, Jimmy Elaine Wilkinson. *Any Friend of the Movement: Networking for Birth Control, 1920–1940*. Columbus: The Ohio State University Press, 2004.

Meyerowitz, Joanne, ed. *Not June Cleaver: Women and Gender in the Postwar Era, 1945–1960*. Philadelphia: Temple University Press, 1994.

Mintz, Morton. *"The Pill": An Alarming Report*. Boston: Beacon Press, 1969.

Mintz, Steven, and Susan Kellogg, *Domestic Revolutions: A Social History of American Family Life*. New York: Free Press, 1988.

Mohanty, Chandra Talpade. "Under Western Eyes: Feminist Scholarship and Colonial Discourses." *Feminist Review* 30 (August 1988): 61–88.

Monk, Diane. "No Pill for the Single Girl." *Chicago Sunday Star*, May 2, 1965.

———. "Our Single Girl Gets Birth Control Info." *Chicago Sunday Star*, May 9, 1965.

Morantz-Sanchez, Regina Markell. *Sympathy and Science: Women Physicians in American Medicine*. New York: Oxford University Press, 1985.

MoveOn.Org on-line petition. http://pol.moveon.org/contraception/ (accessed January 19, 2009).

Naismith, Grace. "The Racket in Contraceptives." *The American Mercury*, July 1950, 3–13.

Nash, Carol K. "Birth Control Clinics." *Birth Control Review* (August 1931): 231.

Nelson, Jennifer. *Women of Color and the Reproductive Rights Movement*. New York: New York University Press, 2003.

"News Notes: A Fight in Chicago." *Birth Control Review* (September 1923): 221.

"News Notes: Illinois." *Birth Control Review* (December 1925): 361.

"News Notes: Illinois." *Birth Control Review* (June 1933): 157.

Nicholl Christine E., and Robert G. Weisbord. "The Early Years of the Rhode Island Birth Control League," *Rhode Island History* 45, no. 4 (1986): 111–25.

Numbers, Ronald L. "The Fall and Rise of the American Medical Profession." In *Sickness and Health in America: Readings in the History of Medicine and Public Health*, 2nd ed., edited by Judith Walzer Leavitt and Ronald L. Numbers, 185–96. Madison: University of Wisconsin Press, 1985.

"Our Correspondents' Column. Letter from E. D." *Birth Control Review* (November 1924): 327.

Palmer, Rachel Lynn, and Sarah K. Greenberg. *Facts and Frauds in Woman's Hygiene: A Medical Guide against Misleading Claims and Dangerous Products*. Garden City, NY: Garden City Publishing, 1938.

Patterson, George T. *The Dread Disease: Cancer and Modern American Culture*. Cambridge: Harvard University Press, 1987.

Peiss, Kathy. *Cheap Amusements: Working Women and Leisure in Turn-of-the-Century New York*. Philadelphia: Temple University Press, 1986.

Petchesky, Rosalind Pollack. *Abortion and Woman's Choice: The State, Sexuality, and Reproductive Freedom*. New York: Longman Press, 1984.

"Planned Parenthood Meeting." *Survey*, November 1948, 343.

"Project Tenants for Birth Control." *Chicago Defender*, December 14, 1962.

Puffer, J. Adams. *The Boy and His Gang*. Boston: Houghton Mifflin, 1912.

Ramírez de Arellano, Annette B., and Conrad Seipp, *Colonialism, Catholicism, and Contraception: A History of Birth Control in Puerto Rico*. Chapel Hill: University of North Carolina Press, 1983.

Reagan, Leslie J. "Engendering the Dread Disease: Women, Men, and Cancer." *American Journal of Public Health* 87, no. 11 (1997): 1779–87.

———. "From Hazard to Blessing to Tragedy: Representations of Miscarriage in Twentieth-Century America." *Feminist Studies* 29, no. 2 (2003): 357–78.

———. *When Abortion Was a Crime: Women, Medicine, and Law in the United States, 1867–1973*. Berkeley: University of California Press, 1997.

Reed, James. *From Private Vice to Public Virtue: The Birth Control Movement and American Society since 1830*. New York: Basic Books, 1978.

Reeves, Harrison. "The Birth Control Industry." *The American Mercury*, November 1936, 285–90.

Rennie, Rose Ann. "Mothers Health Centers." *Birth Control Review* (June 1933): 145–47.

———. "Some Clinic Problems." *Birth Control Review* (April 1934): 52–53.

Reverby. Susan M. *Ordered to Care: The Dilemma of American Nursing, 1850–1945*. Cambridge: Cambridge University Press, 1987.

———, ed. *Tuskegee's Truths: Rethinking the Tuskegee Syphilis Study*. Chapel Hill: University of North Carolina Press, 2000.

Riis, Jacob A. *How the Other Half Lives: Studies among the Tenements of New York*. 1890. Reprinted with a preface by Charles A. Madison. New York: Dover, 1971.

Roberts, Dorothy. *Killing the Black Body: Race, Reproduction, and the Meaning of Liberty*. New York: Pantheon Books, 1997.

Robishaw, Ruth A. "A Study of 4,000 Patients Admitted for Contraceptive Advice and Treatment." *American Journal of Obstetrics and Gynecology* 31 (March 1936): 426–34.

Rodgers, Daniel. T. "In Search of Progressivism." *Reviews in American History* 10 (December 1982): 113–31.

Rodrique, Jessie M. "The Black Community and the Birth Control Movement." In *Passion and Power: Sexuality in History*, edited by Kathy Peiss and Christina Simmons, 138–54. Philadelphia: Temple University Press, 1989.

Rosen, George. *The Structure of American Medical Practice, 1875–1941*. Philadelphia: University of Pennsylvania, 1983.

Rosen, Robyn L. *Reproductive Health, Reproductive Rights: Reformers and the Politics of Maternal Welfare, 1917–1940*. Columbus: The Ohio State University Press, 2003.

———. "The Shifting Battleground for Birth Control: Lessons from New York's Hudson Valley in the Interwar Years." *New York History* 90, no. 3 (2009): 187–215.

Rosenberg, Charles E. *The Care of Strangers: The Rise of America's Hospital System*. New York: Basic Books, 1987.

————. "Social Class and Medical Care in Nineteenth-Century America: The Rise and Fall of the Dispensary." *Bulletin of the History of Medicine* 29, no. 1 (1974): 32–54.

Rothman, David J. *Strangers at the Bedside: A History of How Law and Bioethics Transformed Medical Decision Making.* New York: Basic Books, 1991. New York: Aldine de Gruyter, 2003.

Salomon, Mrs. Henry. "The Rhode Island Clinic." *Birth Control Review* (November 1932): 279–80.

Sanger, Margaret. "Clinics the Solution." *Birth Control Review* (July 1920): 6–8.

————. "Family Limitation." 1914. 2nd ed., New York: [n.p.], 1917.

————. *Motherhood in Bondage.* 1928. Reprint, Elmsford, NY: Maxwell Reprint, 1956.

————. *My Fight for Birth Control.* 1931. Reprint, Elmsford, NY: Maxwell Reprint, 1969.

————. "National Security and Birth Control." *Forum* 93, no. 3 (1935): 139–41.

Sarch, Amy. "Those Dirty Ads!: Birth Control Advertising in the 1920s and 1930s." *Critical Studies in Mass Communication* 14, no. 1 (1997): 31–48.

Schienberg, Jon. "Wal-Mart Dealt Morning-After Pill Setback." *CNNMoney,* February 15, 2006. http://money.cnn.com/2006/02/15/news/companies/walmart_pill/index.htm.

Schneider, Eric C. *In the Web of Class: Delinquents and Reformers in Boston, 1810s–1930s.* New York: New York University Press, 1992.

Schoen, Johanna. *Choice and Coercion: Birth Control, Abortion, and Sterilization in Public Health and Welfare.* Chapel Hill: University of North Carolina Press, 2005.

Scott, Mel. *American City Planning since 1890.* Berkeley: University of California Press, 1969.

Shepherd, Jack. "Birth Control and the Poor: A Solution." *Look,* April 7, 1964, 63–7.

Shore, Elliott. *Talkin' Socialism: J. A. Wayland and the Role of the Press in American Radicalism, 1890–1912.* Lawrence: University Press of Kansas, 1988.

Sies, Mary Corbin, and Christopher Silver. "The History of Planning History." In *Planning in the Twentieth-Century American City,* edited by Mary Corbin Sies and Christopher Silver, 1–34. Baltimore: Johns Hopkins University Press, 1996.

Smith, Helena Huntington. "Enter Planned Parenthood." *Parents' Magazine,* September 1942, 30–31, 45, 79.

Smith, Susan L. *Sick and Tired of Being Sick and Tired: Black Women's Health Activism in America, 1890–1950.* Philadelphia: University of Pennsylvania Press, 1995.

Solinger, Rickie. *Wake Up Little Susie: Single Pregnancy and Race before Roe v. Wade.* New York: Routledge, 1992.

Starr, Paul. *The Social Transformation of American Medicine: The Rise of a Sovereign Profession and the Making of a Vast Industry.* New York: Basic Books, 1982.

"State Organizations for Birth Control: Illinois Birth Control League." *Birth Control Review* (September 1930): 259–60.

Stearns, Peter N., and Mark Knapp, "Men and Romantic Love: Pinpointing a Twentieth-Century Change." *Journal of Social History* 26, no. 4 (1993): 769–95.

Stevens, Rosemary. *In Sickness and In Wealth: American Hospitals in the Twentieth Century.* New York: Basic Books, 1989.

Stix, Regine K. "Birth Control in a Midwestern City: A Study of the Clinics of the Cincinnati Committee on Maternal Health." *Milbank Memorial Fund Quarterly* (January 1939): 69–91; (April 1939): 152–71; (October 1939): 392–423.

Stone, Hannah M. "Clinical Birth Control Abroad." *Birth Control Review* (December 1927): 321–22.

———. "Essentials in Clinic Equipment." *Birth Control Review* (January 1927): 23.

———. "The Vaginal Diaphragm." *Journal of Contraception* 3 (June–July 1938): 123–27.

Strickland, Charles E., and Andrew M. Ambrose. "The Baby Boom, Prosperity, and the Changing Worlds of Children, 1945–1963." In *American Childhood: A Research Guide and Historical Handbook*, edited by Joseph M. Hawes and N. Ray Hiner, 533–85. Westport, CT: Greenwood Press, 1985.

Stubbs, George. "Profits in Birth Control." *New Republic*, February 7, 1934, 367.

Stuyvesant, Elizabeth. "The Brownsville Birth Control Clinic." *Birth Control Review* (March 1917): 6–8.

Sugrue, Thomas J. "Crabgrass-Roots Politics: Race, Rights, and the Reaction against Liberalism in the Urban North, 1940–1964." *Journal of American History* 82, no. 2 (1995): 551–78.

Swann, John P. "Universities, Industry, and the Rise of Biomedical Collaboration in America." In *Pill Peddlers: Essays on the History of the Pharmaceutical Industry*, edited by Jonathon Liebenau, Gregory J. Higby, and Elaine C. Stroud, 73–90. Madison, WI: American Institute of the History of Pharmacy, 1990.

Thompson, Dorothy. "Race Suicide of the Intelligent." *Ladies' Home Journal*, May 1949, 11–13.

Thottam, Jyoti. "Why Wal-Mart Agreed to Plan B." *Time*, March 3, 2006. http://www.time.com/time/business/article/0,8599,1169740,00.html.

Thrasher, Frederick M. *The Gang: A Study of 1,313 Gangs in Chicago*. Chicago: University of Chicago Press, 1927.

"Told by Clinic Nurses." *Birth Control Review* (March 1936): 4.

Tomes, Nancy. "The Great American Medicine Show Revisited." *Bulletin of the History of Medicine* 79 (2005): 627–63.

Tone, Andrea. "Contraceptive Consumers: Gender and the Political Economy of Birth Control in the 1930s." *Journal of Social History* 29, no. 3 (1996): 485–506.

———. *Devices and Desires: A History of Contraceptives in America*. New York: Hill & Wang, 2001.

Tone, Andrea, and Elizabeth Siegel Watkins. Introduction to *Medicating Modern America: Prescription Drugs in History*, edited by Andrea Tone and Elizabeth Siegel Watkins, 1–14. New York: New York University Press, 2007.

Townsend, Tim. "Philosophy, Theology at Issue in Missouri." *Lincoln Journal Star*, August 30, 2010, A5.

Turner, William B. "Class, Controversy, and Contraceptives: Birth Control Advocacy in Nashville, 1932–1944." *Tennessee Historical Quarterly* 53, no. 3 (1994): 166–79.

Uehling, Mark D., with Anne Underwood, Patricia King, and Barbara Burgower. "Clinics of Deception." *Newsweek*, September 1, 1986, 20.

Valien, Preston, and Alberta Price Fitzgerald. "Attitudes of the Negro Mother toward Birth Control." *American Journal of Sociology* 55, no. 3 (1949): 279–83.

Vaughan, Paul. *The Pill on Trial*. New York: Coward-McCann, 1970.

Vogel, Morris J. *The Invention of the Modern Hospital: Boston, 1870–1930*. Chicago: University of Chicago Press, 1980.

"Voice of the People: Ruthless Nature." *Chicago Daily Tribune*, May 10, 1930.

Walker, Juliet E. K. *The History of Black Business in America: Capitalism, Race, and Entrepreneurship*. New York: Twayne, 1998.

Walkowitz, Daniel J. *Working with Class: Social Workers and the Politics of Middle-Class Identity*. Chapel Hill: University of North Carolina Press, 1999.

Walsh, Mary Roth, *"Doctors Wanted: No Women Need Apply": Sexual Barriers in the Medical Profession, 1835–1975*. New Haven: Yale University Press, 1977.

Watkins, Elizabeth Siegel. *On the Pill: A Social History of Oral Contraceptives, 1950–1970*. Baltimore: Johns Hopkins University Press, 1998.

Watkins, Susan Cotts, and Angela D. Danzi. "Women's Gossip and Social Change: Childbirth and Fertility Control among Italian and Jewish Women in the United States, 1920–1940." *Gender and Society* 9, no. 4 (1995): 469–90.

Wembridge, Eleanor Rowland. "The Seventh Child in the Four Room House." *Birth Control Review* (January 1924): 10–13.

Wenocur, Stanley, and Michael Reisch. *From Charity to Enterprise: The Development of American Social Work in a Market Economy*. Urbana: University of Illinois Press, 1989.

"What Do You Think of Birth Control?" *Woman's Home Companion*, July 1948, 7–8.

White, Mary M. "Maintaining Clinic Standards." *Birth Control Review* (October 1936): 9.

Whitfield, Stephen J. *The Culture of the Cold War*. Baltimore: Johns Hopkins University Press, 1991.

Will, George F. "Barbara Boxer in Context: You Can See It on YouTube Today." *Newsweek*, August 9, 2010, 22.

Wille, Lois. "Overpopulation Blamed on 'Selfish' Middle Class." *Chicago Daily News*, February 12, 1965.

Willett, Julie A. *Permanent Waves: The Making of the American Beauty Shop*. New York: New York University Press, 2000.

Wynn, Neil A. *The Afro-American and the Second World War*. London: Elek, 1976.

Yarros, Rachelle. "Birth Control Clinics in Chicago." *Birth Control Review* (December 1928): 354–55.

Young, James Harvey. *The Toadstool Millionaires: A Social History of Patent Medicines in America before Federal Regulation*. Princeton: Princeton University Press, 1961.

Index

abortion, 10; attitudes about in 1930s, 57; business practices v. charity, 153–54, 199n28; and irregular clinics, 63–64; legalized, 15; and loss of clinic supporters, 149; and Planned Parenthood clinics, 141, 161–62n27; Planned Parenthood policy, 141; and post-1973 clinics, 146–49; use as birth control, 50

Addams, Jane, 9, 27

advertising, 56; 1930s, 50–51; deceptive, 66; FTC control over, 83

African Americans, 11–12, 117–20, 123–28; and Chicago affiliate, 191n87; and clinical research projects, 138; entrepreneurs, 25; and 1920s clinics, 162–63n41; and 1960s clinics, 163n42; and Planned Parenthood, 139; and religious opposition to birth control, 193n139

alcoholism, and unplanned families, 92, 120

Allen, L. T., Mrs., 88

AMA (American Medical Association), 15, 48–49, 62–66, 177n100

American Birth Control League, 18, 52, 85

American Health Association, 59

American Bureau of Hygiene, 59

American Medical Association: See AMA

American Mercury, 33, 67

Amsterdam clinics, 26–27, 41

Andelman, Sam, 115

Anderson, Maria H., 104–5, 142

antiabortion clinics, 149–50

antiabortion violence, 144

Arkansas birth control organization, 27

Arnold, Shirley, 118

Associated Charities of Chicago, 32

Atlanta affiliate, abortion policy, 154

Backrach, Joseph, 24

Baird, William, 116

Baker, Dorothy, 97–99, 100, 105

Barclay, Elizabeth, 85

Beecher, Henry, 135–36

Bell, Barbara, 120

Benson, Marguerite, 46, 58, 59, 64, 65

"Big Push, The" 89, 108

birth control: and African Americans, 119120, 124–25; attitudes in 1930s, 49; and consumerism, 11; early radicalization of, 7; early sources of advice, 24; opposition to, 52; and psychological stability, 76–78; and public assistance recipients, 114; and public health reform, 28; as way to cut public expenditures, 33; women's control of, 50, 70, 82–83, 86, 87. *See also* birth control clinics; contraceptives

"Birth Control and the Law" (television documentary), 114

birth control clinics, 6–7; 1930s, 46; atmosphere of, 35–36; clients in 1920s, 11, 162–63n41; clients in 1960s, 12, 163n42; commercial, 15, 54–55, 173nn36–37; early flexibility of, 36; early locations of, 37–38; early success of, 43–44; and Great Depression, 5; locations, 32; names of, 57, 175n55; and Planned Parenthood, 5; professional atmosphere of, 40–41; and Progressive area reform, 7; Sanger's first, 10, 21–22, 36; staffed by women, 39–40; standardization of, 13; and teaching, 13; ties to charities,

32–33, 167n54, 167n57; as women's community, 40
birth control information, and unmarried people, 52, 105–7, 111–15, 140–41
birth control literature, legal disclaimers in, 112
birth control movement, 28; 1960s-1970s, 96–97, 185n2; early conservative views on sex, 8; early distancing from marketplace, 9, 46–48; early years, 20–21; in Illinois, 14–15
Birth Control on Main Street (Hajo), 18
birth control pill: as abortifacient, 150, 152; African American concerns about, 126; and Champaign, IL, clinic, 98; and clinical research projects, 100–101; controversy over, 135; and de-emphasis on diaphragm, 9, 99; demand for, 99
Birth Control Review, 17; attacks on irregular clinics, 64; on clinic staff, 39–40; on clinical practices, 57, 63; on commercialism, 46; on diaphragm, 61; on fees for services, 31; hard-luck stories in, 33; men's contributions to, 79; on patient numbers, 32, 35; on Sanger's first clinic, 22; on women's aversion to hospitals, 38
birth control (term), 7, 80; differentiated from abortion, 46; meanings of, 9, 26, 46–47, 58–59, 67, 143–44; and radical associations, 69; recognition of, 90–91
"Birth Control's Business Baby" (Garrett), 48, 171n6
black market of birth control, 20
Blood, Dennis, 56
Bocker, Dorothy, 1, 159n3
Bogue Project, 108–11, 118, 122
"bona fide" clinics, 58, 64–65
bootleg birth control entrepreneurs, 20–26, 62
Boughton, Alice C., 31, 61
Breon Laboratories, 100
Briggs, Laura, 85, 120
Brightman, Clare, 138–39

Brinckerhoff, George, 24
Brodie, Janet Farrell, 22
Bromley, Dorothy Dunbar, 60, 61
Browne, Jane C., 108, 113, 115, 139
Bundesen, Herman N., 29–30
Bureau of Birth Control Information, 54, 57, 173n35
Bureau of Contraceptive Advice, 57
Bureau of Investigation (AMA), 48, 62–63
Burrell, Curtis, 127
business, assumptions about, 3
Business Week, 99
Buzza, Mildred, 63, 177n95

C-Quens, 103
Calderone, Mary Steichen, 86–87, 93, 102, 110; and clinical research projects, 132–34
California affiliate, 81
Captive Audience Motivation and Education Campaign, 122–23
Caron, Simone, 141, 148–49, 152, 154
Carpenter, Helen, 30, 32
caseworkers, and attitudes toward patients, 34
Catholic Interracial Council, 127
Catholic World, 53
Catholics: criticisms of Planned Parenthood rhetoric, 94; opposition to birth control, 53, 94–95; using birth control clinics, 33
Centralia, IL, affiliate, 44
Champaign County Planned Parenthood, 44, 80, 90, 97–99; and clinical research projects, 100, 105
Champaign, IL, affiliate, 80, 81, 90, 97, 100, 110
charities: and abortions, 143; assumptions about, 3, 4; and birth control clinics, 2, 10, 28–29, 32–33, 159n5, 167n54, 167n57; opposition to clinics, 33–34; and Planned Parenthood, 107. *See also* charitification; charity clinic movement
charitification, 28–29
charity clinic movement, 14; and AMA, 15, 65; attacks on irregular clinics,

58–59; and diaphragm, 61; differentiated from commercial market, 46–47, 51; instability of, 13; and organized medicine, 64–65; propaganda, 67; and scientific medicine, 129–30. *See also* charities; charitification

charity clinics: and black market, 20–21; complaints about, 66; in immigrant communities, 29; and marketplace practices, 30; and organized medicine, 62; patients as research subjects, 12, 103–4, 129. *See also* Parents' Committee of Chicago

Chase, Sarah, 24

Chesler, Ellen, 27, 40

Chicago, IL: African Americans in, 117–18; city clinics in, 114; commercial clinics in, 54; and early birth control movement, 27, 29; locations of clinics, 32

Chicago affiliate: in 1960s, 107–8; and African Americans, 117–28, 191n87; and clinical research projects, 104; decline of, 139–40; growth of, 116–17; rolling board meetings, 121–22

Chicago Board of Health clinics, 115, 190n79

Chicago Daily Tribune, 64

Chicago Defender, 118, 119, 123

Chicago Medical Bureau of Birth Control Information, 54, 57, 62–65; shoddy practice at, 66

Chicago Sunday Star, 115

Chicago Urban League, 118, 119

Chicago Welfare Council, 33

children: happy when planned, 94; postponing and spacing, 78. *See also* unwanted children

Children's Bureau, 79

chiropractors, 55, 65; and irregular clinics, 46, 55; and Women's Bureau of Birth Control Information, 64, 66

Cincinnati, OH, birth control organization, 33; and clinic studies in, 82–84

class bias, 95; post-war, 92–94. *See also* paternalism

class differences: and access to legal abortion, 142–43; and birth control clinics, 41–43, 170nn110–12; and choice of birth control, 49–50

Cleveland, OH, birth control organization, 34, 43, 84, 100, 126, 144; and clinic studies in, 82

clinic: as activity, not place, 13; definition of, 150

clinic waves, 5; first, 7, 15, 44, 67, 170n116; second, 9, 16, 70, 95, 97

clinic work, 81

Clinical Investigation Program (CIP), 102, 104, 133, 134

clinical procedures, 54, 90; 1920s-1930s, 35–36; and invasive treatment, 43

Clinical Research Bureau, 90

clinical research projects, 100–105, 129–34; and Planned Parenthood clinics, 186n24, 187n31; and responsibility to patients, 136, 196n184

"Coffee Sip" program, 108, 118; and African Americans, 123

Cohen, Lizabeth, 11, 106–7

Colliers, 62

Collins, Shirley, 103–4

colonialism: and clinical research projects, 129; and minority birth control, 123

comic book pamphlets, 77

commercialization of birth control: in 1930s, 46–48; and legalization, 5

Commonweal, 53

Comstock Act, 1, 20, 22; and free speech, 44; limiting availability of birth control, 48

condoms, 10, 50, 79, 179n46; and quality control, 60, 83; women's resistance to, 87

"conscientious objection" requirement, 150

consumerism: in 1960s, 106–7; and birth control, 11; and radical political goals, 22–23, 164n7, 164n10

contraceptive industry: and Planned Parenthood, 11; regulation of, 83

Contraceptive Technology, 151

contraceptives, 30–31, 159n5; in 1930s, 50–52, 172n19; commercial, 59–61, 83, 111, 175n67; demonstrations of, 22; distributed by doctors, 108; and immigrants, 24–25, 165n21; for sale early twentieth century, 24; smuggling of, 100; for the unmarried, 15, 141
control, post–World War II enthusiasm for, 73–75
Cook County Hospital, IL, 121; providing contraceptives, 114, 118
Cooper, James, 52
Coronet, 99
court decisions, 10

Danville, IL, affiliate, 44, 88–89
Davidson, Doris, 85
Day, Dr., 115
Decatur, IL, affiliate, 105
delinquency, 78, 127; and unplanned families, 92–93
Dennett, Mary Ware, 44
Depression: and birth control clinics, 5, 8, 170n116; effect on birth control movement, 46
Detroit, MI, affiliate, 101, 103, 132; and Medical Bureau of Birth Control Information, 54
Devices and Desires (Tone), 18, 20
diaphragm, 8, 9; benefits of, 41; and charity clinics, 47, 49–50, 61; continued use of, 182n91; decline of use in Planned Parenthood clinics, 99; dissatisfaction with, 16, 70–71, 82–84, 181n68; early emphasis on, 36; failure in fitting, 66; low sales of, 50; Mesinga type, 26, 30–31; promotion by Planned Parenthood, 86–87, 181n88, 182n92; and women's control of childbearing, 86
Dickinson, Robert L., 38–39, 63, 82, 84–85
Dickler, Susan, 147–48
Dienes, C. Thomas, 114, 122
Dilex Institute of Feminine Hygiene, 51, 172n19
direct action, 25, 166n26

direct marketing, 108–10
Dobbins, Ruth, 98
doctors: and medical hierarchy, 40–41, 148; and pharmaceutical literature, 65; right to provide contraceptives, 30; as sole medical authority, 60; uninvolved with early movement, 24, 165n14; women doctors in clinics, 35–36, 169n90
Doe v. Bolton, 10, 15
douche, 24, 36, 46, 83, 84; caustic ingredients in, 59–60; illustrations of, 165n24, 172n19; inconvenience of, 41; method used by the poor, 50
Dowling, Jennette, 71
drugstores, 24; and immigrant communities, 23, 164n9; price competition from clinics, 100; promoted by Planned Parenthood, 110–11; warnings against, 36, 45. See also over-the-counter birth control products
Du Bois, W. E. B., 119, 125

Ebony, 99, 118
education, and Planned Parenthood clinics, 80–81
educational materials: of Planned Parenthood, 72, 178n6; and post–World War II anxieties, 74–75, 178n16; and race, 92
Eisenstadt v. Baird, 10, 15, 116, 141
Eli Lilly, 103; and clinical research projects, 100
elitist motivations, for birth control, 159–60n6
emergency contraceptive pills, 150–51; and Wal-Mart pharmacies, 155
Enstad, Nan, *Ladies of Labor, Girls of Adventure*, 22
entrepreneurs: African American, 25; and birth control market, 24–25; risks run by, 25–26
Ertman, Martha, *Rethinking Commodification*, 4
"Escape from Fear" (pamphlet), 75–80, 87
Esquire, 99
ethical responsibility, and clinical research projects, 129–32, 133–34

ethnicity, and birth control clinics, 31–32, 41–42
Eugenic Manufacturing Company, 24
eugenics, 159–60n6; and birth control movement, 28
euphemisms, for contraceptives, 83
Evanston, IL, clinic, 81
"Every 10 Seconds a Baby is Born" (pamphlet), 93

Facts and Fraud in Woman's Hygiene (Greenberg and Palmer), 65
"Family Limitation" (Sanger), 7; and confidence in the poor, 34, 109; illustrations in, 25, 165n24; and loss of confidence in the poor, 168n67; and reference to the marketplace, 20–21, 24
family planning, 69; and domestic happiness, 72–73; husband's role, 76–77; postponing and spacing children, 78, 179nn38–39; rhetoric of, 91–95, 112–13
Farr, Gustavas, 24
fathers, 76–77
FDA (Food and Drug Administration), 101–3; and clinical research projects, 134
federal grants, and restrictions, 104–5
fee-based clinics, 30, 167nn49–50
fees for services, as good for clients, 31
feminine hygiene products, 60, 61, 83; advertisements for, 49; as euphemism for birth control, 58–59
Feminine Institute, 51
feminism, influence on clinics, 8, 70
feminist arguments: in advertising, 51; influence on birth control movement, 87
fertilization, as start of life, 150–51, 199n18
financial support: and clinical research projects, 104, 131; from federal government, 104–5
Fishbein, Morris, 52
Food and Drug Administration: *See* FDA
Foote, Edward Bliss, *Medical Common Sense*, 25

Forbes, Betty, 105
Fortune, 60, 61–62
Forum, 62
Frank, Richard, 139
free speech, and Comstock Act, 29, 44
From Charity to Enterprise (Wenocur and Reisch), 34
FTC (Federal Trade Commission), 83

Gabler-Martin abortion clinic, 64
Gamble, Clarence, 60, 85
Garrett, Elizabeth H., 62; "Birth Control's Business Baby," 48, 171n6
Garvey, Marcus, 125
Garwood, Miriam, 88–89, 107
genocide, birth control seen as, 124–25, 126–27
Geyer, Georgie Ann, 122, 123
Ginsburg, Faye, 149, 155
Ginzburg, Olga, 40
Goeckingk, Johanna von, 110
Goldman, Emma, 23
Goldstein, Michael, 152
Goldzieher, Joseph William, 130–32, 194n149
Good Housekeeping, 99
Gordon, Adele, 57, 66, 174n41
Gordon, Linda, 7, 27, 30, 73; on anti-abortion clinics, 149; on Catholic opposition to birth control, 95; on the Clinical Research Bureau, 90; on pro-life movement, 144; *Woman's Body, Woman's Right*, 17, 69, 159n4
Gray, Naomi, 138–39
Greenberg, Sarah K., *Facts and Fraud in Woman's Hygiene*, 65
Greenwich Village radicals, 2, 8; and Sanger, 7
Griswold v. Connecticut, 10
Guttmacher, Alan, 111, 112, 137; advocating abortion, 141, 143; and clinical research projects, 133; and Planned Parenthood abortion policy, 148; and post–1973 Planned Parenthood, 146–47; and Southwest Foundation project, 129–32, 136–37

Hadley, Murray N., 52
Hajo, Cathy Moran, 28, 32, 42, 65; *Birth Control on Main Street*, 18; on dissatisfaction with diaphragm, 82–83; on middle-class paternalism, 84
Hall, Jeannette, 120
Hall, Peter Dobkin, *Inventing the Nonprofit Sector*, 3
Halleck, William, 24
Hampton, Marion, 118
handbills, 23
Hauser, Philip M., 120
health insurance programs, private, 12
"Help Your Neighbor Help Herself" campaign, 118
Hertig, Fred, 121
Hill, John C., 177n95
Himes, Norman, *Medical History of Birth Control*, 38
Hirsch, Arnold, 117
Historical Health Fraud and Alternative Medicine Collection, 1, 17, 48–49
historical perspective, 1–3, 159n5
Hofstra College, 138–39
Holland-Rantos Company, 30, 103, 132
homeopathy/homeopaths, 24, 26, 45, 48, 55
Hon, Antoinette, 23, 25
Houston, TX, affiliate, 27, 104–5, 142
Hulett, Denise, 33–34
Human Fertility, 129
Hunt, Leontyne, 123
Hygienic Company of America, 51

"I Went to a Birth Control Clinic," 37–38, 41–42, 60
Ickes, Harold L., 30
illegitimacy, 120–21
Illinois: and contraceptives for the unmarried, 140; early clinics in, 44; post World War II clinics in, 81; rebellious clinics in Danville, 88–89. *See also* Chicago, IL; Chicago affiliate
Illinois Birth Control League, 40; clients of, 31–32; clinics run by, 54; and publicity, 56

Illinois Department of Children and Family Services, 116
Illinois affiliates, 80–81, 88, 90, 97, 100, 105, 110. *See also names of individual affiliates*
Illinois Public Aid Commission (IPAC) controversy, 113–14, 118, 119, 126
illustrations: in advertising, 56; in birth control literature, 25, 110
immigrants, 23–25; and birth control market, 165n21; and charity clinics, 29; and drugstores, 164n9; limiting populations of, 28; and 1920s clinics, 11, 162–63n41; reluctance to use hospitals, 38
implantation, as start of life, 151, 199n18
Indiana affiliate, 98–99, 104.
Indigenous Neighborhood Worker, 109
infertility programs, 93; and Planned Parenthood, 90, 183n109
information distribution, 1960s, 110–11
informed consent, 134, 135–36, 137
Inventing the Nonprofit Sector (Hall), 3
Iowa affiliate, 105, 115
irregular clinics: and abortions, 63–64; attacks on, 66; and unmarried people, 63, 176n78
irregular providers, 55; and advertising, 56, 58; vilification of, 62. *See also* birth control clinics, commercial; entrepreneurs
Irwin, Rita, 64
IUD (intrauterine device), 24, 101, 106

Jackson, Elsie, 109
Jacobs, Aletta, 26
Jaffe, Fred, 109, 152
Jameson, Frances, 94
Joseph, Miranda, *Against the Romance of Community*, 4
Journal of the American Medical Association, 1, 48, 66

Kaufman, Sherwin, 133

"Keep Your Family the Right Size" (newspaper column), 118
King, Coretta Scott, 119
King, Martin Luther, 119
Knapp, Mark, 79
Kopp, Marie E., 82
Koromex-A, 103

La Dila, 172n19
labor movement, and religious moralism, 95, 185n144
Ladd-Taylor, Molly, 39
Ladies' Home Journal, 94
Ladies of Labor, Girls of Adventure (Enstad), 22
Langmyhr, George, 115, 138–39
Lanteen Laboratories, 54, 56
LaRossa, Ralph, 79
Legal Abortion: A Guide for Women in the United States, 141
Levitt, William, 73
Lewis, Benjamin, 119
Lomax, Louis, 138–39, 197n188
Look, 87, 92
Lucorol, 52
Lysol, 50

Ma and Pa Kettle movies, 94, 184–85n141
Mademoiselle, 99
mail-order catalogs, 52, 172–73n27
malpractice and liability insurance, 138
Mann, David, 127
Mannes, Marya, 123
manuals, on sex and birth control, 52, 60, 61, 172–73n27
manufacturers, ethical, 47
Maremont, Arnold H., 113
Margaret Sanger Award, 119
marketplace, 2; assumptions about, 4
marriage: emphasis on in birth control information, 112–13, 190n69; happiness of and family planning, 94; and sex counseling, 90; teamwork in, 75–77
marriage education classes, 75, 90, 183n112

Martin, Martha, 37, 60, 111. *See also* "I Went to a Birth Control Clinic"
Massachusetts birth control organization, 27 39, 41
Maternal Health Clinic, 57
McCann, Carole, 27, 160n6, 165n14
McCormick, Katherine Dexter, 86
McCroskey, Mr. (Atlanta affiliate president), 154
McFadden, Bernard, 37
McNeill, Jean L., 132
Mead Johnson, 100
Medicaid, 104
medical advisory boards, placing restrictions on clinics, 98–99
Medical Bureau of Birth Control Information, 54, 57, 62–65
Medical Center, 57
Medical Common Sense (Foote), 25
Medical History of Birth Control (Himes), 38
Meldrum, Marcia L., 101, 102, 104
men: as doctors at clinics, 86; hard-luck stories about, 76; interest in family planning, 78–79, 87; and parenthood, 79; as spouses at clinics, 40
mental illness, and unplanned families, 92
Mesinga diaphragm, 26; manufacture of, 30–31. *See also* diaphragm
Meyer, Jimmy Elaine Wilkinson, 33–34, 43, 84, 100
middle-class: and clinic use, 32; early support of clinics, 27–28; and overpopulation, 123
middle-class elitism, 84. *See also* paternalism
midwives, 24, 36, 41, 48, 174n41
Minneola, NY, affiliate, 138
Milwaukee, WI, irregular clinic, 54, 57, 66, 174n41. See also Gordon, Adele; Medical Bureau of Birth Control Information
Minneapolis, MN, birth control organization, 82
Minnesota birth control organization, 27. See also Minneapolis, MN, birth control organization

minorities, and population control, 122. *See also* African Americans; eugenics; genocide

minors: and distribution of information, 111–12; Planned Parenthood policy on, 140, 161–62n27, 197–98n196

mobile-unit service, 108–9, 114, 116

Mollenaro, Francesca, 40

Moore, Vivian, 118

morning-after pill. *See* emergency contraceptive pills

Mothers' Birth Control Clinic, 57

Mother's Guidance Clinic, 57

Mother's Health Clinic, 57

MoveOn.org, 150

multilingualism, in clinics, 40

Naismith, Grace, 67

National Abortion Service program, 147–48

National Committee on Maternal Health, 60

nativist motivations, and birth control movement, 28

Naturol Laboratories, 51

neighborhood action, 109

Nelson, Gaylord, 135

Neo-Malthusian League, 26, 41

Nesbitt, Lendor C., 118, 128

"New Baby is Born, A" (pamphlet), 93

New England Journal of Medicine, 136

New Republic, 62

New York affiliates, 80; and abortion, 141, 147, 154; Albany, 33; New York City, 139

Newsweek, 99, 110, 122

Nichols, George, 64

nonprofits, 3–4, 65

Nordine, Irene, 116

North Carolina birth control organization, 27, 85

nurses, 24; authority of denied, 36, 45, 58, 65; in birth control clinics, 39, 40, 42, 79, 87, 88, 105; as birth control providers, 26, 41; as character in birth control pamphlet, 111; fictional example, 37, 60; image in advertising, 51, 172n21; and irregular clinics, 46, 55, 57, 64, 66, 174nn41–42; and mobile-unit service, 108, 118; salesperson impersonating, 59; visiting nurse programs, 28. *See also* McNeill, Jean L.; Perez, Betty

Office of Economic Opportunity, 104

Ohio birth control organization 27, 43, 121, 66. See also Cleveland, OH, birth control organization and clinic studies done in; and Cincinnati, OH, birth control organization and clinic studies in

oral contraceptives. See birth control pill

oral histories, 18–19

organized medicine: and charity clinics, 47, 62, 64–65, 171n5; fear of competition, 65; opposition to clinic movement, 52–53

Ortho Pharmaceutical, 100, 103

Ortho-Novum, 103

osteopaths, 48, 65

overpopulation concerns, 11, 117, 123, 128

over-the-counter birth control products, 60

Packard, George, 30

Palmer, Rachel Lynn, *Facts and Fraud in Woman's Hygiene*, 65

Paolone, Clementina, 64

parenthood, 76–77, 79–80

Parents' Committee of Chicago, 13; and charity clinics, 29–30, 166n38; and fee-based clinics, 30

Parents' Magazine, 78

Parke-Davis, 100

paternalism, 34, 71, 84–86; in prescribing contraceptives, 181n82

patient consent, and clinical research projects, 133. *See also* informed consent

Patri, Angelo, 80

Pearson, Robert J., 149

pelvic examination, 39, 41, 45, 90

Perez, Betty, 118, 124–25, 128, 191n88
pessary. *See* diaphragm
pharmaceutical companies: and clinical research projects, 100–3; and Planned Parenthood, 2, 9; and scientific breakthroughs, 11
Physical Culture, 37
physical intimacy: and birth control, 79; and planned family, 77
pill, the. See birth control pill
Pill Purchase Plan, 100
Plan B: *See* emergency contraceptive pills
planned family: and physical intimacy, 77; post World War II, 73–74; and psychological stability, 75–80
Planned Parenthood, 1; abortion policy, 141, 147; and African Americans, 125, 139; and birth control clinics, 5, 6; and charity, 107; and commercial birth control methods, 67–68; and contraceptive manufacturers, 11; control of clinics, 136; de-emphasis on clinic services, 89, 156–57; educational materials, 72, 178n6; emphasis on children, not sex, 69; and for-profit abortion clinics, 154; friction between clinics and national organization, 81–82, 88–89, 140, 180n64; and infertility clinics, 90, 183n109; local preference for clinic work, 89, 183n107; and minorities, 139; and nonprofessional workers, 108–9; and oversight of clinical research projects, 132–35, 195n162; and pharmaceutical companies, 2, 9, 99–102; policy on minors, 161–62n27; policy on unmarried clients, 112; post–World War II propaganda, 70–71; promotion of diaphragm, 86–88, 181n88, 182n92; self-protective stance of, 116; and unaffiliated clinics, 115. *See also* Planned Parenthood affiliates; Planned Parenthood clinics
Planned Parenthood affiliates, 14, 163n49; in 1960s, 106, 108, 188–89n53, 188n46; response to legalized

abortion, 141–42. *See also names of individual affiliates*
Planned Parenthood clinics, 67; and abortion, 10, 161–62n27; and choice of method, 84–85, 111, 181n82; and clinical research projects, 102–3, 186n24, 187n31; and education, 80–81; policy changes, 81; post 1973, 146–49; post–World War II numbers, 81, 180n59
Planned Parenthood Federation of America. *See* Planned Parenthood
Planned Parenthood News, 104
Planned Parenthood–World Population, 109, 115
planning, culture of, 73
political revolutionaries, and birth control, 7
population control, 28; and immigrants, 120; and minorities, 122–24
Population Council, 101
post–World War II anxieties, 73–74, 178n16
poverty: and class bias, 95; linked with irresponsibility, 91, 94, 183n118; and population control, 123; seen as lack of character, 92–93
Prero, Sara, 131–32
"Prevention of Conception, The" (Stone), 111
Prinz, Lucie, 116
privacy rights, 10
procedural manuals, 35–36; on advertising a clinic, 91; on birth control methods, 60, 64, 88; on clinic policy, 81; on nurses, 40, 93; on organizing a clinic, 38, 39, 82, 84–85. See also Dickinson, Robert L
Progressive era reform: and birth control clinics, 7, 8; and clinic movement, 27
pro-life movement, 144, 154–55
propaganda: and charity clinic movement, 67; for early clinics, 32–33; post–World War II, 70
psychological stability, and planned family, 75–80

psychology, 70, 73–74

public assistance, and birth control services, 114

public health reform, and birth control, 28

publicity, 56; 1960s, 109–10; and clinical research projects, 133

Puerto Rico: birth control movement in, 27, 85; and early contraceptive tests, 129

quality control, and birth control products, 60, 83

race: and birth control, 126; and birth control clinics, 41–42; and Planned Parenthood propaganda, 91–92; and population control, 123–24; segregated clinic sessions, 43

race genocide, birth control seen as, 126, 135

racial conflicts, 120

racism/racialism: and birth control, 28, 120–22, 128, 159–60n6; and illegitimacy, 121; and population control, 117, 120, 122

radical political goals, and consumer culture, 22–23, 164n7, 164n10

"Read and Remember" (pamphlet), 112

Reader's Digest, 94, 99

Reagan, Leslie, 1, 9, 20, 46, 64, 141, 142

recommendations from other women, 35, 168n72

Reed, James, 11, 27, 60, 83

Reisch, Michael, *From Charity to Enterprise*, 34

religious moralism, and labor movement, 95, 185n144

Restell, Madame (Ann Trow Lohman), 24

Rethinking Commodification (Ertman and Williams), 4

rhetoric of family planning, 69–70

Rhode Island, birth control movement in, 141, 148–49. *See also* Rhode Island affiliate; Rhode Island Birth Control League

Rhode Island affiliate, and abortion policy, 152–54

Rhode Island Birth Control League, 27, 31

R.H.S. (AMA spy), 54, 63

rhythm method, 84, 110, 181n80

Riddlesbarger, Rufus, 51–52, 54, 63; business practices of, 56–57; denouncing abortion, 64; and information distribution, 110. *See also* Lanteen Laboratories; Medical Bureau of Birth Control Information

Robbins, John C., 137, 146–47

Robinson, William H., 118

Robishaw, Ruth A., 82

Rock, John, 93

Rodrique, Jessie, 119, 125

Roe v. Wade, 10, 15, 141

Rosoff, Jeannine, 137

Rothman, David, 130, 135

Rutgers, Johannes, 26

safe period. See rhythm method

San Antonio, TX, affiliate: and clinical research projects, 104, 128–29; and Southwest Foundation project, 130–31

Sanger, Margaret, 1, 69; and birth control clinics, 8; class bias of, 34, 85–86, 93; early days of movement, 26; "Family Limitation," 7, 217, 20–21, 24–25, 34, 109, 165n24, 168n67; and fee-based clinics, 30, 166n41; first clinic, 10, 21; and information distribution, 110; and manufacture of birth control devices, 30–31; rivalry with Dennett, 44, 170n117; smuggling contraceptives, 100; use of the marketplace, 22–23

Sarch, Amy, 46

Schmidt, Julius, 24, 83

Schoen, Johanna, 85

Science Digest, 99

scientific legitimacy, 101, 104

Searle pharmaceutical company, 102–3, 134; and clinical research projects, 100

Septigyn Company, 23
Servex Laboratories, 51
sexual fulfillment, 56
sexuality: advice on, 63; wholesome atti-
    tudes about, 57, 174–75n52
63rd Street Center, 127–28; decline of
    service quality, 139–40
Skinner, B. F., *Walden Two*, 73
Slee, Noah, 30
sliding fee scales, 31, 167n46
Snyder, Mary-Jane, 115
"Soldier Takes a Wife, The" (pamphlet),
    74, 76
Solinger, Rickie, 121
Southern Christian Leadership Confer-
    ence (SCLC), 119
Southwest Foundation research proj-
    ect, 128–31, 136–37, 193–94n145,
    194n148
Speckman, Carl E., 140
Spock, Benjamin, 77
Springfield, IL, birth control organiza-
    tions, 14, 90, 163n48
St. Louis, MO, affiliate, 34, 103, 134
Starr, Paul, 8
Stearns, Peter, 79
Stein, Francine, 136, 149
sterilization programs, 125, 135
Stewart, Douglas, 125, 127, 138–40
Stix, Regine K., 82, 83, 84
Stokes, Walter R., 93
Stone, Hannah, 36, 39–40, 41; "The Pre-
    vention of Conception," 111
Stubbs, George, 62
Stuyvesant, Elizabeth, 21–22
Sunday Afternoon (play script), 71–72,
    74–75, 76, 77, 78, 80, 94
Surete kit, 59
Survey, 78
Syntex Research Project, 130. See also
    Southwest Foundation research project

Tanner, Dr. (Danville, IL, clinic physi-
    cian), 88–89
telephone directories, 54–55, 91
Tennessee birth control organization
    and affiliate, 27, 119

third world analogy, 117, 121–22
Thompson, Evelyn, 118
Tietze, Christopher, 102, 134
Tiffany, Terrance P., 105
Tone, Andrea, 5, 22, 30, 47, 66; on com-
    mercial contraceptives, 83; *Devices
    and Desires*, 18, 20
Trisko, Jean, 107
Tuskegee Syphilis Study, 15, 131, 136,
    163–64n50, 194n153
25-Month Club, 102–3, 133, 134
Twine, Paul, 126–27

unmarried people: barred from early
    contraceptive help, 8–9; and birth
    control, 61–62, 120; and birth con-
    trol information, 52, 111–12; and
    birth control pill, 11, 99; and clinical
    research projects, 105–6, 188n44;
    and irregular clinics, 56, 57, 63,
    176n78; and legalized contraceptives,
    15; Planned Parenthood policy on,
    140, 197–98n196
unplanned families, 91–93, 120; and
    unwanted children, 16, 70
unwanted children; and birth control
    for the unmarried, 11, 107; and
    delinquency, 92–93; and racialist
    rhetoric, 128; and unplanned fami-
    lies, 16, 70, 91, 120
Upjohn, 100
urban slums, 11, 86, 107, 121–22
U.S. v. One Package, 10, 66

Van Cleave, H. J., Mrs., 110, 111
voluntarism, 3
Voluntary Parenthood League, 44

Waco, TX, birth control movement, 27,
    33–34
Walden Two (Skinner), 73
Walkowitz, Daniel, 120
Wal-Mart pharmacies, 155
Ward, Edgar, 118, 123
Washington Post, 122
Washington Post-Times-Herald, 114
Watkins, Elizabeth Siegel, 99, 135

welfare reform, 8
welfare relief, 93
Wembridge, Eleanor Rowland, 34
Wenocur, Stanley, *From Charity to Enterprise*, 34
"What Teenagers Want to Know About Family Planning" (pamphlet), 112
Wheeler, Edith Flower, 52
White, Mary M., 39, 41
Whitfield, Stephen, 73
Williams, Joan, *Rethinking Commodification*, 4
Winslow, C.-E. A., 78
Woman Rebel, 27
Woman's Body, Woman's Right (Gordon), 17, 69, 159n4
Woman's Home Companion, 62
Woman's Journal, 61

women: control over childbearing, 70, 82–83, 86, 87; education and childbearing, 93–94; and sexual fulfillment, 56; staffing clinics, 39–40, 181–82n90
Woman's Bureau of Birth Control Information, 54, 56; and irregular clinics, 64; monitored by AMA, 66–67
"World Eyes Birth Control Project" (newspaper article), 114
worthy poor, 4, 160n8

Yarros, Rachelle, 13, 29, 33, 34, 61
Young, Curtis J., 150
Young, Rebecca, 117–18, 123
Youngs Rubber court case, 10

Zgoda (Polish language newspaper), 23
Zonite Products Corporation, 51